T0205897

Research Ethics:

A Philosophical Guide to the Responsible Conduct of Research

Research Ethics:

A Philosophical Guide to the Responsible Conduct of Research

Gary Comstock

Professor of Philosophy at the Department of Philosophy and Religious Studies,
North Carolina State University,
North Carolina, USA

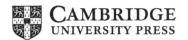
CAMBRIDGE
UNIVERSITY PRESS

CAMBRIDGE
UNIVERSITY PRESS

University Printing House, Cambridge CB2 8BS, United Kingdom

Cambridge University Press is part of the University of Cambridge.

It furthers the University's mission by disseminating knowledge in the pursuit of education, learning and research at the highest international levels of excellence.

www.cambridge.org
Information on this title: www.cambridge.org/9780521187084

© Cambridge University Press 2013

First published 2012
Reprinted 2014

A catalogue record for this publication is available from the British Library

Library of Congress Cataloguing in Publication data

Research ethics : a philosophical guide to the responsible conduct of research / Gary Comstock.
    p.   cm.
  ISBN 978-0-521-18708-4 (Paperback)
  1. Research–Moral and ethical aspects.   2. Scientists–Professional ethics.
I. Comstock, Gary, 1954–
    Q180.55.M67R465 2012
    174–dc23

                                                        2012017172

ISBN 978-0-521-18708-4 Paperback

....

To

Marie Pippert Comstock and Roy Louis Comstock

their lives and their love
an expanding circle

Contents

List of Contributing Authors   xi
Acknowledgments   xiii

Introduction   1
The goal of this book is to welcome researchers into the community of question-askers   1
The problem facing new researchers is that research pressures undermine vocations   2
The solution is not RCR training or a series of unconnected lectures and online exercises   4
The solution is a vibrant moral community and a coherent introduction to ethical thinking   7
Research means asking questions and looking for answers   8
Ethics means asking questions and looking for answers about right and wrong, and good and bad   10
The plan of this book is to introduce the RCR topics organized as an expanding moral circle   14

Part A − Protect my interests   21
Graduate students have diverse interests   21
. . . yet all have a common set of duties   22
. . . including the duty to avoid research misconduct   22
Case study: "Can of worms," by John Allen   24
. . . and to blow the whistle   30
But is whistle-blowing really in an egoist's interests?   31
Kinds of interests   32
Rational egoism is the view that one should always act to best satisfy one's categorical interests   34
How to proceed as an egoist   35

1   **Report misconduct**   39
What is cheating?   39
Is cheating unethical for egoists?   41
No: egoists have reasons to cheat   41
Yes: egoists have stronger reasons not to cheat   43
. . . because they have their own internal filters   44
. . . and are surrounded by cheater detectors   47
. . . cheater detectors who disapprove of cheaters   49
. . . and punish cheaters   51

... and, furthermore, the community requires whistle-blowing 53
So, in situations of confusion and ambiguity, honesty seems the best policy – even for egoists 54

2 **Avoid plagiarism** 58
Protect myself against charges of plagiarism 58
Can I get away with it? 61
Exercise: "Recognize plagiarism," by Charlotte Bronson and Gary Comstock 62
Why words matter to the egoist 64
Conclusion 66

3 **Beware intuition** 68
Egoists must be conscious of observation bias 68
... wary of misleading heuristics 69
... and on guard against self-misunderstanding 71
... not to mention probability ineptness 72
Case study: "Monty Hall," by Keith Devlin 72
To safeguard judgments against prejudice and intuition, engage others 76

4 **Justify decisions** 79
Give reasons to justify your decisions 79
... especially in borderline cases 79
Case study: "What's in a picture? The temptation of image manipulation," by Mike Rossner and Kenneth M. Yamada 80
Conclusion: some reservations about egoism 87

Part B – Promote our interests 91
Graduate students sign diverse contracts 92
Yet all are part of one contractual community 93
... in which giving reasons comes naturally 95
... because we are emotional, social animals 97
... and yet the community is constantly threatened by unreasonable decisions 99
Reason-giving contractualism is the view that a person should always act in accord with principles that no free and equal person could reasonably reject 100
How to proceed as a contractualist 102

5 **Articulate reasons** 105
Professional codes articulate two types of rules 106
Common rules that members should internalize 106
Specific rules that members should examine critically 107
... and be able to justify 108
Case study: The Ecological Society of America Code of Ethics 108
Background essay: "Utilitarianism and the evolution of ecological ethics," by Gary Varner 111
Conclusion 117

6 **Write cooperatively**   118
Background essay: "Responsible authorship," by James R. Wilson, Lonnie Balaban and Gary Comstock   118
Case study: "Authorship: new faculty," by James R. Wilson, Daniel J. Robison and Gary Comstock   124
Guidelines: "Publication ethics: a common sense guide," by Wesley E. Snyder   130

7 **Protect manuscripts**   133
A peer reviewer is an implicit contractor   133
Background essay: "Peer review," by James R. Wilson   133
How to proceed as a peer reviewer   142

8 **Clarify statistics**   144
Collect data responsibly   144
. . . and guard its confidentiality   145
Case study: "What educated citizens should know about statistics and probability," by Jessica Utts   146
Conclusion: some reservations about contractualism   152

Part C – Respect strangers' rights   155
Graduate students have various legal rights   157
Yet all have the same moral rights   158
Moral rights theories are views that hold that one should always respect the dignity of others   162
Case study: human pesticide toxicity testing   163

9 **Inform subjects**   169
Introduction   169
What informed consent is   170
Why it's complicated   170
Why it's hard to get   172
Why it matters   176
Background essay: "Informed consent and the construction of values," by Douglas MacLean   177
How to get experimental subjects' informed consent: sample form   181

10 **Mentor inclusively**   184
A mentor is a counselor   184
Background essay: "Mentoring,"
by Ellen Hyman-Browne (Deceased), Michael Kalichman and Daniel Vasgird   185
Exercise: "Interview your mentor," by Gary Comstock and Charlotte Bronson   195
Case study: "Why 'female' science professor?" by Female Science Professor   197
Case study: "NIH uncovers racial disparity in grant awards," by Jocelyn Kaiser   199
Conclusion   201

11 **Recognize property**   202
Introduction   202

Who owns your data? 202
Background essay: "Intellectual property," by Adam Cureton, Douglas MacLean, Jami Taylor and Henry Schaffer 203
Case study: "DNA patents and human dignity," by David B. Resnik 212
Conclusion 216

12 **Reveal conflicts** 218
Introduction 218
Background essay: "Shared responsibility, individual integrity: scientists addressing conflicts of interest in biomedical research," Federation of American Societies for Experimental Biology 221
Conclusion: some reservations about rights 226

Part D – Honor all interests 229
Research aims at a variety of good consequences 231
Naive utilitarianism requires maximizing good consequences 231
... while assigning all like interests an equal weight 232
But not all good consequences are acceptable 234
Two-level utilitarianism is the view that one should habitually act to respect rights but when thinking critically should maximize good consequences 235
... including good consequences for sentient animals 238
Conclusion: how to proceed as a utilitarian 240

13 **Treat humanely** 243
Everyday rules for treating animals humanely in research 243
Critical thinking about using animals in research 246
Background essay: "The case for the use of animals in biomedical research," by Carl Cohen 247
Background essay: "Util-izing animals" by Hugh LaFollette and Niall Shanks (Deceased) 253
Conclusion 265

14 **Preserve environments** 267
Ecosystems have utility for future people and animals 268
Background essay: "The ethics of climate change," by John Broome 269
Conclusion 273

15 **Cultivate responsibility** 274
Background essay: "Wingspread declaration on renewing the civic mission of the American research university," by Harry Boyte and Elizabeth Hollander 276
Conclusion: some reservations about two-level utilitarianism 281

Conclusion 285

Index 288

List of Contributing Authors

John Allen
Senior Editor, On Wisconsin Magazine,
Wisconsin Alumni Association,
Madison, WI, USA

Lonnie Balaban
Editor and writer, Cary, NC, USA

Harry Boyte
Co-Director, Center for Democracy
and Citzenship, Minneapolis, MN, USA

Charlotte Bronson
Professor of Plant Pathology and Associate
Vice President for Research, Iowa State
University, Ames, IA, USA

John Broome
White's Professor of Moral
Philosophy and Fellow of Corpus
Christi College, University of Oxford,
Oxford, UK

Carl Cohen
Professor of Philosophy, University of
Michigan, Ann Arbor, MI, USA

Adam Cureton
Assistant Professor of Philosophy,
University of Tennessee, Knoxville, TN, USA

Keith Devlin
Executive Director, Human-Sciences and
Technologies Advanced Research Institute,
Stanford University, Stanford, CA, USA

Female Science Professor, a full professor
in a physical sciences field at a large
research university, Monty Hall

Elizabeth Hollander
Senior Fellow, Tisch College of Citizenship
and Public Service, Tufts University,
Medford, MA, USA

Ellen Hyman-Browne (Deceased)
Formerly Research Compliance
Officer, Children's Hospital, Philadelphia,
PA, USA

Michael Kalichman
Director, Research Ethics Program,
University of California, San Diego,
CA, USA

Jocelyn Kaiser
Staff Writer, Science, Washington DC,
USA

Hugh LaFollette
Cole Chair in Ethics, University of
South Florida St. Petersburg,
St. Petersburg, FL, USA

Douglas MacLean
Professor of Philosophy, University
of North Carolina, Chapel Hill,
NC, USA

David B. Resnik
Bioethicist and Institutional Review Board
Chair, National Institutes of Health
Sciences, NC, USA

Daniel J. Robison
Professor of Forestry and Associate Dean
for Research, College of Natural Resources,
North Carolina State University, Raleigh,
NC, USA

Mike Rossner
Executive Director, Rockefeller University
Press, New York, NY, USA

Henry Schaffer
Professor Emeritus of Genetics and
Biomathematics, North Carolina State
University, Raleigh, NC, USA

Niall Shanks (Deceased)
Formerly Curtis D. Gridley Distinguished
Professor of History and Philosophy
of Science, Wichita State University,
KA, USA

Wesley E. Snyder
Professor of Electrical and Computer
Engineering, North Carolina State
University, Raleigh, NC, USA

Jami Taylor
Assistant Professor, Political Science and
Public Administration, University of
Toledo, Toledo, OH, USA

Jessica Utts
Professor and Chair, Statistics, University
of California, Irvine, CA, USA

Gary Varner
Professor of Philosophy, Texas A&M
University, College Station, TX, USA

Daniel Vasgird
Director, Office of Research Integrity and
Compliance, West Virginia University,
Morgantown, WV, USA

James R. Wilson
Professor of Industrial Engineering,
North Carolina State University, Raleigh,
NC, USA

Kenneth M. Yamada
NIH Distinguished Investigator and Chief,
Laboratory of Cell and Developmental
Biology, National Institute of Dental and
Craniofacial Research, Bethesda, MD, USA

Acknowledgments

In the second half of this century's first decade, I was privileged to participate in a wide-ranging conversation about the teaching of research ethics. The conversation or, more accurately, conversations occurred primarily among those scholars involved in a project known as the Model Curriculum for Land Grant Universities in Research Ethics (LANGURE). More than a hundred faculty and graduate students contributed to LANGURE, and their creativity and imagination inspired me to write this book. Our goal was to develop a novel curriculum in the responsible conduct of research (RCR), a curriculum that would take a philosophical approach to the topic and emphasize the centrality of senior members of the community in RCR pedagogy. I'll say more about these goals and assumptions in the Introduction. Before proceeding, however, I wish to acknowledge those who helped to shape the ideas expressed in these pages. There are many and – at the risk of forgetting someone – I venture to acknowledge them all.

Christine Grant and Brenda Alston-Mills served with me as LANGURE's co-principal investigators. It is a privilege to acknowledge their contributions. Two brilliant and creative scholars, each was an indefatigable source of critical insight and good humor. It was an honor and a delight to work alongside them. As this book is one of the "deliverables" of our project and supported by the National Science Foundation (NSF Grant 0530217), we are required to add that any opinions, findings and conclusions or recommendations expressed in this material are those of the author and do not necessarily reflect the views of NSF.

For fixing some of my mistaken views about moral philosophy and helping me to get right whatever is right in the overall structure of the book, four philosophical tutors deserve special credit. Gary Varner persuaded me of the virtues of R. M. Hare's two-level utilitarian ethical theory years ago and he commented extensively on many of these chapters. Doug MacLean helped me to sharpen the exposition of contractualism, argued vigorously with me about the plausibility of egoism, and registered more complaints about the pedagogical wisdom of featuring egoism – as I do – as the first ethical theory that a reader will here encounter. Rob Streiffer and Terry McConnell read almost all of the manuscript, pointing out passages where the argument needed clarification and strengthening. Both saved me from numerous errors. Rob has also helped me to appreciate the role that ethicists may play in public policy discussions. I am deeply indebted to these four exemplary scholars and honored to call them friends.

Others helped too. David Resnik, Dan Vasgird, and Jami Taylor commented on several chapters. Spencer Muse saved me from making more than one gaffe in the discussion of statistical methods. Members of the OpenSeminar in Research Ethics made numerous contributions. It's imperative that I say a further word about this productive informal research group because I invoke it, and even presume to speak as a representative of it, throughout the book.

The OpenSeminar in Research Ethics (openseminar.org/ethics) is a repository of open-source courses in responsible conduct of research. The courses are created, maintained, and updated by senior scholars. These scholars, experts in mentoring junior researchers as they prepare to become professionals, constitute a diverse, informal online community. I gratefully acknowledge the contributions of the OpenSeminar group, especially those who serve on its Advisory Board: Brenda Alston-Mills, Chi Anyansi-Archibong, Alan Beck, Dian Dooley, Christine Grant, Douglas MacLean, Terrance McConnell, Mildred Pointer, David Preston, Rob Streiffer, and Clark Wolf. The managing editors are Anita Gordon, Carol Fedor, David Edelman, Jamaal Pitt, Jorge Ferrer, and Sadashiva Naik. Members who contributed overviews of ethical issues in their disciplines to the website include: Man-Sung Yim, Jun Li, and Tatjana Jevremovic; Tom Wentworth and Kristen Rosenfeld; Brooke Edmunds, Eric Davis and Gerald Holmes; David Wright; Emily Vollmer, Nancy Creamer and Paul Mueller; Michael Paesler; Martha Scotford and Traci Rose Rider; Abigail Cameron, Stephanie Teixeira and Michael Schulman; and David Johnston, Billy Williams, and Phil Lewis. Members who made indirect contributions to this volume include David Musick, Janet Malek, Gene Spafford, George Bodner, Mulumebet Worku, Veronica Nwosu, Robin Liles, Bruce Harmon, Michael Peters, A. G. Rud, Andrew Hirsch, Jothi Kumar, James Svara, Surya Mallapragada, and Tom Wentworth. I have benefited from conversations about research ethics with Mark Sagoff and Rachelle Hollander, but never as thoroughly as when we worked together on a grant proposal for an online research ethics center. To everyone mentioned here, thank you.

I am also grateful to other scientists, engineers, social scientists, and humanists with whom I have worked in various collaborative efforts to institutionalize the teaching of research ethics education. I must especially recognize Michael Paesler and Jim Wilson. Under Paesler's leadership, the North Carolina State University Physics Department began to require a one-credit course in research ethics of all of its doctoral students. Under Wilson's leadership, the NC State and engineering communities have come to understand better the moral dimensions of authorship and peer review practices. Jim's work is the basis of Chapters 6 and 7.

I learned about various aspects of ethical issues in different scientific disciplines when serving on the editorial committee of the third edition of On Being a Scientist (2009). Thanks to the members of that group: Carolyn Bertozzi, John Ahearne, Francisco Ayala, Andrea L. Bertozzi, David Bishop, Frances Houle, Deborah G. Johnson, Michael Loui, Rebecca R. Richard-Kortum, Nick Steneck, and Michael J. Zigmond.

I worked on the book while in residence at the National Humanities Center as an Autonomy, Singularity, Creativity Fellow (2007–09) and am deeply indebted to the NHC staff, the other Fellows and, especially, to Geoffrey Harpham, Director, for their unflagging encouragement. Thanks, as well, to Ruben Carbonell and Raj Narayan of the Kenan Institute for Engineering, Technology, and Science, and Michael Pendlebury, Head of my Department, for arranging the material conditions that made it possible for me to complete the manuscript. The Kenan Institute provided assistance during 2009–11, and my Department contributed more than one off-campus research assignment.

Jennifer Manion provided critical editorial feedback and incisive suggestions to improve the arguments of Parts A–D. Her sharp eye identified many a grammatical jumble, her sharp pencil untangled the messes, and the result of her work was dramatic improvement in the clarity of my prose. Jane Seakins at Cambridge University Press cheerfully kept the project on track.

Finally, thank you to my mentor and confidant, Tom Regan. Tom first encouraged me to study research ethics, helped me to refine my understanding of moral rights and, among many other things, stood by me through more than one difficult day. It is unusual to find great courage, intelligence, and kindness in a man. Tom has them all in equal measure. I am glad to have the opportunity to recognize his virtues and salute his lifetime of achievement.

§§§

I dedicate the book to Mom and Dad. I suspect that they have no idea how much their support has meant to me, especially during the last few years. Children are fortunate when they believe with reason that their parents are the best parents in the world. But I am more fortunate still, because everyone I know says *my* parents are the best parents *they* know of, too.

Introduction

Thomas Edison is often credited with creating the first research laboratory. Legend has it that when a new hire asked about the rules of the lab, Edison responded with a wisecrack. "We don't have rules. We're trying to accomplish something."

This book, in part, is about the rules of research – but those of you who find such rules burdensome, don't put the book down yet. We have some empathy with you. We understand the sentiment behind Melissa Anderson's assertion that it's "no secret that researchers tend to view instruction in the responsible conduct of research as an annoyance" (Anderson 2009). That said, we must immediately add that the policies and regulations governing research are critical to your – to our – success. If someone tries to conduct research in ignorance of the rules they are headed for trouble. And that said, we return to our opening theme, Edison's quip. In this book we will not take a traditional approach to what is now called RCR "training." Rather than emphasizing the rules, we emphasize what we're trying to accomplish.

And what is that? In a phrase, it is a philosophical task, the asking of good questions.

The goal of this book is to welcome researchers into the community of question-askers

But let's start with who "we" are. The book is addressed primarily to graduate students beginning their careers as researchers, people who ask and try to answer good questions. Because there are all kinds of good questions, the book features the contributions of scholars from diverse disciplines within the so-called knowledge industries. So "we" usually means the so-called author's we – me and you. Sometimes, however, I use the editorial we and cast myself in the role of a spokesman for a larger group of people all of whom – you must take it on my authority – agree with my opinions. I'll let the context convey which form of "we" I mean.

When I presume to speak on behalf of others, the others I have in mind are a loose ensemble of dozens of researchers known as the OpenSeminar in Research Ethics. This informal scattered group consists of faculty and graduate students from the physical and biological sciences, mathematics and engineering, and the social sciences and humanities who participated in one way or another in the creation of the pedagogical approach found in this book. I hasten to add that members of the group have varying degrees of philosophical agreement with the consequentialist theory around which the book is organized. That, of course, is a polite way of saying that some strongly disagree with consequentialism. Given the fact that disagreement about theoretical matters is a good thing in research, however, it's also an indication of the scholarly health of our community.[1]

---

[1] See the Acknowledgments for more information about the OpenSeminar and its predecessor, LANGURE. Members of both groups helped to shape the way in which the RCR topics are presented in the 15 chapters and the way in which the expanding circle decision-making method is laid out in the four

---

Research Ethics: A Philosophical Guide to the Responsible Conduct of Research. Gary Comstock. Published by Cambridge University Press. © Cambridge University Press 2013.

What does this group have in common? We ask questions and search systematically for answers, look for reasons as to why one answer is better than another, and then pose more questions. We identify problems, articulate questions, try on various answers for size, and demand comprehensive and satisfying explanations for why this answer is better than that one. On the basis of accumulated explanations, we construct theories, submit these abstractions to scrutiny, and try to identify the overall theory with the greatest explanatory power, usefulness, elegance, and beauty. We form hypotheses and test them. We examine evidence and analyze arguments. We try to decide which of the competing explanations is the best justified. But we do not rest there. Our work invariably leads to new questions, and we begin again.

The problem facing new researchers is that research pressures undermine vocations

Research is a personal activity requiring individual dedication and perseverance. Max Weber called research (he specifically had scientific research in mind) a vocation, a word taken from the Latin *vocare*, a verb meaning to call (Mills & Gerth 1946).[2] In the medieval Christian context, *vocare* was used to refer to the invitation God issued to select men to join the priesthood. In a secular context, a vocation simply means a line of work to which one feels particularly drawn, as if one had been created to be a physicist, chemical engineer, or a scholar of religion.

Mark Sagoff argues that research is inherently value-laden insofar as it is a process of self-examination and self-clarification. He writes,

> As a vocation, research insists on intellectual honesty, trustworthiness, candor, and clarity; and anything less is to that extent not research. These virtues are what Weber describes as the inward conditions of research. The outward conditions – the business of research – may not fully cohere with the inward conditions but for research to thrive they cannot depart too widely from them.[3]

There is no doubt that research is a business activity and a source of income. Nor could many of us pursue it if we weren't paid a stipend or a salary and benefits. But how, asked Weber, can a graduate student pursue his or her vocation while also navigating through these financial waters? Can one remain true to one's calling while being consumed by the business of paying off one's student loans, much less the task of being the first one to submit a patent application on one's discovery? Compounding these challenges is the fact that research occurs in a university culture that may very well regard research instrumentally – as a means to a paycheck – a culture that seems at times almost to encourage mercenaries and cheaters.

More and more, graduate students are products of an educational system telling them that being a good professional simply requires state-of-the-art technical expertise. Something is missing here, the message that research is a vocation. And there is a cost for this omission. In 1997, Robert McGinn asked his Stanford undergraduate engineering

---

parts (A, B, C, and D). Disciplines represented in the OpenSeminar and LANGURE included the physical and biological sciences, engineering, the social sciences, and humanities. I recount these points to emphasize that "we" encompasses a broad swath.

[2] I thank Sagoff for bringing Weber's lecture to my attention.

[3] This paragraph is taken from the grant proposal Sagoff and I drafted with Rachelle Hollander.

majors whether their instructors had given explicit information about what it means to be ethically responsible as an engineer. Less than two-thirds of the students – 63% – said they had received the information. Four years later, in 2001, the number dropped to 60%.

We shouldn't be surprised, then, that scientists are engaging in questionable conduct, although perhaps we should be surprised that they admit it. A headline in *Nature's* News pages proclaims, "One in three scientists confesses to having sinned" (Wadman 2005). An article in the same issue reports that, in a poll of more than 3000 scientists, 15% admitted to having changed the design, methodology, or results of a study in response to pressure from a funding source (Martinson *et al.* 2005). Twelve percent said that in the past 3 years they had overlooked another scientist's use of flawed data. Faculty, meanwhile, pay less attention than they should to their own practices when writing up the results of their research. According to a study in *Nature*, "up to 20% of published papers contain some degree of self-plagiarism." It's bad enough when professors pad their résumés. However, as *Nature* goes on to note, when an author publishes the same paper in multiple venues, life-threatening consequences may follow. If another author conducts a meta-analysis of publications on a certain topic and one author has duplicated his or her paper in the record, the meta-analysis may be fooled into making dangerous errors (Giles 2005).[4] For instance, in a meta-analysis of 84 randomized clinical trials conducted between 1991 and 1996 that studied the ability of a drug to suppress postoperative vomiting, the author's inclusion of duplicated papers "led to a 23% overestimation" of the drug's efficacy (Tramèr *et al.* 1997).

Other ethical pitfalls, such as prevarication and evasion, are also not foreign to research. Here are two examples.

Marc Hauser, a psychologist at Harvard University, conducts research on the moral lives of animals. While coding video of primates listening to novel sounds, Hauser consistently coded the animals' responses differently than had his two graduate students who were handling the same data. Hauser's coding supported his hypothesis that the monkeys exhibit responses to novelty that are similar to those of human children. When the graduate students questioned his methods, the university investigated his actions and eventually found him solely responsible for the fabrication of data (Bartlett 2010).

In March 2006, at the University of Vermont, a research assistant suspected Professor Eric Poehlman, an exercise physiologist studying aging, of switching data points to exaggerate patients' deteriorating health. An expert on metabolism in menopausal women, Poehlman was found guilty of misrepresenting his data so that they fit with his favored interpretation. He was barred from receiving additional funds from any US research agency. He admitted to having made material false statements in grant applications, stating that in one case, since he did not have access to preliminary test results needed to complete his proposal, he simply made up the numbers (United States Department of Health and Human Services 2005a and Kintisch 2005).

Do graduate students enter a community that winks at wrongdoing as often as it exposes it? Donald McCabe, a sociologist at Rutgers, has studied student misconduct for decades. McCabe has found that more than 40% of faculty report that they have ignored cheating. More than half of all faculty members have never reported a single case of cheating to anyone

---

[4] Giles cites (Tramèr *et al.* 1997).

else (McCabe *et al.* 2006). As we shall see in Chapter 1, most of us allow a certain amount of dishonesty in ourselves, if not in others. Dan Ariely's experiments with students on Ivy League campuses suggest that students have a fudge factor; they allow themselves to inflate their own scores by as much as 10 or 20% when they self-report scores under conditions of anonymity. That is, rather than reporting, correctly, that Mark got four answers right out of a possible 20, Mark will help himself to an extra point or two and report that he actually got five or six right – if he believes he won't be caught. Is it simply "human nature" to improve one's score when one is given the chance? The data suggest that it is. And that's the problem.

In the face of these grim facts about the competitive nature of research, its financial pressures, the human tendency to cheat, and the apparent paucity of moral support for young researchers, can graduate students afford to treat their research as anything other than a self-interested business endeavor? Weber thought not. He called the academic life "a mad hazard" because he was convinced it would ruin most of the students who tried to succeed in it. And he told them so.

The solution is not RCR training or a series of unconnected lectures and online exercises

The RCR field – if it is a field – is confused and muddled. Instructors in the area have not paid adequate attention to its foundations. Institutions responding to federal demands for education in the area have produced unimaginative programs with a familiar and unpromising face. According to the conventional model, young researchers are required to attend a series of lectures by local or national experts on each of the nine RCR subjects identified by the Office of Research Integrity as "core topics":

1. Data Acquisition, Management, Sharing and Ownership
2. Conflict of Interest and Commitment
3. Human Subjects
4. Animal Welfare
5. Research Misconduct
6. Publication Practices and Responsible Authorship
7. Mentor/Trainee Responsibilities
8. Peer Review
9. Collaborative Science

But what is the relationship between these topics? What makes them individually necessary as members of the list? Are they mutually exclusive of each other or do they overlap? What makes them jointly sufficient to cover all the main topics? Answers to these critical questions are not easy to find.[5] Typically, lecturers invited to address RCR rarely comment

---

[5] Each of the nine topics on the list is important, but neither the number of items nor their order is sacred. In 1994, NIH listed six topics (NIH 1994). Recent enumerations often add two topics – science in society and safe laboratory practices – for a total of 11. The Council of Graduate Schools (CGS) adds five and comes up, apparently, with 14 (The Council of Graduate Schools 2008). If the teachers are so confused conceptually, how can we expect students to understand? Ironically, the CGS document asserts that "a comprehensive approach" should include, as two of its additional five topics, "ethical decision-making and deliberation processes" and "ethical principals [sic]." But shouldn't these two so-called additional areas be considered part and parcel of the original nine?

on the field as a whole. Instead, new topics seem to be added to the list as this or that historical scandal erupts and some authority decides training must be offered for the new area, too.[6]

In too many universities, so-called RCR training consists of a set of exercises in which students passively listen to a series of lectures by a procession of experts, each of whom explains the regulations governing their area but not the connections between the areas.[7] The result is that students are exposed to rules but they are not offered the opportunity to discuss the moral principles on which the rules are based or the connections between the various RCR topics. Is there a moral decision-making procedure that one could use to think through issues arising not only in the canonical list of areas but also in novel situations?[8]

Research has evolved its own set of rules and regulations. We – the OpenSeminar group – share the view that research regulations can impede progress and we worry that the rules are becoming increasingly burdensome, perhaps even counterproductive (Grady 2010). Minimally, we – you and I – should question the value of the traditional response to the federal requirement to provide RCR training. Why, for example, should we call it training rather than education?[9]

How could one discuss any of the first nine topics even superficially without explaining the processes and principles of ethical decision-making? (How, we are tempted to add – assuming that you could discuss RCR without discussing ethics – could you discuss "ethical decision-making and deliberation processes" without discussing ethical principles?) CGS no doubt has good intentions, but its confused discussion exemplifies and exacerbates the conceptual disarray of the field.

[6] For example, the US Public Health Service syphilis trials in Tuskegee, Alabama, gave rise to the topic of informed consent and the use of humans in research. The use of monkeys in Silver Springs Maryland in head injury experiments spurred the emergence of animals in research as a topic. The controversy swirling around David Baltimore's lab prompted discussion of issues related to falsification of data and whistle-blowing. At some point questions were raised about proper storage of data and interpretation of statistics. Disrespect of research assistants and abuse of mentoring relationships added even more subjects to the agenda. And so on. The topics on the list, in other words, have no obvious relationship to each other. The list itself is nothing more than a bunch of topics lassoed together largely as the result of historical accident.

[7] So, for example, the head of the Institutional Review Board (IRB) visits the seminar and explains the rules regarding the use of human subjects – but nothing about how the rules regarding the use of animals are related to the use of humans. The head of the Institutional Animal Care and Use Committee (IACUC) visits to discuss the regulations governing the use of animals – but does not explain why these rules differ so dramatically from those governing the use of humans. Then the Director of Sponsored Programs visits to explain university rules about intellectual property but doesn't explore the question of whether the claim that these rules are justified because they spur innovation and economic development has any basis in fact. The director of Student Conduct provides statistics on the number of undergraduate plagiarism cases but does not ask about the moral psychology of the student who cheats occasionally – which is most of them – nor the philosophical justification of the claim that cheating is always wrong. And so on down the line.

[8] Is it necessary for RCR training programs to cover every item on the canonical list? Do graduate students in electrical engineering or ancient philosophy, for example, need to be trained to use human subjects? And are there topics not on the ORI canonical list that ought to be on it (e.g., we'll add intellectual property, environmental ethics, and the social responsibilities of researchers)? The problems here are two-fold. First, the relevance of ethical theories to each of the RCR topics may not be explained. Second, after the lecture on ethics, the theories may never be coherently spoken of again.

[9] And why should we put up with a process that consists of little more than a set of rote online activities designed to satisfy an administrative check-off requirement (cf. Comstock et al. 2007)?

RCR books do not serve researchers well if they represent a printed form of a compliance exercise. Such exercises allow students to sit alone in front of a computer screen and mechanically regurgitate rules. Despite the fact that the conventional model may be successful in introducing students to relevant policies and regulations, it is not designed to convey the idea that ethical reflection itself is a systematic endeavor. Nor do students come away from online click-through "training" exercises feeling that they are part of a community of moral discourse. Teachers of RCR should approach the subject as a research area in itself. That means taking seriously relevant literature amassed over the past few decades in the areas of normative ethics and meta-ethics. This book takes a step in that direction, showing how ethical theories and methods can bring coherence to the canonical topics.[10]

---

[10] Adil Shamoo and David Resnik (Shamoo & Resnik 2009) helped to begin rectifying the problem with the first edition of their textbook. Now in a second edition, the book begins with an introduction to ethical theory and decision-making and proceeds to discuss as a linked pair the issues of authorship and peer review. They also follow their discussion of the use of animals with the protection of humans, another natural alliance. The book does not, however, structure itself according to a decision-making method that readers could use in resolving moral dilemmas in different areas. In his brief introduction to the subject, historian Nicholas Steneck (Steneck 2004) discerns a different order in the topics. He begins with ethical issues arising in the planning of research, moving on to consider the questions that arise in conducting research, and concludes with issues that come up in reporting and disseminating research. Putting on a historian's hat can bring temporal order to the topics.

These two works are notable as viable alternatives to the received "RCR training" paradigm. Our book differs from theirs in four ways. First, we adopt a single, straightforward, philosophical approach to the material. Second, we use this approach to group the various topics in more natural ways. Third, we sustain our general, consequentialist, vision throughout the treatment of particular issues in a way that shows the intellectual cohesion of RCR. Fourth, we structure the book as an exercise in moral imagination, an exercise that moves from the good of the individual to the good of the whole.

Our approach does not reinforce the mistaken idea that ethics is a matter of memorizing regulations and obeying authorities. The conventional model approaches RCR education as an exercise in rule-teaching and rule-following, but there is no evidence that this model works. This conclusion comes as no surprise to those who work in the area because the model assumes an impoverished notion of the professions. Professionals don't memorize rules and follow them. Rather, we form vibrant communities of moral discourse. We question our procedures and probe the foundations of our rules. We come to know how to behave by reasoning about what we do, behaving conscientiously because we have the freedom to exercise independent judgment. We know that professionals are society's conscience. When society faces a new ethical question, professionals must figure out what is the right thing to do even though no one has yet discovered the right rule for the situation.

The OpenSeminar approach is critical of the received view. We find it ineffective at best and self-contradictory at worst. Part of the reason for this state of affairs is that when the first government agency began to require RCR training decades ago, it did not provide benchmarks by which the success of efforts could be evaluated. Consequently, it is disquietingly unclear what works and does not work in this critical area. We note, for example, that the number of RCR training programs overall is increasing, as is the absolute number of graduate students so "trained." The obvious expectation, therefore, would be that the number of research misconduct reports would decrease. However, to the contrary, the number of institutions reporting misconduct cases to ORI has not decreased year to year (Titus et al. 2008; Wells 2006).

The solution is a vibrant moral community and a coherent introduction to ethical thinking

In this book, we depart in two ways from the conventional model.

First, whereas RCR training aims at compliance with rules, we aim to welcome students into the community of scholars – people who ask questions systematically when a new ethical challenge arises. We aim to nurture interests in critical inquiry and self-motivated responsible behavior, believing that individuals invested in and closely supervised by their communities will not only follow rules they have autonomously adopted for themselves. They will also be prepared critically to examine and on occasion revise such rules.

Second, whereas the received approach relies on a framework cobbled together from a hodge-podge of topics (Heitman & Bulger 2005), we sort the topics philosophically so as to reveal their coherence and systematicity. In footnote 10 we saluted the advances represented in the work of Shamoo and Resnik, on the one hand, and Steneck, on the other. Might there be an even better way to organize the material?

We think so, and we think the right organizing principle is philosophical. We start by introducing egoistic self-interest as a way to motivate right behavior, expanding the moral circle beyond the self in the next step to include one's group. In a third step, we recognize the moral rights of those outside our contractual arrangements. The fourth and final step acknowledges the claims on us of animals and, perhaps, of future generations and even nature itself. Our approach aims, as we say, first and foremost to welcome junior researchers into academic communities and to hone their skills of critical inquiry. We strive to provide them with a method by which to resolve complex and changing ethical questions. We draw insights from educational psychology, evolutionary biology, and the moral development literature, to confront student apathy. We take seriously the fact that when it comes to research ethics many graduate students think "Really? Who cares?" We do not pretend that this thorny question does not hover over all of our endeavors. We choose to address it directly and at the very start by introducing cases in which students have been harmed by misconduct. Yes, we appeal initially to self-interest. But then we expand the circle outward – from oneself to others – motivating this move by citing the role of the moral emotions in personal identity. Our approach is conceptually coherent, research based, and focused on imagination and question-asking rather than compliance and rule-following.

This book also focuses on the intrinsic rewards of research, the inherent pleasures of what we're trying to accomplish. The chapters are designed to help you hone your talents as you gain knowledge and experience and to introduce heroic folk who have overcome significant obstacles and helped to advance research in responsible, admirable ways. They also introduce people who, by taking shortcuts or engaging in outright fraud, have undermined the fabric of trust that's so essential to the health of our community. Along the way, we will direct you to read your professional code, and you will learn steps you can take to help restore confidence in our essential practices: authorship and mentoring, honoring of intellectual property, responsible gathering and use of statistics, avoidance of potential conflicts of interest. The book is intended to help you – the serious younger scholar of the natural, biological, or social sciences, or of engineering or the humanities – to "read" your environment, size up the contingencies that threaten the achievement of your goals, and steer around them.[11] The authors will have achieved their goal if the book helps to make "normal misbehavior" less normal and the idea of research as a vocation more normal.

As you prepare to enter your research community, we emphasize self-awareness and clarity about your values, as well as effective mentoring, as methods for achieving your goals. Along the way, you may meet researchers who are unwilling to play by the rules. A central objective of this volume is to help you take a realistic approach to them. We suggest that you strike up conversations with those more advanced in their careers, for an isolated researcher is a vulnerable researcher. The OpenSeminar in Research Ethics sponsors a Facebook group and we encourage you to join us (http://www.facebook.com/group. php?gid=15680283403). Our online group promotes discussions of ethical concerns that arise in the daily work of senior scientists, mathematicians, engineers, social scientists, humanists, and their doctoral and postdoctoral students. But it only aims to stimulate and support moral discourse by and about researchers engaged in their own self-clarification, self-criticism, and self-education. Neither the group nor this book is meant to replace the primary research community, for only in face-to-face communities can we truly pursue the vocation of research.

If it is face-to-face contact with people that I need – you may now be asking yourself – why should I read this book? Why read a book about research ethics when one can learn the rules much more quickly from one's mentor and peers, codified in your discipline's code of ethics, and when there is so little time in a graduate student's life for activities not directly related to their degree program? What fledgling researcher has time for abstract philosophizing?

The answer is three-fold. First, your mentors and peers probably cannot teach you all that you need to know. Second, sometimes the rules we seek are not found in the code; without additional guidance, we'll remain at a loss, not knowing how to behave. Yet as professionals, we must do the right thing. Third, if anyone should make time for philosophizing, it should be those who wish to earn a *philosophiae doctor* degree.

But the short answer is this: read this book to protect yourself. As a new researcher, you will encounter many obstacles in your attempt to build a successful career. Your mentor cannot possibly cover all of the problems or tell you how to deal with all of the temptations to take shortcuts, to free ride on others' work, or to adopt a purely instrumental attitude toward your project. This book can help you focus on the intrinsic rewards of research and meet others who share your interests.

Research means asking questions and looking for answers

Speaking generally, research begins in wonderment, when we are puzzled by how something works or what a certain proposition means or whether a correlation suggests a causal

---

[11] The research community must constantly acculturate new members, acquainting them with its norms and aspirations and thereby reinvigorating and perpetuating the best version of itself. And newcomers must be able to trust established mentors, mentors who in turn empower them, as well as others, to be as autonomous as is appropriate. Toward that end – renewing the research community by welcoming you into it – this book seeks to introduce you not only to research ethics, but also to people whom you can trust and who share your objectives and puzzles, your desire for knowledge and your values.

relation. We then discuss our questions and form a hypothesis. We go on to gather data, run experiments, try out our explanations on others and test our answers in whatever ways we can think of.

Defined more formally, research is

a systematic investigation, including research development, testing and evaluation, designed to develop or contribute to generalizable knowledge (Dept. of Health and Human Services 1992, p.45 CFR 46.102).

So construed, research includes activities in the basic and applied fields of science, engineering, and mathematics, as well as the social sciences and humanities. Yes, research involves the formation and testing of hypotheses whether the subject matter is DNA, a software code sequence, or an electrical engineering design. And yet, research also refers to a wider set of practices and institutions. For example, research in the humanities and arts, traditionally known as scholarship, involves other sorts of activities, including the systematic search for explanations of the imaginative expressions we find in literature, music, and the creative arts.

We must keep an open mind about the breadth of activities that qualify as research if we are to understand the multitude of practices that legitimately fall into the category. As a point of departure, however, we might think of research as an organized family of activities that begins in wonderment and questioning, proceeds with methodical searches for generalizable answers supported by good reasons, and continues with the generation of new questions.

Research is inherently a human activity involving not only our reasoning capacities, but also our emotions and attitudes. Just think about the act of asking a question. Any time a peer of yours raises her hand during a class discussion or waits urgently for a conversation partner to finish his sentence so that she can press an objection, she embodies a range of virtues: wonder, humility, honesty, self-confidence, and integrity, to name a few. To ask questions is to risk the possibility that others will think you ignorant. But it also brings the possibility that others will admire your commitment to pursue the truth. To express these attitudes to another, especially publicly, demonstrates courage and resolve. Asking questions requires and rewards persistence, skepticism, and self-examination. Without those traits, you may not have the staying power necessary to steer clear of the obstacles that will likely arise.

Posing questions, and the emotions this involves, is central to science. Without questions, our search for the truth lacks motivation, drive, persistence. Systematicity is also important, because the process must be directed and cumulative. Without a designed, orderly way of learning from previous mistakes and successes, the process will lack comprehensiveness and direction, and we will be unable to extend it, build on prior successes and failures, and generate generalizable knowledge.

Successful research results not in arcane bits of trivia, meaningless streams of data, or idiosyncratic observations about random events. It results in broad ideas and overarching syntheses that are portable, casting light on matters beyond the matters for which they were originally developed. Sometimes, the results of research produce observations or breakthroughs leading to revolutionary new principles or exciting theories. Breakthroughs, however, must be justifiable. The results of our experiments, which allow us to separate good hypotheses from bad ones, must be replicable by others and explanations of observations must pass muster before juries of academic peers.

How can we distinguish between stronger and weaker hypotheses? Generally, the best hypotheses in experimental fields are consistent with each other, and result in predictions that can be confirmed or disconfirmed by empirical tests. The best hypotheses are fecund, giving rise to new predictions and ideas for experiments in other areas. When scientific disciplines such as astronomy and geology are involved, or any of the social sciences and humanities where empirical confirmation may not be possible, generalizations that lend coherence to diverse phenomena and observations are important. Simple and lower-level explanations are better than complicated explanations that unnecessarily appeal to higher-order domains. All things being equal, elegant, simple, and beautiful theories are preferred over excessively complex and pedantic ones.

Ethics means asking questions and looking for answers about right and wrong, and good and bad

The study of ethics is a field of research in which we ask questions about harms and benefits, virtues and vices, choices and dispositions, conflicts and agreements, and the justifications of decisions. The three central branches are:

- descriptive ethics, the empirical study of what people actually do, believe, and value;
- normative ethics, the evaluative study of how we should behave in particular cases;
- metaethics, the philosophical study of the foundations of moral language.

Descriptive ethics involves psychological, sociological, and anthropological inquiry into ethical values as evidenced by what people say they ought to do, as well as by what they actually do. This book focuses primarily on normative ethics, which analyzes the development of moral standards, and applies them to the following kinds of questions: what topic ought I to choose for my dissertation research? What should I do if I witness someone cheating? What policies and regulations concerning research would be the best for my institution to adopt? Finally, metaethicists study questions such as: where does morality come from? How do we ultimately justify ethical judgments? Is the basis of ethics found in God's will? In evolutionary adaptations? In moral intuitions? All of the above? None of them?

One way to begin our venture into normative ethics is to consider a paradigm case of unethical behavior. Jan Schon, a promising young physicist, won awards for his work in organic molecular crystals; in February 2002 he was named outstanding young investigator by the Materials Research Society. But by April of that same year, Bell Labs had fired him for falsifying data. Why would his fabrication be considered wrong? One reason would be the harm it caused. And who was harmed? Himself, obviously. His employer. His friends and colleagues, who had believed in him. The Materials Research Society, which had honored him. Those who read his work and redesigned or redirected their research because of his (false) findings. And indeed the entire community of physicists, which was embarrassed and chagrined by his misdeeds.

Harm is a moral concern; where there is harm, there may be a breach of moral duty. Can beings other than humans be harmed? What is the scope of the prohibition against harm? Does it include animals? Plants? Ecosystems? Future generations? Artificial intelligences? Our regulatory bodies acknowledge that vertebrates are sentient and can experience pain, and so our research regulations include protections for some, although not all, animals. Perhaps we should say, then, that ethical considerations typically arise whenever any action involves harm or potential harm to sentient individuals.

Theories of normative ethics help us to figure out how to behave, giving guidance and recommendations when we face conflicting interests. They do this by giving us the means to make moral judgments, which are prescriptive rather than descriptive. That is, moral judgments tell us not how we in fact act, but how we ought to act. This is important, since we aren't always inclined to do what is right. To further complicate things, we often don't know what interests take precedence. For example, say I can spend $5.00 to satisfy my friend's desire for a cappuccino or give the $5.00 to Oxfam to help provide clean drinking water for a stranger in another country. Which interest should take precedence? This is a difficult question and different ethical theories give conflicting answers. The point here is that a good ethical theory yields answers that are normative, action-guiding answers.

Normative ethics doesn't just provide one standard according to which one can determine what one ought to do or whether a certain situation is morally good or bad. It posits a number of ethical theories, each with its own standard or standards, and these theories sometimes yield different answers to practical problems. Just as scientific claims are grounded in scientific theories, moral judgments are grounded in ethical theories. Therefore, when considering normative questions, we need to know which theory is in play. A good theory has four characteristics.

1.   It is serious

In trying to decide whether an ethical theory is a good one, evaluate it with these issues in mind. Ethical issues bother us. Think of the emotional investment you have in your response to legislation that deals with preventive war strikes, discrimination on the basis of race or religion, abortions, gay marriages, sport hunting, or human embryonic stem cell research. When we raise such issues we believe that they deserve to be taken seriously. And we want to be taken seriously when we engage in reasoned argument about them. If a theory makes light of all of these issues – or claims to have a ready solution for every one of them, a solution that turns out on examination to be nothing more than a dismissive sleight of hand – then we have a good reason to wonder whether the theory is a theory about ethics at all.

2.   It is fair

Ethical theories should give rise to similar judgments about similar cases. That is, they are characterized by fairness. If a theory lets me decide that it is morally wrong for Carrie to drop an outlying data point in a particular paper, but it doesn't have me apply the same judgment to Kwame in similar circumstances, then something is wrong with the theory. It shouldn't matter that Kwame is a friend whereas Carrie is a stranger. Similar circumstances call for similar judgments. If I don't use language in this way then I am probably not making a moral judgment. If I say dropping data points is ok when my friends do it but not ok when anyone else does it, I am making a claim of preference or taste, not morality. Should I go on to insist, oddly, that my judgment is an "ethical" one after all, then I am using the language of ethics in a very unconventional way. To call an action "unethical" or "morally wrong" simply is to say that the action is wrong for all persons facing similar circumstances.

3.   It is overriding

As suggested in the previous paragraph, moral judgments are sometimes confused with judgments of taste or etiquette. If I say that I prefer bananas to mandarin oranges on my breakfast cereal and that you're wrong to prefer oranges, I don't mean "wrong" in a moral sense. I am not making a moral claim because my claim is not meant to be universal or overriding. It applies only to me. On the other hand, if I say that consuming bananas in the United States is wrong because it supports an ecologically unfriendly and monopolistic form of international agribusiness, I am making an ethical claim. It is a claim that applies to everyone and it is meant to override their preferences. Should we support companies with harmful practices? This is a difficult question and different ethical theories give conflicting answers. The point here is that whatever theory or source one regards as most fundamental in such matters is one's ethical basis, because it takes precedence over other sources of authority, even religious sources.

4.   It is systematic

A good moral theory tells us, in a detailed and comprehensive way, what things are good and bad. What might a theory consider good? Typical candidates include justice, the virtues, pleasure, happiness, human flourishing, a good will, the satisfaction of desires, human rights, obedience to divine commands, and keeping one's word. Likewise, each theory has a corresponding view about ultimate badness. What might be some candidates? The vices, pain, unhappiness, human destitution, and suffering. Because even good theories can differ substantively, they may yield different answers to the following questions: where does the satisfaction of desires or happiness figure in? The cultivation of virtue? Respecting human rights?

In sum, any ethical theory worth its salt will be serious, fair, overriding, and systematic. Many theories that meet these criteria – virtue theory, nihilism, relativism, divine command theory, objective list approaches, and various feminist and environmental theories – are worth considering, but we do not have time or space here to do so. In the chapters that follow, we'll focus on three theories that have attracted the most attention from English-speaking moral philosophers: two forms of deontology – contractualism and rights-based deontology – and utilitarianism, or consequentialist-based ethics. We'll begin, however, with a fourth theory, egoism, because it describes a minimal moral commitment that every psychologically healthy person has.

Egoism holds that a person ought to do what is in his or her own long-term best interests. Egoism provides a ready answer to the question: why should I be moral? For among the many interests that you have, having a successful research career is one of them, and being caught in violation of professional standards will derail your career. In Part A, we use the egoistic perspective to explain the reasons that research misconduct is contrary to one's interests. Throughout the book we'll point out weaknesses with each of the four ethical theories. As each Part (A, B, C, and D) deals with a different theory, look for criticisms of a theory at the end of the chapter that concludes the Part. The relevant chapters are 4, 8, 12, and 15. For example, a major problem with egoism is that it fails our first two criteria of good ethical theories. It seems to be neither serious nor fair because it seems to make light of difficult ethical questions and it is arbitrarily prejudiced toward one group's interests (mine). This point is explained at the end of Chapter 4.

Contractualism, a deontological theory, provides a strong answer to a second question: what is goodness? Contractualism's answer is: reasonableness. The good is found in our nature as rational animals who do things like make promises, and who can be counted on to perform the actions we have pledged to do for each other. Loving parents, friends, instructors, and other mentors teach us to speak and act with courage and honesty – and to give reasons for our actions when we haven't acted appropriately. Contractualists urge morally good people to justify to others what they do. Such justification is usually as simple as pointing out that one's action coheres with the terms of a compact one has entered. Since the research careers to which graduate students aspire are governed by norms and principles, we will use contractualism in Part B to explore professional codes, authorship, peer review, and the collecting, managing, and communicating of data. A reservation about contractualism is that it seems to make it impossible to criticize the rules and reasons of the group to which one belongs (see end of Chapter 8).

Rights theories are forms of deontology, like contractualism. They provide a powerful answer to a third question: what counts as a right action? The answer is that right actions respect the dignity of individuals. Rights theorists hold that people are autonomous, have the ability to make our own choices and others must respect this capacity. Even if someone is using their freedom to make sub-optimal decisions, their decision-making ability must not be over-ridden. Rights theories advise us not to harm individuals even if our aim is to secure much greater benefits for many others. Because research often involves human subjects, rights theories will be the foundation in Part C for an exploration of the use of humans in research, mentoring, intellectual property, and conflicts of interests. The major weakness of the theory is that it seems to have a difficult time justifying the grounds of human rights (see end of Chapter 12).

Utilitarianism provides a different answer than contract theory to the question: what is goodness? Here, the good is pleasure or happiness or the satisfaction of interests. Utilitarianism holds that a person ought to do what will maximize or optimize the good, which amounts to the overall best consequences for everyone concerned and it counsels us to consider equally the like interests of all individuals affected by our actions. Since research sometimes involves nonhuman subjects, we'll employ the theory in Part D to review the use of animals in research, our duties to the environment and future generations, and the wider social responsibilities of researchers. Utilitarianism's major weakness is that it seems to undervalue the weight of our special attachments to those nearest and dearest to us (see end of Chapter 15).

Why look at four separate theories? Can't all four be blended into one over-arching theory? Most philosophers think that the answer is no because each theory gives different answers to critical questions, the questions of what things are good and bad and which actions are right and wrong. Each theory, then, is a rival of the others because each has different theoretical commitments and normative implications. Indeed, each theory has a school populated with moral philosophers who defend it, a school that also seeks to expose the weaknesses of the competitors. This is not a situation we should lament because disagreements concerning foundational matters exist in every discipline. Healthy research fields are marked by vigorous theoretical arguments. That said, a promising proposal by the late-twentieth-century Oxford philosopher R. M. Hare suggests a way to tap into the strengths of all four theories.

Hare, a utilitarian, recognized the significance of egoism and interpreted utilitarianism in a way favorable to contractualism and rights theories (Hare 1981). Influenced by Hare, Princeton ethicist Peter Singer, Hare's student, in a book called *The Expanding Circle*, draws on evolutionary theory to develop a hybrid picture (Singer 1981). In the following chapters, morality begins with self-interest, extends to one's immediate family and friends, and works outward from there as if in a widening circle of moral consideration in the direction of all human beings and sentient animals. The Hare–Singer picture not only serves as the backdrop for this book. It also describes a heuristic to bring order to the scattered RCR topics as well as a method for moral decision-making – a practical device that calls to mind the diverse factors relevant to moral decisions.

The plan of this book is to introduce the RCR topics organized as an expanding moral circle

The book teaches a method of ethical decision-making based on four theories just described. We introduce details of the method in the surveys that introduce each of this book's parts: Part A focuses on egoistic, self-interested concerns; Part B takes up contractual, communal interests; Part C focuses on the rights of strangers; and Part D extends moral consideration to other animals. You'll see that we have assigned each of the 15 RCR topics to a different theory. Please note that the assignment of topics to theories is somewhat arbitrary. While we choose, for example, to cover plagiarism after introducing egoism, we could have discussed plagiarism after introducing contractualism – or after introducing rights theories or utilitarianism, for that matter. We trust, however, that our assignment of topics to theories will help to illustrate the expanding circle method of decision-making. The method is meant to be "portable," to be of help in thinking through ethical decisions in other areas of your life.

The canonical RCR topics are discussed in the chapters (1, 2, and 3, continuing to 15). You can read the chapters without reading the philosophical material found in the four parts (A, B, C, and D), but a word of caution is in order. If you skip the four parts, you may have a hard time understanding the details of the expanding circle metaphor.

A word about that scheme. The expanding circle begins at home, with a consideration of what is in my best interests, my own egoistic concerns. Each of us has many interests, and identifying which of your interests is most important to you is not an easy task. It requires rigorous and ongoing self-examination. You'll need to ask: who am I? What do I most want to do with my life? Honest introspection will reveal that the satisfaction of your professional interests is impossible without the satisfaction of the interests of others. To satisfy your desire to obtain an advanced degree and begin your career requires that others satisfy their desires and do their jobs competently, too.

So ethics might start with egoistic concerns (and note that this is a controversial suggestion in itself), but anyone who is a member of a group – and this is all of us – will see that being loyal to oneself entails being loyal to the groups whose memberships give one's life meaning. After all, some of our interests are inevitably tied up with others' interests. As children, we want to satisfy our own desires, but we also naturally care about our parents and learn to show respect for our siblings. Nor does the circle end there. Singer (Singer 1981) summarizes the basic idea with a passage from the nineteenth-century Irish historian of morals, William Lecky:

At one time the benevolent affections embrace merely the family, soon the circle expanding includes first a class, then a nation, then a coalition of nations, then all humanity, and finally, its influence is felt in the dealings of man with the animal world. (Lecky 1879)

Our interests entail others' interests in part because we use language and seek affiliation with other language users. Excluding pathological cases, humans are linguistic beings who learn from each other that words refer to objects and can be ordered grammatically and rhetorically to communicate hopes, dreams, and passions. Our implication in the interests of others is a gift; even our ability to introspect about ourselves is a capacity we would not possess if our parents and teachers did not give us the conceptual tools essential for self-examination.

Humans need language and want companionship with those who teach it to them. Hardwired for empathy toward those nearest and dearest, we naturally feel empathy with those like us. Furthermore, we can learn to care about humans who are not so intimately related to us, and even to care about strangers. While it is perhaps not easy to feel genuine concern for those outside one's in-group, it is not impossible, either. And the emotional connections we experience can cause a shift in understanding. With proper upbringing, we may come to understand that the physical and psychological pains of others hurt them just as much as ours hurt us, that others value their lives as much as we value ours. Believing that all humans are entitled to equal rights is the foundation for laws protecting humans used in research. The same argument can be given for taking account of the needs of the homeless and hungry, wherever they are. The expansion of the circle continues outward toward future human generations.

But it does not end with our species. For we also protect animals – at least those used in research, at least to some extent, with welfare laws that require that we replace sentient creatures with mathematical models or in vitro models whenever possible. Nor does the circle necessarily end there; some argue that it includes natural ecosystems, recognizing the intrinsic values of the earth and its systems. Arguably, then, even nature itself – its endangered species and habitats – deserves consideration. Where should we draw the line? The answer is up for grabs and a question that moral philosophers conduct research on. The only point we need to insist upon here is that researchers may begin with their own egoistic concerns but they cannot reasonably end there. The logic of our commitments as professionals requires that we take seriously the interests of others.

In this book, we use Singer's notion of an expanding circle to lend coherence to the usual hodge-podge of canonical RCR topics.[12] As it is in a person's own interest to report

---

[12] Other ways of organizing the topics of research ethics include the Committee on Science, Engineering, and Public Policy, National Academy of Sciences, National Academy of Engineering, and Institute of Medicine, *On Being a Scientist*, 3rd ed. (National Academies (US) 2009), a short and widely used pamphlet in the sciences; Francis Macrina, *Scientific Integrity: An Introductory Text with Cases*, 3rd ed. (Macrina 2005) a comprehensive discussion of RCR in science; Robin Penslar, *Research Ethics: Cases and Materials* (Penslar 1995), another early collection, still useful; National Academy of Sciences, National Academy of Engineering, IOM, *Responsible Science: Ensuring the Integrity of the Research Process* (Committee on Science, Engineering, and Public Policy 1992); Bruce Sales and Susan Folkman, eds., *Ethics in Research with Human Participants* (Sales & Folkman 2000) for researchers in psychology; and Elliott and Stern, *Research Ethics: A Reader* (Elliott & Stern 1997).

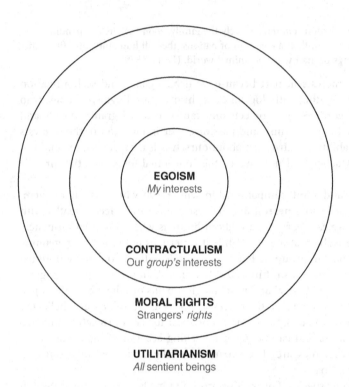

Figure 1. The expanding moral circle.

falsification, understand fabrication, avoid plagiarism, beware of intuition, and justify one's decisions, we explore in Part A the principle that we ought to do what is in our own long-term best interests. As it is in the interest of each person in a research group to articulate their reasons for their conclusions, to write cooperatively, review manuscripts profession-ally, and report statistics transparently, we consider in Part B the principle that we ought to keep our promises and contracts. As it is a basic matter of rights to respect human subjects, mentor inclusively, recognize intellectual property, and reveal both conflicts of interests and collaborations with private industry, we investigate in Part C a principle that has emerged in the last two centuries as one of the most robust and promising in all of ethical theory: we ought to respect each individual's moral rights. Finally, as many animals can feel pain, are subjects of their own lives, and have interests of their own, we must take seriously our role in the welfare of non-human animals as research subjects. In this last step, we expand the circle fully, considering in Part D animal experimentation, duties to future generations and the natural environment, and the larger social responsibilities of researchers. In the last Part, then, we adopt the utilitarian idea that we ought to do what will maximize aggregate happiness.

A reminder before we move on. As explained, we will lay out the expanding circle in Parts A through D while discussing the standard RCR topics in Chapters 1–15. Skipping the parts is permissible, of course, but doing so may be a handicap if you are unfamiliar with the expanding circle method. That said, neither the four Parts nor 15 chapters presume that you have a background in philosophy or familiarity with ethical theory. We've written the book in a style meant to introduce difficult ideas in a way that newcomers can grasp.

Part A. Protect my interests

    1. Report misconduct
    2. Avoid plagiarism
    3. Beware intuition
    4. Justify decisions

Part B. Promote our interests

    5. Articulate reasons
    6. Write cooperatively
    7. Protect manuscripts
    8. Clarify statistics

Part C. Respect strangers' rights

    9. Inform subjects
    10. Mentor inclusively
    11. Recognize property
    12. Reveal conflicts

Part D. Honor all interests

    13. Treat humanely
    14. Preserve environments
    15. Cultivate responsibility

Figure 2. RCR topics organized according to the expanding moral circle metaphor.

Figure 2 summarizes the approach.

Take home lessons

- The goal of this book is to welcome researchers into the scholarly community.
- Problem: career pressures undermine research vocations.
- Solution: a vibrant moral research community.
- Research is a systematic investigation including research development, testing and evaluation, designed to develop or contribute to generalizable knowledge.
- Ethics is the field of research that studies arguments about right and wrong, and good and bad.
- The expanding circle decision-making method has four stages: my interests, our interests, strangers' rights, all interests.
- These stages correspond to four ethical theories: egoism, contractualism, moral rights, and utilitarianism.
- A normative ethic should be serious, fair, overriding and systematic.
- This book organizes the standard RCR topics in terms of the expanding circle.

Bibliography

Anderson, M.S. 2009. Supply and demand in RCR instruction. *PSI (Project for Scholarly Integrity) Blog.* Available at: http://www. scholarlyintegrity.org/Blog.aspx?blogmonth=5&blogyear=2009&blogid=544.

Bartlett, T. 2010. Document sheds light on investigation at Harvard. *The*

Chronicle of Higher Education. Available at: http://chronicle.com/article/Document-Sheds-Light-on/123988/ [Accessed August 30, 2010].

Committee on Science, Engineering, and Public Policy (US). Panel on Scientific Responsibility and the Conduct of Research. 1992. *Responsible Science, Volume I: Ensuring the Integrity of the Research Process* (bound photocopy). National Academies Press.

Comstock, G., Alston-Mills, B. & Grant, C. 2007. Research Ethics Education: Beyond RCR Training. *FCTL Newsletter,* **2**(1), 4.

Dept. of Health and Human Services, U.S. 1992. *Protection of human subjects⍰: Title 45, Code of federal regulations, part 46, revised June 18, 1991.,* Bethesda, MD: Dept. of Health and Human Services, National Institutes of Health, Office for Protection from Research Risks,. Available at: http://www2.lib.ncsu.edu/catalog/record/NCSU1257084.

Elliott, D. & Stern, J.E. 1997. *Research Ethics: A Reader* , 1st edn. Institute for the Study of Applied and Professional Ethics at Dartmouth College.

Giles, J. 2005. Special Report: Taking on the cheats. *Nature,* **435**(7040), 258–259.

Grady, C. 2010. Do IRBs protect human research participants? *JAMA: The Journal of the American Medical Association,* **304**(10), 1122–1123.

Hare, R.M. 1981. *Moral Thinking: Its Levels, Methods and Point.* New York: Oxford University Press.

Heitman, E. & Bulger, R.E. 2005. Assessing the educational literature in the responsible conduct of research for core content. *Accountability in Research,* **12**(3), 207–224.

Kintisch, E. 2005. Scientific misconduct: researcher faces prison for fraud in NIH grant applications and papers. *Science,* **307** (5717), 1851a.

Lecky, W.E.H. 1879. *History of European Morals from Augustus to Charlemagne,* 3d edn, rev. New York: D. Appleton.

Macrina, F.L. 2005. *Scientific Integrity: Text and Cases in Responsible Conduct of Research,* 3rd edn. American Society for Microbiology.

Martinson, B.C., Anderson, M.S. & de Vries, R. 2005. Scientists behaving badly. *Nature,* **435**(7043), 737–738.

McCabe, D., Butterfield, K. & Treviño, L.K. 2006. Academic dishonesty in graduate business programs: prevalence, causes, and proposed action. *Academy of Management Learning and Education,* **5**(3), 294–306.

National Academies (US). 2009. *On Being a Scientist: A Guide to Responsible Conduct in Research,* 3rd edn. Washington DC: National Academies Press.

NIH. 1994. *Reminder and Update: Requirement for Instruction in the Responsible Conduct of Research for Institutional National Research Service Award (NRSA) Research Training Grants.*

Penslar, R.L. 1995. *Research Ethics: Cases and Materials,* annotated edn. Indiana University Press.

Sales, B.D. & Folkman, S. 2000. *Ethics in Research with Human Participants,* 1st edn. American Psychological Association (APA).

Shamoo, A.E. & Resnik, D.B. 2009. *Responsible Conduct of Research,* 2nd edn. New York: Oxford University Press.

Singer, P. 1981. *The Expanding Circle: Ethics and Sociobiology.* New York: Farrar, Straus & Giroux.

Steneck, N.H. 2004. *ORI Introduction to the Responsible Conduct of Research.* University of Michigan Library.

The Council of Graduate Schools. 2008. *The Project for Scholarly Integrity in Graduate Education: A Framework for Collaborative Action.*

Titus, S.L., Wells, J.A. & Rhoades, L.J. 2008. Repairing research integrity. *Nature,* **453**(7198), 980–982.

Tramèr, M.R. *et al.* 1997. Impact of covert duplicate publication on meta-analysis: a case study. *BMJ (Clinical Research Edn),* **315**(7109), 635–640.

United States Department of Health and Human Services. 2005a. *Press Release – Dr. Eric T. Poehlman.* Available at: http://ori.hhs.gov/misconduct/cases/press_release_poehlman.shtml [Accessed August 29, 2010].

Wadman, M. 2005. One in three scientists confesses to having sinned. *Nature*, **435**(7043), 718–719.

Weber, M. 1946. Science as a vocation. In C.W. Mills & H.H. Gerth, eds. *From Max Weber: Essays in Sociology.* New York: Oxford University Press, pp. 129–156.

Wells, J.A. 2006. *Final Report: Observing and Reporting Suspect Misconduct in Biomedical Research.* Available at: ori.hhs.gov/research/intra/documents/gallup_finalreport.pdf.

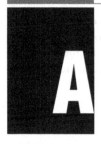

Protect my interests

Deans will often make two points when they welcome graduate students on orientation day. The first point has to do with the diversity of the class; students have a wide variety of backgrounds. The second point has to do with something all of the students, despite their differences, have in common: a core set of values and responsibilities. Let's listen in on the dean's speech.

Graduate students have diverse interests

"You are an intriguingly varied lot," she begins. "I suspect that many of you have values similar to a student I know, Elliot, Mr. All-Business. Elliot is dedicated to networking aggressively with important figures in his field. Elliott's primary goal is to rub elbows with luminaries who can help him obtain a high-powered job and excellent salary. Elliot once told me, 'Who cares if my research topic does not thrill me? I just want to get my publications and move on up.' Now, if you have goals similar to Elliot's, look for a mentor who can help you build your reputation. We will help you to do this."

"On the other hand," the dean continues, "others are very different. Some are probably like another young friend, Jay, Mr. All-Scholarship. Jay wants to meet scholars who can help him perfect his knowledge of the nuances of cellular processes, thoughtful people who will help him push forward the frontiers of knowledge concerning malignant tumor growth. First and foremost, Jay told me, he wants a mentor who can help him develop excellent academic judgment and superb bench skills. 'If my research is not inherently valuable,' Jay said, 'why would I invest my life in it?' Now, if you are like Jay, look for a mentor to help you examine your work critically, tackle problems creatively, and engage the public in your results. We will help you to do this."[1]

As the dean surmised, other graduate students have motivations, interests, and purposes that differ from Elliot's and Jay's. Some might be pursuing a research career to improve understanding of the neural causes of spina bifida. Others may be working to develop an algorithm for new software that can speed communication between portable electrical

---

[1] I am here drawing on the names and circumstances of two fictional characters portrayed in "Choosing a Lab: The Students' Perspective," a segment of a video, "In the Lab: Mentors and Students," produced by the National Institutes of Health.

Research Ethics: A Philosophical Guide to the Responsible Conduct of Research. Gary Comstock. Published by Cambridge University Press. © Cambridge University Press 2013.

devices. Yet others are studying to explain the cultural forces blocking access of the rural poor to microlending businesses. Still others may want to discover the most efficient ways of turning sustainable forest products into paper while simultaneously using the forests as places to sequester carbon. Graduate students have a variety of research ends and a variety of reasons for pursuing them.

. . . yet all have a common set of duties

And yet all have at least one shared responsibility – to conduct their research responsibly. And what does that mean? The specific expectations are spelled out in each university's documents. For example, if you were entering the Department of Food Science and Technology at Virginia Tech University, you would receive the "Graduate Student Contract," an explicit and representative statement of the duties and expectations of that department's graduate students. The 21-page document states that, among other things, all graduate assistants must, for example, act "in a mature, professional, courteous manner toward students, staff and faculty regardless of their race, gender, religion, sexual orientation, or national origin."[2]

We will explore the implications of rules such as this rule throughout this book. And we will revisit the Virginia Tech document in Part B. Meanwhile, we should emphasize the importance of the rules. Those who disobey rules face consequences. For example, if students in this department let their GPAs drop below 3.0, they may find themselves facing probation. If they are on full assistantship yet spend less than 20 hours in the lab, they may receive a letter threatening withdrawal of support. To protect yourself, pay attention to all of the documents that you are instructed to read.

. . . including the duty to avoid research misconduct

Conducting research responsibly is no doubt among the most important duties you have. In your role as student, you can subvert your own research not only through neglect but also by intentional acts of subversion, such as gaining academic credit by purposely reporting inaccurate results, copying another's data, pretending someone else's words are yours, or using other unapproved means to get academic credit. All of these are instances of academic dishonesty, which occurs whenever students get credit for work that is not really their own.

As researchers, we may be tempted to gain academic or professional credit by fabricating or falsifying data or figures, or by pretending that another's words are our words. And the consequences are hardly trivial. In the United States, the three most egregious instances of misconduct are federal crimes. Any serious case of falsifying or fabricating data or plagiarizing texts may result in penalties from being declared ineligible for government grants to losing one's job.

The Office of Research Integrity (ORI) at the U.S. Department of Health and Human Services defines research misconduct as follows:[3]

---

[2] Retrieved 11/9/2010 from www.fst.vt.edu/graduate/handbook/appendices.pdf.
[3] The definition of research misconduct is found at http://ori.dhhs.gov/misconduct/
definition_misconduct.shtml. Accessed Sept. 12, 2010. Cf. National Science Foundation regulation 45 CFR 689 http://www.nsf.gov/oig/resmisreg.pdf.

- Fabrication – making up data or results and recording or reporting them.
- Falsification – manipulating research materials, equipment, or processes, or changing, or omitting data or results such that the research is not accurately represented in the research record.
- Plagiarism – appropriating and using as one's own another person's documented ideas, processes, results, or words without giving appropriate credit, including those obtained through confidential review of others' research proposals and manuscripts.

Notice that the definitions of fabrication and falsification cover data you generate during your research as well as the actual data you publish. And notice that the definition of plagiarism does not confine itself to ideas and words found in published papers; it extends as well to unpublished manuscripts that you may be peer reviewing. The policy explains that three conditions must be satisfied to justify a finding of research misconduct. The suspect action must:

(1) have been committed intentionally, or knowingly, or recklessly,

(2) be proven by a preponderance of evidence, and

(3) represent a significant departure from accepted practices.

The US National Science Foundation and other federal agencies have adopted these definitions, clarifying that "differences of opinion or errors of judgment" are not misconduct, nor are unintentional or careless mistakes in recording and selecting data, or exercising poor judgment in analyzing or interpreting data. Overinterpreting the results of your research or engaging in other questionable practices may undermine the success of your project, but overreaching and sloppiness do not rise to the level of acts punishable as federal offenses.

How much misconduct is there? Donald McCabe *et al.* surveyed more than 5000 graduate students in 2002–04 and asked them to report whether in the past year they had engaged in any of 13 behaviors ranging from cheating to plagiarism to "submitting work done by someone else."[4] Segregating by discipline, here were the results:

- Business   56%
- Engineering   54%
- Physical sciences   50%
- Medical and health-care   49%
- Law   45%
- Social science and humanities   39%

These numbers suggest that roughly half of all graduate students cheat in some form or fashion every year. But what, exactly, are they doing? Do their actions actually qualify as misconduct as defined by ORI? These are important questions to answer, for several reasons. If we overestimate the amount of cheating that is actually taking place, we are suffering from false beliefs. These false beliefs might in turn have the indirect effect of encouraging cheating: if many of your peers are gaining an unfair advantage by cheating, then you will be at even greater disadvantage if you choose to follow the rules. And if

---

[4] McCabe *et al.* 2006.

cheating expands because the research community believes it is more widespread than it is, then that community will have an even more difficult time managing it.

We will take up these questions in Chapter 1. Meanwhile, if you are in doubt about how to avoid misconduct, speak with your mentor. Become active in your research community, which you can find in many places, including online at the OpenSeminar in Research Ethics Facebook group. Why do we stress so often the importance of acculturation into the wider community? Answer: because local communities can be imperfect, as the incidence of cheating among graduate students suggests. But the situation is even more dangerous than these figures suggest. For your mentor may be engaging in conduct that could ruin your career.

Consider the story of a group of graduate students in the genetics community at the University of Wisconsin. To most appearances, Professor Elizabeth Goodwin's worm genetics lab was healthy – or so thought doctoral students Amy Hubert, Garrett Padilla, Chantal Ly, and Mary Allen. Unfortunately, things were not as they seemed.

Case study: "Can of worms," by John Allen[5]

On September 20, 2006, Irwin Goldman received an email with good news – "exceptional news," he wrote at the time – he'd never expected to hear, at least not from anyone at UW-Madison. Graduate student Amy Hubert PhDx'08 had made a breakthrough in her research, successfully identifying the piece of DNA in the nematode worm *Caenorhabditis elegans* that corresponds with a gene called *laf-1*.

Laf-1 is important in sex determination among nematodes, which are typically hermaphroditic. Those that have a single *laf-1* gene mutation develop as females. Those that have two die – thus "laf," which stands for "lethal and feminizing."

No one ever said a worm's life is easy.

But, then, neither is a graduate student's, and Amy Hubert's has been harder than most.

Seven months earlier, she was working and studying in the lab of Elizabeth Goodwin, then a leading researcher in *C. elegans* genetics, when Goodwin was accused of scientific misconduct – essentially of misrepresenting her work in an application for federal funding. It was one of the most serious scandals in UW science, and even today those connected to it are reluctant to talk about it. The university launched an investigation, and Goodwin soon resigned. UW-Madison had to give up thousands of grant dollars and still faces the possibility of sanction by the federal government.

The chief evidence against Goodwin came from Hubert and her graduate student colleagues, and the aftermath of the scandal has taken nearly as heavy a toll on them as it did on Goodwin. Of the seven people working in her lab – six graduate students and one research specialist – five are no longer at UW-Madison. Hubert hopes to complete her doctorate soon, which would make her the first member of the lab to do so.

Her success may illustrate her academic skill, but the fact that she's the only one from that team nearing graduation to date shows something else: the vulnerable position in which graduate students find themselves in the modern scientific world of grant-based research. Wholly dependent upon their faculty mentors for educational, financial, and career support, grad students lead a perilous life. And the increasingly competitive struggle among professors to win research grants only makes that peril more acute.

---

[5] Reprinted from *On Wisconsin*, Spring 2008. John Allen is Senior Editor, *On Wisconsin* Magazine, Madison, WI. jallen@waastaff.com.

Chasing phantoms

C. elegans is a model organism, one of a handful of species that scientists study closely to learn about general biological principles. There are a few others: several bacteria and yeasts, Arabidopsis plants, fruit flies, zebra fish, rats, and mice. Nematodes are useful as a model organism because they're among the simplest creatures to possess a nervous system, they can be frozen and thawed without damaging their viability, and they reproduce rapidly – even more quickly than fruit flies. Nobel Prize-winner Sydney Brenner pioneered studies of *C. elegans* in the 1970s, making it a relatively recent entry into the roster of model species. As a result, says CALS associate dean Irwin Goldman PhD'91, "the *C. elegans* community is still relatively small and tight-knit."

That closeness is highlighted at WormBase, an online database that keeps records of the researchers who are working on *C. elegans*, cross-referencing mentors to protégés. Sydney Brenner, for instance, is listed as WB (WormBase) Person77. He was the mentor for David Hirsh, WBPerson259, a professor at Columbia who mentored Judith Kimble, WBPerson320. A biochemistry professor at UW-Madison, Kimble supervised Elizabeth Goodwin, WBPerson213, when she was a postdoctoral fellow. And Goodwin was the mentor to WBPerson3474, Amy Hubert.

Hubert came to UW-Madison in 2001 from the north-central Kansas town of Concordia. Like many graduate students, she'd earned her previous degree elsewhere – a bachelor's at the University of Kansas. She'd been attracted to the UW by its reputation as a leader in genetics, but she didn't join Goodwin's lab until spring 2002.

"I liked Betsy [Goodwin] as an adviser," Hubert says. "She was very friendly, very hands-on, always checking in with us about how our work was going."

Goodwin was then one of the rising stars of the UW's genetics department. "She was an extremely good citizen," says Phil Anderson, another *C. elegans* expert (WBPerson21) and a professor of genetics. "She did more than her fair share of committee work, and she was very involved socially. She entertained prospective graduate students and helped recruit new faculty. She brought a genuine sense of joy to working here."

Goodwin's lab was then one of only two or three in the world that were doing such advanced research into sex determination among nematodes, aiming to shed light on the importance of sexual reproduction in evolution. She was developing a hypothesis that *laf-1* affected sex determination in *C. elegans* because it encoded a strand of "small RNA" – ribonucleic acid – instead of a conventional protein, which most genes encode. Such a discovery would have been a major coup, had she been able to prove it.

"Within the last five or ten years," says Anderson, "small RNAs have become very fashionable in research. There's been a lot of exciting progress around small RNAs, and there's a lot of mystery there."

But Hubert quickly lost conviction that Goodwin's small RNA hypothesis was the right track. "When I first joined the lab," she says, "I was getting the same results that Betsy and the others were. But I began to see that the *laf-1* mutants weren't all matching the prediction. Some of the results were just – well, they weren't all that strong."

While Goodwin continued to pursue the small RNA hypothesis, Hubert turned to more traditional approaches. She decided to revisit the question of *laf-1*'s identity by continuing to map its location in the *C. elegans* genome. "And the more mapping I did, the more it showed me that *laf-1* was in a different spot from where everyone else [in the lab] was looking."

"Amy's a real geneticist, while the rest of us were molecular biologists," says one of her former lab partners, Mary Allen MS'06. "She was willing to take a long time and go back through the *laf-1* work from the beginning, redoing the experiments and looking for inconsistencies. She was willing to go through the tedious process of looking at each generation of worms to see the phenotypes. I can remember her spending up to twelve hours in the lab, even on Saturdays. It was a lot of hard work, and a lot of time, but it paid off for her."

It was this difference of opinion that ultimately saved Hubert's career at the UW. When the Goodwin affair blew up at the beginning of 2006, Hubert's colleagues, whose work had all been intertwined with Goodwin's search for small RNA, saw their years of labor vanish.

"The project that Betsy was so committed to turned out to be a phantom," says Anderson. "Laf-1 does not encode small RNA. And because that was a phantom, it wasn't producing results, and it never would. The students who were chasing this phantom, they weren't making any progress. Amy had the foresight – almost from when she first joined the lab – she had the good sense to challenge Betsy on this. She went back to the tried-and-true methods of mapping the DNA. Because of that, she was able to survive Betsy's departure. That's why she was able to make her breakthrough."

Trying to do good

The Goodwin affair became public on February 23, 2006, when Goodwin resigned from the UW, bringing to a close 3 months of tension and quiet recriminations that had infected the members of her lab. She slipped quietly out of town and hasn't spoken publicly about the allegations since, leaving her lawyers to respond to the charges. But her departure didn't bring the affair to a close. In many ways, the difficulties were just beginning.

The misconduct allegations leveled against Goodwin were, according to Bill Mellon, associate dean of the graduate school and head of the UW's research compliance, among the most serious he's heard in his 29 years at UW-Madison, and certainly the most serious involving a tenure-track faculty member. But the university couldn't just drop the issue upon Goodwin's departure.

"We had an obligation to investigate the charges," says Mellon. "There were at least two federal grant applications involved, a renewal and an application for new funding, and we have to show the government that we're serious about our honesty and the honesty of our scientists. So we had to carry out a long and detailed process – and I must say, Professor Goodwin's absence made the process all the more difficult."

Without Goodwin to answer the charges or explain her actions, investigators have struggled to determine just how far the damage goes. Mellon is confident that Goodwin wasn't guilty of fraud – "she used the federal money to run the experiments she said she was going to run," he says – and so far, no one has challenged the validity of the articles Goodwin has published. But the university had to report its findings to the federal government, and it hasn't yet heard what the government's Office of Research Integrity has to say about the Goodwin case.

Still, if the process has been difficult for the university, it's been even harder on Goodwin's former students.

At the time of the allegations, Goodwin's lab employed six graduate students – Hubert, Allen, Garett Padilla MS'06, Chantal Ly MS'06, Sarah La Martina'00, MS'06, and Jacqueline Baca – and one research specialist, Maya Fuerstenau'04. In November 2005, Padilla discovered a discrepancy in the data that Goodwin was reporting in her grant renewal application. The application made it appear that the lab was producing favorable results, when in fact the data were incomplete, inconclusive, or worse. He brought this to the attention of his colleagues and to Goodwin.

"At first, all we saw was that the data were wrong in one figure on one of the grants," says Hubert. "After Garett talked to Betsy about it, she told him it was just a mistake, that the data had been placeholders. But the more we looked, the more we saw that seemed wrong. She was saying some experiments had been done that hadn't been, and the figures that were being used to illustrate her results weren't the correct figures. The conclusions she gave, in some cases, weren't correct. Things had been relabeled, and we concluded that it couldn't have just been a mistake. It had to be deliberate."

The graduate students then faced a difficult decision – whether to report Goodwin to the university, knowing that, if they were wrong, it would ruin their relationship with their mentor and boss, and if they were right, it would destroy the research they'd been conducting for years.

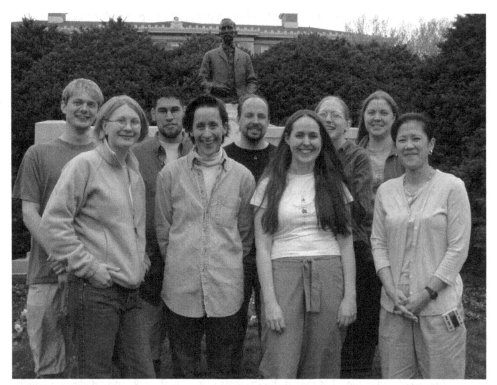

Figure A.1. Professor Goodwin's lab in 2005. Front row: Goodwin (second from the left), Sarah LaMartina (second from the right), and Chantal Ly (far right). Back row: Garett Padilla (second from the left), and Mary Allen (second from the right). (Photo by Mary Allen, used with permission.)

"We had a lot of discussion about what to do," says Allen. "A lot of discussion. We were grappling with a big decision, and some people were afraid that they'd have to start over."

Eventually, however, the students came to a unanimous decision. "When we looked at it, though, there wasn't really a choice," says Hubert. "We wanted to believe [Goodwin]. We felt she was trying to do good for the lab. But we had to report it."

In December, they informed Mike Culbertson, chair of the genetics department. He reported the allegations to Mellon, and Mellon asked Irwin Goldman from CALS and Paul DeLuca, an associate dean of the School of Medicine and Public Health, to begin an informal inquiry to determine whether there was any merit to the students' allegations.

"We met with the students and with the professor, and we looked at the grant proposal and the data provided by the students, and it seemed clear that there was some attempt at deception," says Goldman. "Betsy was giving one set of numbers to NIH [National Institutes of Health] and another to the students. This was clearly not a frivolous accusation."

While Goldman and DeLuca were gathering information, the lab environment was deteriorating. "We didn't really know what was going on," says Hubert. "We had spoken with the investigators, but were asked not to speak about Betsy to anyone else. At the same time, she was free to defend herself, and we had the feeling that she was bad-mouthing us around the department, saying that we were making mountains out of molehills and that we were out to get her. For a while, we got the feeling that we were the ones who were in the wrong."

As the situation progressed, the students felt increasingly betrayed and isolated. "It's like there were two Betsys," says Hubert. "The one who was my friend and who was so helpful, and then the one who had done this thing on her application. I couldn't believe they were the same person. I still can't."

Goldman and DeLuca issued their recommendation to Mellon, reporting their opinion that the students' charges had merit. Mellon then referred the matter to a formal investigative committee. And just as they began their work, Goodwin resigned. The committee finished its work a month later, concluding in a report to the Office of the Chancellor that Goodwin was guilty of the charges the students had leveled. The UW submitted its report to the Department of Health and Human Services, which oversees NIH, and returned what remained of her grant money.

Within a few weeks, news about the misconduct spread through both the local and the scientific community, as major stories appeared in the *Wisconsin State Journal* and in the journal *Science*.

"Once the report was delivered, I think it was clear that we'd been in the right," Hubert says.

But if they were vindicated, they were hardly safe. In reporting their mentor's misconduct, they'd endangered their own careers as well.

Heroes

For Irwin Goldman, the key to the Goodwin affair isn't ultimately what happens to Goodwin, but rather what happens to her former students. Hubert and her colleagues, he says, "displayed professional heroism. They put their careers at great personal risk for the sake of scientific integrity. That's exactly the kind of people we want to attract into the sciences. These students risked a lot for the truth. They didn't deserve to suffer for the actions of their mentor."

And yet when the students decided to come forward, it seemed likely that they would be punished nearly as severely as Goodwin. When she resigned and the university forfeited her funding, her lab closed down. That meant the students were out of work – no salaries, no tuition reimbursement, and, perhaps worst of all, no research. That would mean no progress on their degrees, and possibly starting over. That, Goldman feels, is a poor reward for honesty.

Unlike undergrads, graduate students are often more like apprentice academics, breaking into careers in science and research. Many parts of the university, including the College of Agricultural and Life Sciences, where Goldman works, are dependent upon them for carrying out research. Protecting these students from dishonest faculty isn't just an issue of justice, he maintains; it's a matter of the UW's self-interest.

"We have almost a thousand graduate students in this college alone," he says. "We try to get the best students to want to spend five or more years here. And if we want to attract and keep them, we have to care about them and their vulnerability."

So Goldman convinced his colleagues within CALS to guarantee that Goodwin's students would receive funding for at least the remainder of the semester, and he began looking for avenues through which they could continue their studies. For Hubert, who was far advanced in her work, he found a home in the lab of Phil Anderson. Another student, Jacqueline Baca, who was nearer the beginning of her work, was also placed in a different lab. But the others, facing the realization that they would have to start over, left the UW. Allen left Madison to study worms under Tom Blumenthal at the University of Colorado-Boulder; Ly and La Martina found laboratory jobs in other states; and Padilla departed for law school.

"We can't give [students] back the time that they lose," says Bill Mellon, "but we can try to protect them from financial disaster."

That's what Goldman set out to do. After Goodwin resigned, he began work drafting a policy for CALS that would protect graduate students in the event of scientific misconduct by their mentors. It demands that the college "use its best effort to secure funding for CALS graduate students, including Research Assistants, Fellows, and Trainees, and research associates whose positions and funding may be jeopardized by his/her good faith disclosure of scientific misconduct." Adopted last year, the policy "is the only one I know of in the country," says Goldman, and it's since become a model for a university-wide attempt to improve the grad-student safety net.

"If there's a hero in all this, it's Irwin," says Anderson. "He not only did everything he could to do right by Betsy's students, but he also pushed the rest of us to try to do right by them."

Still, there's only so much that a college can do to protect its students from faculty upheaval. The policy only covers scientific misconduct, not any of the other ways that a professor might depart – death, for example, or by taking a position at another university or in government or industry. In those cases, the students are still left to scramble.

"It's depressing," says Goldman, "and perhaps it's a flaw in the university system that's developed over the last hundred and fifty years. But we're doing our best to protect these students, because they're the future of science."

In a few short months, an experienced researcher's act of mislabeling photos seriously undermined the careers of at least six promising young scholars. It also affected their general well-being. Mary Allen, one of the few members of the Goodwin lab who stayed in science, writes that some members began to lose weight while others gained weight; some could not get out of bed in the morning. They ran themselves in circles with worry. Their mental health deteriorated as they battled depression and anxiety.[6] Mary Allen said that the episode cost her 2 years of her life. Even though they may not have known the degree to which they'd suffer by reporting their advisor, they knew that doing so would put them in jeopardy. All things told, neither foresight nor hindsight suggested that this decision was in the students' best interests.

What are the lessons of the Goodwin case? First, excellent research does not necessarily mean ethical research. Kind and caring researchers are not above misconduct. Second, the lives of graduate students are so tied up with the lives of their mentors that both parties must keep their eyes on each other. Neither mentor nor mentee should be shy about raising questions at the first hint of trouble. Third, the longer the clock ticks when fraud is suspected the deeper the trouble may become. Fourth, students should ask questions early and often. If principal investigators are not conducting conversations about research ethics in the lab, students can initiate the conversations by mentioning the Elizabeth Goodwin case and asking questions. Who does the PI think was responsible for the mistakes in the case? Should Goodwin have discussed lab procedures more regularly and intensively with her students? Did Goodwin lean too heavily on senior students to guide newcomers?

Ethical lapses such as Goodwin's give rise to soul-searching in the community because they evoke such powerful emotions in us. We are chagrined about the misbehavior of a rising star in biology. We are cheered by the courage of her students. We admire the fact that the students were not intimidated by faculty whispering about them in the hallway. We're happy that they did not settle to take the easy way out. When folks implied that they ought to relax and look the other way, they found strength in each other. Told to lighten up, they chose instead to encourage each other. We find ourselves hoping we would do likewise in similar circumstances.

In June 2010, Elizabeth Goodwin admitted to having falsified data in a grant progress report "to convince reviewers that more scientific progress had been made with her research than was actually the case," according to the Department of Justice.[7] Goodwin received

---

[6] Personal correspondence with Mary Allen, November 28, 2006, quoted with permission.
[7] Couzin-Frankel 2010b.

2 years probation, voluntarily agreed not to receive federally funded research for 3 years, and was ordered to pay a $500 fine plus $50,000 in restitution to the Department of Health and Human Services and $50,000 to the University of Wisconsin.[8]

. . . and to blow the whistle

A quick review. Using egoism as our standard, we began to explore the question of whether research misconduct is unethical and whether egoistic graduate students have a duty to report it. The research community believes that observers of misconduct should usually report what they see. But for egoists out to protect themselves from harm, that sounds like bad advice. Goodwin's students told on her and look what happened to them! What egoist would conclude from the Goodwin affair that Goodwin's students did the right thing? Doesn't prudence dictate *not* blowing the whistle in this case?

It appears that to protect oneself one should keep one's head low. If Amy Hubert had not rocked the boat, she would have made out better, no? Don't draw attention to yourself; keep quiet; don't make a fuss – isn't that what egoism would recommend?

The question demands an answer and we will try to supply it in Chapters 1 through 4. To begin, however, we need to have a clearer picture of egoism. Here is an initial stab at a definition.

Simple egoism: one should always act to satisfy one's own interests.

Simple egoism (SE) is a consequentialist theory, because in SE the morality of an action depends on the kinds of effects it has. Right actions are those with good effects and bad actions are those with bad effects. For an egoist, good effects are those in which one's interests – which are defined as one's desires – are fulfilled. Suppose Mary Allen wants to finish her dissertation by March 1, but doing so would mean that she'd have to shirk other responsibilities. If she sincerely and honestly thinks she can meet that deadline, and doing so would serve her long-term goals, then she should try to meet it. She should try even if it entails that she will fall short of fulfilling her other duties along the way, simple egoism requires it.

So according to Simple egoism, Allen is unethical if she does not do what's in her best interests. Suppose Allen knows that to meet her deadline she must finish collecting her data by January 1 and submit a final draft to her advisor by February 1. If she does not take the intermediate steps necessary to achieve her final goal – because, say, she suddenly chooses to follow through on another responsibility – then she is not really sincere in aiming at her goal. For choosing not to do what she knows she must do is, given her goals, to frustrate herself in the act of trying to become herself.

Simple egoism thus provides a persuasive, if instrumentalist, answer to the fundamental question of ethics: why should I be moral? Egoism's answer is this:

I should be moral because being moral will best satisfy my own interests.

Not to perform some action when it is required to best satisfy your own interests is forbidden by simple egoism, since, by failing to act, the egoist defeats herself in trying to get what she wants. After all, simple egoism requires only that egoists adopt the means that best satisfy their ends.

---

[8] Couzin-Frankel 2010a.

Let us analyze another case from an egoistic perspective. Suppose Garrett Padilla had walked into the lab one day and found himself with a strong reason to drop some data points. Suppose he had worked for months on an experiment, had not gotten the results expected, and had to finish his report that day so that Professor Goodwin could finalize the paper she would be presenting at a conference the next week. Padilla would find himself with two conflicting interests:

(a) drop the points to produce the "right" results – the results Goodwin needs, or
(b) do not drop the points and so obey a cardinal rule in data collection.

If Padilla's deepest desire is to become a credentialed researcher in the worm genetics community, he should opt for (b) and follow the rules. For young researchers who break rules are liable to be found out, and often suffer dire consequences as a result. On the other hand, if Padilla's deepest desire is to please Goodwin, his mentor, and he knows Goodwin wants him to get a certain result, then (perhaps) he should decide to opt for (a) and break the rule. In either case, the important point (for an egoist) is that there is no one correct decision, no "objective" answer. There is only Padilla's decision, and he must make his decision in light of what he thinks is best for him.

A simple egoist in Goodwin's lab, then, depending on his goals, would not be morally wrong to blow the whistle. But neither would there be anything wrong with another simple egoist, given her interests, sealing her lips and letting Goodwin go about her business while the egoist goes about hers. The morality of the decision all depends on what best satisfies the egoist's desires.

But is whistle-blowing really in an egoist's interests?

We might think that laying low would have been in the students' interests in the Goodwin case. Is that not the lesson of the episode? Didn't they make what the egoist would consider the morally *incorrect* choice? Each of them was scathed, if not destroyed, by their whistle-blowing. One can argue that they all emerged from the episode worse off than they would have been had they said nothing. Perhaps they should have said nothing, fulfilled their duties at the university, used its resources to secure their futures, and then quietly moved on?

SE could lead to this answer. But not so fast. Failing to blow the whistle – as the students clearly saw – also has its costs. And they realized that the consequences of not reporting misconduct might carry even worse consequences for them than reporting it. That is, they saw that they might hurt themselves more by *not* whistle-blowing than by whistle-blowing. They agonized over the difficult decision of what they ought to do as well as over the difficulty in assessing the possible consequences. So what, in the end, convinced them to report the misconduct?

They came to believe that continuing to remain silent would make them complicit in Goodwin's actions. Rather than being those who were wronged, they would become compatriots in wrongdoing, perhaps having to face charges similar to those facing Goodwin. The consequences to them could be devastating: loss of their assistantships, expulsion from the university, hefty fines, criminal charges, court proceedings, sanctions against them by federal agencies – and their names in the newspapers for their parents and friends to read.

We might think SE instructs us to do whatever feels good now, whatever we happen to want to do at the moment. But matters are more complex than that because the egoist cannot always easily see what ultimately serves his interests. And to complicate matters, the egoist typically has more than one thing that he wants. He must not only figure out how to calculate the likely consequences, good and bad, of various actions. He must also figure out how to decide what to do when he has competing interests. Which interests should take precedence for him?

Kinds of interests

Some of our interests are short-term; others are long-term. We can sometimes pursue multiple interests without any conflict, but at other times our interests compete with each other, vying for our allegiance and potentially knocking other interests out of the running. Thoughtful egoists recognize this. They know that they must sort out several kinds of interests if they are to figure out what they really want to do.

First, we have proximal interests, minor interests that do not much matter to us. Should I wear dark or light brown socks today? Use a 45 or 60 watt light bulb? These are trivial choices–make up your mind and go. We are constantly making such "mindless" decisions in matters that make almost no difference to our well-being.

Second, we have intermediate or significant interests that matter a great deal. We all need to keep our weight under control if we want to stay healthy. Suppose you decide to lose 20 pounds. You commit to go running several evenings a week, but one night you are tempted to play video games instead. If losing weight is still a significant interest of yours, you'll likely have to remind yourself of your commitment and then take the steps necessary to avoid temptation. If you somehow lose the ability to exercise control over your significant interests (say, you become injured) or you fail to exercise control, then your well-being may be compromised.

Third, we have overriding interests – let's call them categorical interests – that give our lives meaning and significance. They differ from significant interests in the degree of satisfaction they carry: achieving categorical interests is more rewarding than achieving significant interests. What are these interests about and why do we have them? They are interests that result from seizing opportunities to shape our lives into the kind of lives we want to have – lives that include consciously chosen vocations and careers. And we have these long-range, difficult-to-achieve, interests by virtue of the fact that we are self-conscious, intentional, self-reflective animals that can decide our own values, enjoy memories of our pasts and control our futures.

Whether you ultimately want to shape yourself into a chemistry researcher, plant manager, health professional, or string bass player, you must at some point decide to take the intermediate steps necessary to achieve it. We have the capacity to make ourselves into the person we want to be because we can reflect on where we have been in the past, the present state of our talents, and where we are likely to be in the future. If you decide to devote your energies to becoming a good parent, you might have to sacrifice the amount of time you spend watching football or helping to build homes for victims of natural disasters. And given the consequences to your children, for good or ill, of your parenting skills, and the sacrifices you have made in other areas to pursue parenting as your categorical interest, if you then fail at parenting you may have done others lasting damage and done debilitating harm to yourself: harm to the children you failed to parent well and harm to yourself when

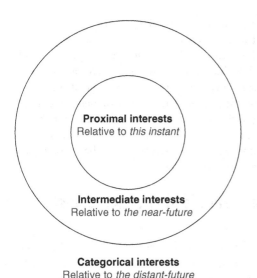

Figure A.2. Three kinds of interests.

Proximal interests
Relative to *this instant*

Intermediate interests
Relative to *the near-future*

Categorical interests
Relative to *the distant-future*

you see the damage you have done to them and the opportunities you have skipped in order to pursue parenthood. Pursuing categorical interests can be rewarding – and dangerous.

How can you tell if your desires or interests are categorical? The deathbed test may help. Imagine yourself with only a few days to live. If, reflecting on a particular desire, you say, as did Scottish philosopher David Hume (d. 1776), that you are dying "as easily and cheerfully as my best friends could desire" since you will have "done every thing of consequence which I ever meant to do; and I could at no time expect to leave my relations and friends in a better situation than that in which I am now likely to leave them," then your desire is categorical.[9]

We have the ability to rank our interests and reassess them, determining whether they are trivial, significant or categorical. Note that the category into which a given interest falls depends on the individual whose interest it is. Becoming a parent, for example, is not always and everywhere a categorical interest. Each of us decides how much of ourselves to invest in certain activities. Further, we each determine our own hierarchy of interests through careful self-examination.

Even now, as you pursue your graduate studies, you may not yet have determined what you most want to do with your life. Should you try to become a professional researcher in physics at a major university or teach physics at a small college? You may not know the answer, but even if you do, you will almost certainly encounter obstacles en route to your goal. For the process of trying to make yourself into this or that kind of a person is an adventure, fraught with opportunities to succeed or fail.

With this in mind, let's return to our discussion of the Goodwin case, and the students' ultimate decision to report their advisor. Our initial analysis suggested that, from the perspective of an egoist, the students, intent as they were on keeping their positions in the university, may have made the morally incorrect choice by blowing the whistle. For

---

[9] Smith 1776.

blowing the whistle seemed to jeopardize their ability to achieve their desire to earn a PhD. However, we then realized that assessing what was in their best interests was a complicated affair. We can now ask: as difficult as it is to know who one is and where one is going, could it be that the safe route is always to report misconduct. The answer is yes. This answer will not surprise us if we are mindful at the vagaries surrounding our knowledge at ourselves and our futures. For even the rational egoist must figure out which of her categorical interests is most important to her and, having decided that matter, how to order her short- and longer-term interests in light of her overarching goals. In the midst of such shifting uncertainties, a general policy of always reporting misconduct seems like the best strategy to achieve one's own self-interests – whatever they turn out to be.

Rational egoism is the view that one should always act to best satisfy one's categorical interests

If categorical interests provide the overarching frame by which we order our ends, then they take precedence over other interests. They are the goals and desires of overriding import- ance to us. Let's say that you've been working hard all afternoon on an engineering software algorithm that you must get done before tomorrow; you're exhausted, and you just want to take a nap. Of course, you want to satisfy that interest, but you also know that to get what you really want – what you want for yourself over the long haul – you must be ready to override short-term desires. To finish your algorithm on time, you will have to forego the nap and, if things get thorny, maybe also forget the beer with friends later tonight.

> Rational egoism: one should always act to best satisfy one's categorical interests.

Rational egoism cannot be reduced to the simple formula of simple egoism, to do whatever you want, nor does it instruct us to pursue whatever interest feels most urgent. We must rank our interests, identify those that rise to the top of the list, and then order our desires so as to pursue those that are most important. If Elliot's categorical interest is to complete a doctorate, then he owes it to himself to perform the actions necessary to accomplish that end. If, for example, he will diminish his chances of achieving the goal by cheating or mislabeling photos then, on pain of being irrational, he ought not to cheat. Cheating stands in the way of his getting to his goal.

Let us return to the Elizabeth Goodwin case a final time. Thinking as a rational egoist, Goodwin could (and probably should) have objected to her mislabeling of the figures because it did not serve her long-term interests. In fact, pursuing an intermediate interest (getting the grant) thwarted one of her categorical interests, pursuing academic research as a life-long career. Whenever the consequences and risks of being caught are worse than the consequences of not cheating, egoists should not cheat. And just why is that again? Because rational egoists should not act in ways that will prevent them from achieving the goals they have decided they most want to achieve.

Second, we've already begun to see why, as egoists – and we mean rational egoists, here and henceforth – the students might have done the right thing. Obviously, they sacrificed much by reporting Goodwin. But they also recognized that they might suffer much more by not reporting her. They may well have thought that they would sacrifice their long-term goals of being successful academics or professional researchers or persons without criminal records had they kept silent and had she been found out. By reporting Goodwin, they may have reasoned, we might have to sacrifice our goals of remaining students at this university and we'll have to scrap years of research, but at least we'll preserve a shot at reaching the goal we really care about, namely becoming respected members of our communities, whether that includes the research community or some other.

If the students reasoned as we have done here, would they be reasoning well? We will try to answer this question as we move through Chapters 1 through 4. Before moving on to those issues, let us note several strengths of rational egoism. The first is the power of rational egoism's instrumental rationality to explain why one ought to be moral; one is obliged to be moral because doing so is necessary to achieve one's goals. Rational egoism also requires integrity. To achieve your categorical interests, you must be honest with yourself, guarding against weakness of will and self-deception and other challenges that threaten to undermine your progress toward your goals. Without consistency in focus and relentlessly honest self-examination – without self-clarification and self-clarity – you will not achieve your goals.

A rational egoist might also try to argue that an implication of their theory is that all individuals have the right to pursue the good as they conceive it. (Whether they could make good on this claim is a matter we won't have time to discuss.) Insofar as you should best satisfy your own interests and not worry about others, the egoist might reason, you will, almost by default, leave others free to try to best satisfy their interests. Unless Jay (remember him from the dean's speech?) thinks Elliot's motivations for attending grad school or his behavior while in school are unethical, Jay has no justification to argue with Elliot from a rational egoist's perspective about those matters. Jay has no stake in Elliot's life and interfering in it would be patronizing and condescending. Furthermore, Jay has no good egoistic grounds to think his motivations are inherently superior to Elliot's.

Rational egoism is not without its drawbacks and we will discuss some of its problems at the end of Chapter 4. Yet the theory has a clear virtue; it recognizes that our psychologies and identities differ. We are each our own best expert on our own wants and needs. Consequently, the particulars of what will count as a good internal reason for me to perform some action may differ from what counts as a good internal reason for you.[10] In secular democracies, we place a premium on constructing institutions that protect freedoms and liberties. No ethical theory seems to allow as much space for the flourishing of individuals as rational egoism, which allows all persons to solve for themselves the problem of their competing self-interests.

How to proceed as an egoist

First, identify your categorical interests. The deathbed exercise we suggested earlier is one way to try to do this. Imagine yourself again nearing your last breath. During your final hours, will you take the most pleasure from thinking of how well you did as you tried to fulfill your role as a researcher, parent, daughter, teacher, friend, or colleague? Will you want to dwell on the accomplishments represented in the degrees you attained or the papers that cited your work? Or will it be more important to you that you empowered students, designed solid and interesting buildings, improved soil, or enriched a third grader's life by volunteering at your local elementary school? Whatever answers you give to these questions will be the right answers because no one else is positioned to provide you with a vision of the good life for you.

---

[10] Egoism only tells me how to act; it does not try to legislate for others. Strictly speaking, others' interests only enter the egoist's deliberations if the others can help the egoist advance his projects – or if others are in the way of his projects.

Second, reassess your goals from time to time. Some of our interests, such as pursuing a research career, should not change – or not change very often. They are central to us; they define our identities. Other interests are more transient – even if significant – and we can suffer them changing more rapidly. How do you distinguish overarching interests that should be abandoned only rarely from less important but still significant interests that may be changed with less risk to your sense of self? This is a difficult question that only you can answer, and only after much self-scrutiny.

Third, prepare for frustrations and failures. Since becoming a person is a project, an adventure that is to varying degrees under your control, it is your responsibility to make yourself into a person who fits the vision of the person you want to be. Egoists must be on guard, therefore, against psychological threats to integrity: a lack of will to follow through on one's plans, dishonesty with oneself, self-deception, and insincerity with oneself or others about one's accomplishments. They must be acutely aware, too, of how social conditions are stacked against them: humans are typically not skilled at getting away with cheating, or at assessing probabilities of various consequences, or at justifying misconduct to others. If you are honest with yourself and live a life of integrity – and if you have a bit of luck to boot – you will not only live a long and a fulfilling life, but will live a life you can be proud of.

Why should researchers follow the rules of responsible conduct? Really – who honestly cares about this stuff? As we have seen, this is a complex, difficult, and fundamental question. But we can begin to make progress on it by noting that we care, the research community cares. What's more, whoever aspires to come into the group needs to convince the community gatekeepers that they care too. So, doing the right thing in research is, at a minimum, an expected behavior. To put it bluntly, it is in your self-interest to know and obey the rules if you want to join this profession. And, as we shall now see, those who choose not to follow the rules face dangers that they probably cannot anticipate. For many matters around here – around the research world – are beyond one's control and rule-following can help to minimize one's exposure. Responsible conduct, then, is good advice for all of us, but it is especially good advice for those who are concerned first and foremost with their own success.

Take home lessons

- To protect yourself, watch for signs of fabrication and falsification.
- If you see something, say something.
- Examine your categorical interests with an eye on deciding whether you really own them and, if you do, think carefully about how best to satisfy them.

Bibliography

Allen, J. 2008. Can of worms. *On Wisconsin*. Available at: http://www.uwalumni.com/home/alumniandfriends/onwisconsin/owspring2008/owspring2008.aspx [Accessed June 7, 2011].

Couzin-Frankel, J. 2010a. Probation for Biologist Who Admitted to Misconduct. *ScienceInsider*. Available at: http://news.sciencemag.org/scienceinsider/2010/09/probation-for-biologist-who-admitted.html [Accessed June 8, 2011].

Couzin-Frankel, J. 2010b. Scientist turned in by grad students for misconduct pleads guilty. *ScienceInsider*. Available at: http://news.sciencemag.org/scienceinsider/2010/06/scientist-turned-in-by-grad.html [Accessed June 8, 2011].

McCabe, D., Butterfield, K. & Treviño, L.K. 2006. Academic dishonesty in graduate business programs: prevalence, causes, and proposed action. *Academy of Management Learning and Education*, 5(3), 294–306.

Smith, A. 1776. Letter from Adam Smith, LL.D. to William Strachan, Esq. Kirkaldy, Fifeshire. Available at: http://www.ourcivilisation.com/ smartboard/shop/smitha/humedead.htm [Accessed June 13, 2011].

Chapter

Report misconduct

Fabricating, manipulating, changing, making up, falsifying, omitting: what do these verbs have in common? All are part of the Health and Human Services definition of research misconduct and all may be used, given the right context, as synonyms for cheating. As noted in Part A, the research community disapproves of cheating but an egoist need not if a particular act of cheating is in the egoist's own best interests. So what reasons, if any, does an egoist have not to commit falsification or fabrication of data, or plagiarism?

To answer this question we must understand the complexity of the research context in which the egoist operates, and then ask how likely it is that an egoist's actual interests will be served by surreptitious corner cutting in research. These are the goals of the next four chapters.

What is cheating?

According to the saying, it takes two to tango. It takes more than one to cheat, too, because cheating is a social act in which one person deceives another. Although we occasionally say that someone "cheats himself," ordinarily cheating requires one who deceives and another who is deceived (Gert 2001). To deceive is to mislead or lie, to manipulate another's expectations falsely and so to gain unearned benefits for oneself.

Not all acts of deception are objectionable. Some we not only enjoy but praise. When the basketball player Derrick Rose feints right, crosses over his opponent and drives left around him to the basket, he has definitely misled his defender. But he hasn't cheated. Basketball rules encourage misdirection. If D. Rose sees that no official is in position to make a call and gains an advantage by touching the ball with both hands while dribbling it, his deception is now illicit because he has harmed others. That is cheating. But when he gains an advantage by deception within the rules he harms no one. His deception is legitimate.

So deception is only objectionable cheating when it is a harmful act of rule-breaking. With that introduction, we are in a position to provide a set of conditions to define cheating.[1] Cheating is, first:

1. An act of rule-breaking

Cheaters seek rewards by illicit means. Consider another example. Spades is a game played with a 52-card deck in which Spades are trumps, meaning any numbered Spade (e.g., the

---

[1] In formulating this analysis of cheating I rely on Doug MacLean's analysis of lying in "Lying: An Ethical Introduction" (unpublished manuscript). Also see Gert (2001) and Bok (1999).

Research Ethics: A Philosophical Guide to the Responsible Conduct of Research. Gary Comstock.
Published by Cambridge University Press. © Cambridge University Press 2013.

2 of Spades) will beat any card of another suit (e.g., the King of Hearts). Play begins when the first player lays down a card. The other three players must then follow suit. Following suit is a rule that requires the second, third, and fourth players to play a card of whatever suit the first player plays. If Hearts is led, all other players must lay down Hearts if they have one. If not, they can toss off a lower card and rid their hand of unwanted items or play a Spade and potentially win the hand and its points. If Hearts are led and player two plays a Spade, then player two wins the hand with her trump card and the other players assume that she does not have a Heart.

Now, experienced players can easily cheat those who are playing the game for the first time. The card shark can cheat by not following suit because other players have no way of knowing whether the card shark is cheating until the last card is played. Therefore, to catch a cheater requires that one keep track of every card played right up until and through the final round. As the novice Spade player is unlikely to be able to remember who has played which card, cheating is relatively easy.

When an experienced Spade player breaks the follow-suit rule they do so in order to win the hand's points or to get rid of a weak card that would otherwise hurt them later on. Obviously, the cheater's goal is to trick the others, gain unfair advantage, and not be discovered. This leads us to the second condition, that the cheater performs the act:

2. With the intention not to be caught

If someone breaks a rule unintentionally, perhaps because they did not know the rule, then they have not cheated. They have revealed their ignorance and their need for instruction. A third condition is suggested by returning to D. Rose's cross-over, a move that proves that deception is sometimes not only expected but also admired. Because feints and bluffs are a part of many games, we must now add a third constraint. The deception in question must occur:

3. In a context in which permission to break the rule has not been granted

Imagine you're playing cards with three others players. Two of them are, like you, old hands at the game. But the fourth player is a youngster who does not know the rules. In this case, a well-meaning adult might break the follow-suit rule under special circumstances. Suppose that the child is getting frustrated because she never wins a hand. You might wink at the other two adults, secretly signaling to them that you are going to break a rule in order to encourage the newcomer. The child does not suspect you of "cheating," you fail to follow suit in a few key instances, and the child, grinning, wins a hand. Have you cheated? Perhaps not if your game mates have given you permission to break the rule.

Card players are a various lot, and not everyone agrees that it is permissible to break the rules in order to encourage children to stick with the game. If I know that the other two adults at the table think my methods are inappropriate, I may decide not to break the rule – or may break it only after taking every precaution that I will not be caught. If the community does not give permission for rule-breaking, then rule-breaking is cheating even if performed for what the cheater considers an acceptable – or even noble – purpose. On the other hand, if the community is apprised of all the circumstances surrounding an action and approves of the action, then the action may not count as cheating in this case even though it would count as cheating under normal circumstances.

Is cheating unethical for egoists?

Easy question. No act is intrinsically unethical for egoists because acts are only unethical if they hinder egoists from achieving their categorical interests. An egoist might legitimately adopt the goal of cheating as often as possible and, in such a case, frequent acts of misbehavior might be in their interest. One might disagree with the vision of the good life chosen by the egoist, but one could not argue with her chosen means of attaining it. For if your goal is to get ahead by whatever means necessary, and your moral theory tells you that any means to your goal is ethical, then others cannot object to your means if they accept the legitimacy of your moral theory. So, it seems that cheating is not unethical for egoists.

No: egoists have reasons to cheat

There are many practical reasons for the self-interested person to live and let live, cheat and let cheat. First, cheating may help the egoist achieve their goals. Second, blowing the whistle on others may bring unwanted attention to themselves; witness what happened to Garrett Padilla when he squealed on Professor Goodwin. It is one thing to suspect misconduct of your superior and let it go – and a far different thing to report it to someone else. For Padilla's actions caused him untold agony and self-doubt. Was he seeing the evidence objectively? Was he unconsciously biased against Goodwin for some unacknowledged reason? Was he motivated by some past minor disagreement with her? Was he perhaps envious of her? Was he sure that he properly understood the scientific standards she was supposedly violating? Padilla could have saved himself much trouble by closing his eyes to what Goodwin had done.

Were Padilla an egoist (we have no evidence, by the way, that he was – we're just making the assumption for the sake of the argument), what reason would he have to report his mentor's misbehavior? If his goal was to stay out of trouble, finish his degree, and get on with his life, he'd have little motivation to take the risk. For his career was at stake, and he faced so many unknowns. How would his mentor react to his accusation? Who would come to his side? What in fact had he seen Goodwin do? What in fact could he prove to others? Would his institution support him? He wrestled with the fact that there were so many uncontrollable variables.

The egoist might appeal to the awful consequences that beset Goodwin's students as an argument against whistle-blowing. After the Goodwin incident had been reported in the papers, a researcher wrote to *Science* wondering whether the University of Wisconsin had left its students twisting in the wind. Rachel Ruhlen observed that "most of the students involved scattered, leaving UW, leaving graduate school, leaving academia, even leaving science . . .. Did UW do everything in its power to find labs for these students? Or were they all too happy to see the last of them?" (Ruhlen 2006).

It seems to the egoist – and perhaps to all of the rest of us, too – that the deck is stacked against the whistle-blower. The members of departments and the administrators of colleges and universities have powerful incentives to look the other way when their star performers misbehave. Why, then, would any student in their right mind – much less an egoist concerned only with his own welfare – report a superior's misconduct? Even the committee on research ethics assembled by the National Academies of Science recommends proceeding very cautiously:

> The circumstances surrounding potential violations of scientific standards are so varied that it is impossible to lay out a checklist of what should be done. Suspicions are best raised in the form of questions rather than allegations (National Academies (US) 2009).

Given the magnitude of the risks involved, it is hard to see what reasons an egoist has to think that reporting falsification and fabrication would be in their interests.

It is true that federal law prohibits institutions from creating an atmosphere of distrust in which whistle-blowers will not feel secure to come forward with information. In fact, institutions must have safeguards in place to protect whistle-blowers from retribution by the accused, any form of retaliation by others, and loss of job. That said, it is widely acknowledged to be exceedingly difficult to protect whistle-blowers in many instances. Consider what happened at UW. In spite of the bad press that followed the Goodwin incident and the steps the university took to respond to that press, the policies it developed did not satisfy all critics. In 2007, Goodwin's College adopted this policy (University of Wisconsin, College of Agricultural and Life Sciences 2007):

> The Dean's Office of the College of Agricultural and Life Sciences will use its best effort to secure funding for CALS graduate students, including Research Assistants, Fellows, and Trainees, and research associates whose positions and funding may be jeopardized by his/her good faith disclosure of scientific misconduct. Graduate and postdoctoral study represents unique endeavors that cannot always be supervised by interchangeable advisors. There may be circumstances where considerable research time is lost and/or when it becomes necessary for students to find a new advisor or research associates to find a new supervisor or advisor and in some cases, it may not be possible for the Dean's Office to provide an advisor or supervisor at UW-Madison or to secure funds to support the affected students and research associates. However, it is our goal to support and protect our students and research associates from circumstances arising because of their good faith disclosure of wrongdoing and misconduct that is not their fault and to encourage them to step forward and report misconduct that they may witness. It is, however, important to recognize that unfounded or bad faith allegations of scientific misconduct have a serious impact on the individual accused of the wrongdoing even when the allegations are proven wrong. Students are reminded that under UWS 17, "Student Nonacademic Disciplinary Procedures", disciplinary sanctions may be imposed for knowingly making a false statement to any university employee or agents regarding a university matter.

Does this statement provide adequate protection? The institution is trying to make good on its promise to protect future graduate students. But is the policy likely to make future graduate students think that they will not lose their positions, as several of Goodwin's students did, if they blow the whistle? Refer to the last two sentences that invoke "unfounded or bad faith allegations" and that express a worry about the "serious impact on the individual accused." Such concerns are no doubt appropriate and well-founded. But do they belong in this policy? Why is nothing said about what the university owes to whistle-blowers as remedies for its failures? What message is sent to the student trying to decide whether to alert someone about their supervisor's misconduct?

So an egoist might read the Goodwin case and decide it presents very few reasons to blow the whistle on cheaters. And the egoist can easily find other reasons to be less than forthcoming when it comes to cheating and cheaters, for lots of cheating is going on. As we noted in Part A, half of all graduate students admit to doing it.

And apparently it's easy to get away with cheating. A national expert on academic misconduct, Donald McCabe, has studied the subject for decades. He reports that many faculty members turn a blind eye on cheating. More than 40% of faculty surveyed reported that they had ignored cheating. And more than half of faculty had never reported cheating to anyone else (Cloward 2005).[2] We know that some faculty pay less attention than they

---

[2] Cloward attributes the numbers to McCabe, Donald L. "Presentation at the Annual Conference of Center for Academic Integrity," Kansas State University (2004).

should to their own practices in writing up the results of their research. According to *Nature*, "Studies in certain fields have estimated that anything up to 20% of published papers contain some degree of self-plagiarism" (Giles 2005).

Nor are the faculty always telling students what morality requires in research. In an informal survey of Stanford undergraduate engineering students by Robert McGinn in 1997, approximately 20% reported that their engineering instructors had conveyed specific information about what it means to be ethically responsible in engineering. Four years later, this percentage had dropped to 12% (McGinn 2003).

Another reason: the problem inside the academy is just a mirror of a wider cheating culture. Ignoring the rules is part of business as usual among well-known public figures in politics, business, sports, or music. The scandals are legion: Enron, Bernie Madoff, WorldCom, and so on. McCabe finds students offering many kinds of rationalizations, including:

- What's important is getting the job done. How you get it done is less important.
- All I'm doing is emulating the behavior I'll need when I get out in the real world.

In light of all of these reasons to cheat, perhaps we can forgive egoists for thinking that they can get away with rule-breaking and that they need not to get involved with whistle-blowing. In the rest of this chapter and the three chapters to follow, however, we will find reasons that add up to a different conclusion, reasons that should convince even the hardboiled egoist to think twice. Egoists should weigh carefully the fact that they have far less power and information than do faculty, that they are poor calculators of risk and probability and that they are supervised by individuals who not only disapprove of cheating but are very good at sniffing it out. In short, there may be numerous circumstances in which egoistic researchers will find themselves with powerful reasons not to cheat. Let's look at some of these possibilities.

Yes: egoists have stronger reasons not to cheat

We have been entertaining the twin ideas that cheating is never wrong for an egoist and that egoists should rarely, if ever, feel that it is in their self-interest to engage in whistle-blowing. But perhaps neither claim is true. For cheating will always be wrong for egoists if it interferes with their categorical interests. Perhaps egoists can tolerate a significant amount of cheating and lying on their own part. Still, some of their misbehavior could be so egregious that they themselves are incapacitated by it. Egoists can feel just as guilty as non-egoists and when they do, they must consider the behaviors that produced this bad consequence. It's true, egoists only have to worry about the consequences to themselves of their actions. But it's quite possible for an egoist to desire to think of himself as an honest man. And it's possible for him to become frustrated with himself in the achievement of his goals. So cheating is unethical for all egoists who wants to think of themselves as honest people.

Egoists should object to cheating whenever it has bad consequences for their psychological equilibrium. If an egoist is to succeed in a society that prizes honesty and punishes dishonesty, she will have to internalize a value system of checks and balances that matches her society's balance sheet. And once she does, she will have to keep her acts of deception and lying within the range allowed by society or run two dangerous risks. The first risk is that others will smoke her out as a cheater. The second risk is that she herself will be unable to maintain a conception of herself as a person of integrity. Whenever an egoist sees little to gain from cheating and has an internal reward system that discourages cheating, that egoist has good reasons not to cheat above the socially and personally accepted levels, whatever they are.

To be slightly more precise, we might say that lying is wrong for the egoist in circumstances in which the lie is likely to lead to more harm than good for the egoist. But this account suggests that whenever the consequences of lying are on the whole good for someone, then lying is permissible. We have to be careful here, however, to distinguish the principle that explains why lies are wrong (when they are wrong) from a practical or action-guiding rule that we want to see people apply and teach to others. Thus, even if egoists accept that it is only the bad consequences for them that result from lying that makes lying wrong, they would probably reject an action-guiding rule that said, "Don't lie if and only if the expected consequences of lying are likely to be worse for you than those of not lying." The problem with that rule is that it requires each individual to calculate the likely effects in every situation. How good are we at calculating the probabilities of various consequences? And how good are we at being impartial and objective when it comes to such calculations?

We'll examine these questions soon. Meanwhile, it's worth observing that it's possible that cheating would rarely be in an egoist's self-interest given the realities of the research environment. The main lesson of this chapter is that egoists have reasons to inculcate epistemic humility. Even if they think they will not get caught, a little objectivity suggests otherwise.

Let's summarize. When would cheating be clearly unethical for egoists? Whenever the act would prevent them from attaining their goals. Should one of their goals be to take care of those they love, they may not want to cheat if their cheating has the consequence of shaming their loved ones. If they want to be upstanding members of a profession known for honesty and integrity, or if they want their paychecks to keep coming, or if they think that their cheating will encourage their acquaintances to cheat and that consequence will diminish the profession's reputation, then cheating is not advisable. Whenever an egoist has a goal that might be thwarted by the egoist's cheating or the cheating of others, then the egoist has a reason not to cheat.

So, egoism can account for the wrongness of cheating in some circumstances – but which circumstances? The answer will depend on a number of factors: whether one's conscience can tolerate it, whether the likelihood of being caught is significant, whether the probable punishment for being caught is onerous, whether the rewards for not being caught are sizable, whether the transaction in which one may cheat involves cash, and so on (Ariely 2008b). Let's look at some of these factors.

. . . because they have their own internal filters

Whether we are egoists or not, we typically would like to think of ourselves as people of integrity. Toward that end we seem to have internal governors, self-imposed filters limiting the amount of misconduct we tolerate in ourselves. The internal negative consequences of cheating for an egoist's self-image may well outweigh whatever external benefits the act might bring. How much cheating might graduate students allow themselves before they exceed their limits? We do not have research on this question but we do have some preliminary work on undergraduate students. Based on investigations conducted by the behavioral economist Dan Ariely and his group, there is some reason to think that typical undergrads have a fudge factor in the range of 12.5–20%.

1.69	1.82	2.91
4.67	4.81	3.05
5.82	5.06	4.28
6.36	5.19	4.57

Figure 1.1. A sample matrix of the adding-to-10 task.

Here's how Ariely reached his conclusion. He, Mazar, and Amir handed 229 students two pieces of paper, a test sheet and a bubble sheet for their answers. The test page had 20 matrices on it and each matrix required circling two numbers that added up to 10 (Figure 1.1 Hint: one of the numbers is 4.81.) After four minutes, the proctor ended the trial and told each student to transfer their answers to the bubble sheet and hand it in for grading. Students were paid 50 cents for each right response (Ariely 2008b). Under these conditions, the average correct was 3.1 so, on average, each subject pocketed $1.50. End of experiment..

In a subsequent trial, the team was interested to discover whether conditions of anonymity would increase cheating. In this iteration, students were allowed to retain their test sheets among their belongings, thus giving the students the opportunity to shred their answers. When students knew no one could see their answers, "they got smarter," as Ariely puts it. The average increased to 4.1, and the average payment to $2.00 (Mazar et al. 2008c).

Method of grading	Number correct
Graded by proctor	3.1
Graded by self, answers shredded	4.1

The evidence suggests that when the average student is convinced they will not be caught, they will inflate their scores from three to four. Four is a third larger than 3 (3×1.33), so we might conclude that the students' fudge factor is 33%. However, as Ariely observes, students had the opportunity to claim as many as 17 extra points and did not take that advantage. Why would they decide to lie only about one point? Commenting on another trial in which students had earned four points of 20 but claimed they had gotten six, Ariely notes that they have claimed only two of 16 possible extra points, or "12.5% of their cheating opportunity" (Mazar et al. 2005d).

Another experiment involved 50 multiple-choice general knowledge questions and Harvard students who were paid 10 cents for each correct answer, Ariely's group found that under conditions of anonymity the average correct score rose from 32.6 to 36.2, or an extra 3.6 points. Since students could have claimed an extra 17.9 points ($50 - 32.6 = 17.9$) and yet they restricted themselves to taking only an extra 3.6, Ariely concludes that their fudge factor was 3.6/17.9, or "only 20% of the possible average magnitude" (Ariely 2008b). Having completed many iterations of this experiment involving hundreds of students, Ariely reaches two conclusions. First,

> most of us, when tempted, are willing to be a little dishonest, regardless of the risks. [Second]. . .
> even when we have no chance of getting caught, we still don't become wild liars – our conscience
> imposes some limits. (Ariely 2008a)

To overgeneralize and oversimplify, we might think of the typical US undergraduate as a 12–20% cheater. That is, these students will allow themselves to cheat up to a point somewhere in this range, but not beyond it. This is true even if the students are certain they can get away with more shenanigans.

Now, Ariely did not control for philosophical orientation among his subjects and, given an egoist's narrow interest in her own welfare, there may be reason to think that egoists will cluster toward the upper end of this range, or even go above it. But there is little reason to think that they would lack a fudge filter altogether. For egoists are not creatures from another planet or animals of a different species. Barring pathological cases, egoists have consciences like the rest of us and even if they might allow themselves to cheat more, they too must deal with the fact that, at some point on the cheating spectrum, they may come to think of themselves as cheaters and for that reason come to disapprove of themselves. Wherever the egoist draws that line, there is where misconduct, by definition, becomes wrong for her.

Can we draw any generalizations from Ariely's work about the question: how much cheating do we tolerate? Apparently not, because the answer may vary from culture to culture. In an online comment responding to Ariely's *Harvard Business Review* interview, a Bill Rhyne reports having conducted an experiment "using Dan Ariely's test methodology in China and the USA in the Spring of 2008" in which the Chinese students acted in virtually identical fashion to the US students. Neither group cheated when they were likely to be discovered and both groups inflated their scores, up to 27%, under conditions of anonymity (Rhyne 2008).

But here's anecdotal evidence that individuals in other academic cultures might have more lenient tolerances for cheating. A group of 30 Russian academics in the social sciences and humanities gathered for a conference outside Moscow in 2009 were asked how much copying and pasting they allowed their students. One volunteered that Russian students had much more leeway in this area than their Western counterparts. How much leeway? Students are generally allowed, one of the faculty members volunteered, to copy up to 30% of their term papers, or up to three pages in a 10-page paper. May we conclude that Russian undergraduates are 30% cheaters? Perhaps not, although none of the professors disagreed with the suggestion. But if so, then tolerances for misconduct may vary significantly between academic groups. More research, as the saying goes, is needed.

We do not have sufficient data to draw uncontroversial conclusions about the fudge factor that comes "naturally" to human beings. That said, Ariely's work suggests a provisional, admittedly oversimplified, beginning point. We – that is, academics in the United States – seem to tolerate at least for ourselves a level of cheating that improves our own performance by roughly a factor of 12–20%. We don't, that is, seem to require absolute honesty of ourselves, but neither do we take full advantage of situations. We allow ourselves and others a fudge factor that varies. How much it varies depends on a multitude of considerations: our assessment of how much we stand to gain from cheating, the likelihood of being caught, the size of the reward if successful, the distastefulness of the penalties if we're found out, the anonymity of the conditions of the transaction, and how far removed the transaction is from actual cash.

Let us underline three important qualifications. First, the results of the study by Ariely and colleagues are not applicable only to egoists as the team studied a range of undergraduates and did not segregate them by philosophical commitment. Second, the team did not probe the amount of cheating we allow others to do; they focused only on the amount of cheating one is willing to tolerate in oneself. Third, the team produced empirical results. Just what normative conclusions we ought to draw from the data is another question. For even if we are persuaded that Ariely's research findings are robust for undergraduate students, the results still tell us only how much people do in fact cheat when they are reasonably convinced that they will get away with it. The results do not address the question: "How much cheating should we tolerate?"

Suppose we polled university faculty in the USA and asked them this question: do you think it is acceptable for your students to cheat to the extent that Ariely's subjects cheated? We suspect the vast majority would say no. We can without contradiction, that is, accept Ariely's results (and even acknowledge that we might be a cheater in his experiments) and still believe that we should not tolerate that much cheating.

A footnote. When we ask how much cheating we should tolerate, we might mean "how much should we tolerate under ideal conditions," in which case we might reply: "None!" Or we might interpret the question more realistically, as asking how much cheating we should tolerate before blowing the whistle on a student, promulgating new standards, or mounting a campaign to change student attitudes. Thus, we might say: "All cheating is wrong, but if plagiarizing 30% of a paper is widely accepted in some academic cultures and if education and research can be successful while allowing such a fudge factor, then so be it. As long as the academic mission is not threatened, we can perhaps tolerate this amount of cheating." Or, in opposition to that conclusion, we might argue instead: "A 30% tolerance for plagiarism is outrageous and should be brought down to 10–20%, or whatever." This is to take the "should" in our question – how much should we tolerate? – in a practical rather than normative sense.

Egoists, like non-egoists, may tolerate a lot of monkey business in themselves. Still, they have reasons not to be maximal cheaters. These reasons include the dictates of their own conscience and the fact that they face formidable uncertainties in accurately assessing their chances of being caught.

There is another hurdle standing in the way of all cheaters, a hurdle to which we now turn our attention. We are surrounded by people who are very good at identifying free riders.

. . . and are surrounded by cheater detectors

Humans are animals who have evolved nuanced and subtle mechanisms for detecting cheating. Our species is skilled at identifying individuals trying to skirt the rules and take advantage of us. This is true in spite of the fact that we are not particularly good at deductive reasoning. The psychologist Peter Wason developed a test that highlights our relative skills in these two domains.

In the Wason test, you are shown a set of four cards and told a story such as this one:

David planted a lovely garden with flowers of every color. He has not been able to enjoy it, though, because deer from the forest nearby have been nibbling on his plants, killing some of them. He would like to keep the deer out of his garden. His grandmother said that in the old days, she kept deer away by spraying an herbal tea – lacana – in her garden. She said:

"If you spray lacana tea on your flowers, deer will stay out of your yard."

This sounded dubious. So David convinced some of his neighbors to spray their flowers with lacana tea, to see what would happen. You are interested in seeing whether any of the results of this experiment violate Grandma's rule.

And then you are given the following instructions about the cards.

> The cards below represent four yards near David's house. Each card represents one yard. One side of the card tells whether or not lacana tea was sprayed on the flowers in a yard, and the other side tells whether or not deer stayed out of that yard.

sprayed with lacana tea	not sprayed with lacana tea	deer stayed away	deer did not stay away

> Which of the following cards would you definitely need to turn over to see if what happened in any of these yards violated Grandma's rule:
>
> "If you spray lacana tea on your flowers, deer will stay out of your yard."
>
> Don't turn over any more cards than are absolutely necessary.

Did you figure out that you only need to turn over two cards to see if Grandma's rule holds? If not, you are not alone. Only 20% of undergraduates at the University of California Santa Barbara knew the answer (Psychology Department n.d.).

You will be much more likely to solve the problem if it is posed in terms that ask you to find the cheater.[3] Here is Daniel Dennett's formulation.

> You are the bouncer in a bar, and your job depends on not letting any underage (under 21) customers drink beer. The cards have information about age on one side, and what the patron is drinking on the other. What cards do you need to turn over?

drinking beer	drinking Coke	25 years old	16 years old

> The first and the last, obviously, the same as in the first problem.

According to Cosmides and Tooby's version of evolutionary psychology, the human mind is like a Swiss-army knife, equipped with special cognitive components for specific purposes (Cosmides & Tooby 1992). If they are right, one of these components is a module dedicated to sniffing out contract breakers. When resources are scarce, groups of humans cannot afford to have pilferers in their midst. When the shifty-eyed are siphoning off the goods, individuals who can quickly identify the thieves are of enormous value to the group. If evolutionary theory tells us to expect the spread of valuable traits throughout a population,

---

[3] Why are we so much better at solving the second problem than the first? Both problems, logically speaking, are structurally the same. Both assume the rule "if p then q" and both require checking any statement claiming p or $\sim q$. In both examples, the rule can be checked by turning over only two cards, the first and last. But why is it so much easier to identify the p (drinking beer) and $\sim q$ (not over 21) statements in the second formulation? Dennett follows Cosmides and Tooby in arguing that the explanation is not in the fact that the second example is more concrete or simply couched in familiar terms. Nor is it that the first formulation is more abstract and logical. It is rather an evolutionary explanation:

> ... the easy cases are all cases that are readily interpreted as tasks of patrolling a social contract, or, in other words, cheater detection. (Dennett 1995)

then we should expect to find that most of us have a cheater detector, too. And, apparently, most of us do have it, as the Wason test suggests. For the Wason tests suggests the following conclusion. If we are presented with a problem that requires us to identify the individual who is trying to get away with something, we can solve the problem much more quickly if it is presented to us in a way that requires us to follow a story than if it requires us to use deductive logic. And – since everyday situations in the lab present themselves to us in the form of narratives, plots, and characters – cheaters run the risk of sticking out like a sore thumb.

. . . cheater detectors who disapprove of cheaters

But the prevalence of cheater-detector mechanisms may not suffice to deter the egoist who knows that half of all graduate students cheat and that 40% of all faculty do not report them. On the basis of this latter information, one might think that cheating is so widespread that cheater-detectors are overburdened and unable to properly enforce anti-cheating measures. Why not conclude, therefore, that one can get away with cheating no matter how skilled the community might be at detecting it?

It's important that aspiring cheaters obtain a reliable answer to this question because their ability to achieve their own best interests rides on it. As we shall now see, however, there is little support for the idea that researchers can deceive others over the long haul. For while we have seen some reasons to think that the senior research community winks at misconduct, there are even stronger reasons to think that it does not.

In 2005, *Nature* published an article with the headline, "One in three scientists confesses to having sinned" (Martinson *et al.* 2005). The headline certainly seems to support the egoist's sense that misbehavior is widespread. But the paper, reporting the results of an anonymous mail survey of 3247 scientists, tells a different story.

The study by Brian Martinson, Melissa Anderson, and Raymond De Vries asked a cross section of US researchers, from early- to mid-career, to respond to a series of questions about their own research conduct. All respondents were recipients of NIH grants. And, indeed, as the writers of *Nature*'s headline proclaimed, fully a third of the respondents reported that they themselves had "engaged in at least one of the top ten [mis-]behaviours [as identified by authors of the study] during the previous three years." Sounds bad for those who care about the reputation of the community – and good for cheaters who want to be surrounded by other cheaters. But let's look in more detail at the study.

Martinson *et al.* described the top ten misbehaviors as follows: Falsifying or "cooking" research data; ignoring major aspects of human-subject requirements; not properly disclosing involvement in firms whose products are based on one's own research; relationships with students, research subjects or clients that may be interpreted as questionable; using another's ideas without obtaining permission or giving due credit; unauthorized use of confidential information in connection with one's own research; failing to present data that contradict one's own previous research; circumventing certain minor aspects of human-subject requirements; overlooking others' use of flawed data or questionable interpretation of data; and changing the design, methodology or results of a study in response to pressure from a funding source. These activities also sound objectionable, but is it possible that respondents might have misinterpreted some of the questions?

The devil is in the details. Take the question about whether the respondent has used "another's ideas without obtaining permission or giving due credit." Could a researcher be guilty of this offense without having done anything seriously wrong?

Here's a thought. Suppose you overhear a good idea at lunch, forget it, innocently include it in a paper months later, and do not acknowledge the source. Later, you remember what happened and record it among your answers to Martinson's survey questions. The community does not recommend that you proceed in this fashion and if you do it habitually you are acting outside the norm. Nonetheless, we would not ordinarily call a person who does it once a plagiarist – and yet they would have used another's ideas without obtaining permission or giving due credit. This definition of plagiarism – if that's what it is – therefore, is quite broad. Perhaps overly broad. Even so, only 1.4% of respondents admitted to having done it.

An even smaller number, 0.4%, admitted to falsifying or fabricating data. Assuming the two categories are distinct – asssuming, that is, that no one who admitted to plagiarism admitted to falsification or fabrication – and adding them together, we have a total of 1.7% admitting to one of the three acts of official research misconduct. That seems a far cry from the "one in three" figure of the headline. What gives? To make sense of the headline, we'll have to look elsewhere, into the other categories with bigger numbers. Let's do that now.

Between 12.2 and 12.8% of respondents said they had "overlooked another scientist's use of flawed data or questionable interpretation of data." Sounds ominous but, again, consider a more innocent interpretation. What if a respondent was admitting that she had once read a poorly constructed argument in an article or happened upon an exaggerated conclusion in a journal title and done nothing? Many of us, I suspect, have found ourselves in the position of encountering mistaken inferences, suspect interpretations of data, or poorly justified headlines and simply not had the time or energy to call attention to them. In order to meet other major responsibilities, all of us, occasionally, must let offenses go unre-marked. Are we sinning?

Or consider another category, the one with the largest number. Between 9.5 and 20.6% of respondents admitted to having "changed the design, methodology or results of a study in response to pressure from a funding source." Again, sounds bad. But consider different ways the question might have been interpreted. Suppose you receive feedback on your rejected grant proposal in which a reviewer suggests changing an element of your design or adopting a slightly different method. You think about the criticism, decide it's valid, and rewrite the proposal. This is what you're supposed to do. Then you read the Martinson question. If you interpret your normal behavior in revising proposals to fall under the Martinson description, then you answer the question affirmatively – you have changed a project in response to "pressure" from a funding source. But did you mean to report a serious research offense? This seems implausible.

In two other categories, 6.0% of respondents admitted "failing to present data that contradict one's own previous research," and 7.6% reported "circumventing certain minor aspects of human-subjects requirements." Again, neither practice is encouraged, and yet it is not difficult to imagine circumstances in which respondents were self-reporting practices that are neither harmful to their individual integrity nor threatening to the health of their group. For example, suppose that both Robertson and Robinson independently produce data sets that contradict mine, and in the same way. I might in my article cite Robertson's study while ignoring Robinson's because the quality of the one is so far superior to the other. I have failed to present data (Robinson's) that contradicts my previous research, but have I erred in my research? Or, I might conduct a clinical trial at an institution that clearly stipulates that no one is to work on the study until every person working on the project has completed an online tutorial concerning the use of human subjects. However, my graduate student Roger tells me he has completed 90% of the tutorial, will finish it tomorrow, but wants to get started today working on the project. I let him. I am circumventing a minor aspect of human-subjects requirements, but am I engaged in research misconduct? Doubtful.

We have reviewed the four categories in the Martinson study with the largest numbers: between 10 and 20% for changing studies in response to funding source pressures; roughly, 12% for overlooking a colleague's questionable interpretation of data; about 6% for not reporting contradictory data; and around 7% for overlooking minor aspects of human-subjects requirements. Compare these numbers to the 1.7% who admitted research misconduct. If one is skeptical (as I am) that behaviors in the categories with big numbers are necessarily serious offenses, then one must re-think the journal's conclusion that one in three scientists sin. A more nuanced judgment is called for.

Here is the upshot of this section. The egoist's thought – *I can get away with cheating because everyone's doing it* – is not justified by the available evidence. While sensational headlines might make egoists, not to mention the general public, think that the research community tolerates a great deal of chicanery, that conclusion is not justified by the data.

. . . and punish cheaters

What happens to researchers who are caught cheating? They may have their names and offenses discussed in newspapers and posted on public websites. For example, the Office of Research Integrity updates its summary of misconduct findings annually (Figure 1.2).

Is the egoist ready for the repercussions? Ready, that is, to be debarred from contracting with any agency of the US government and prohibited from serving in advisory or consulting capacities to the Public Health Service? Ready to be placed on probation and fined? Goodwin was assessed a $500 penalty plus ordered to pay $50,000 in restitution to Health and Human Services and $50,000 to a university scholarship fund (Couzin-Frankel 2010).

In spite of all of these practical reasons not to commit misconduct, the egoist might still think she could fly below the radar and, if caught, beg for forgiveness. In the past, such a strategy might have worked because faculty were once given freedom to deal with wayward students on a case by case basis. Without a consensus understanding of what constitutes misconduct and without a requirement that all misconduct be reported to a central office, the door is open for student serial cheaters to escape notice. As a result of serial cheating, institutions now require faculty to report all cases. Policies have been enacted, too, to protect student rights by providing uniform procedures for students accused of cheating to receive a fair hearing.

As the previous remarks suggest, misconduct policies have a practical basis. They also have a basis in theory. For experiments in iterated prisoner's dilemma games show that roughly a third of all players will either not cooperate with their partners or will break the rules. Over time, as a given game is repeated and players are allowed to get to know each others' moves, cheaters and defectors can be punished. Indeed, if bad actors are not punished, all players will eventually defect, become cheaters, or in other ways bring the game to an inconclusive and unsatisfying end. This result will surprise no one. When cheaters escape unnoticed, everyone else starts to lose their motivation to abide by the rules, too. In the end, folks will lose any motivation even to play the game. Punishing cheaters is necessary to keep the game from deteriorating. When players agree to play for an indeterminate length of time so that no one knows when the last hand will be played, and if cooperating players are able to interact with each other often while defectors are put in positions where they must interact with other defectors often, and if cooperators are

Findings of Scientific Misconduct

Notice Number: NOT-OD-10-130

Key Dates
Release Date: August 30, 2010

Issued by
Department of Health and Human Services (DHHS), (http://www.hhs.gov/)

Notice is hereby given that the Office of Research Integrity (ORI) and the Assistant Secretary for Health have taken final action in the following case:

Elizabeth Goodwin, PhD, University of Wisconsin-Madison: Based on the report of an investigation conducted by the University of Wisconsin-Madison (UW-M) and additional analysis conducted by ORI in its oversight review, the U.S. Public Health Service (PHS) found that Elizabeth Goodwin, PhD, former associate professor of genetics and medical genetics, UW-M, engaged in scientific misconduct while her research was supported by National Institute of General Medical Sciences (NIGMS), National Institutes of Health (NIH), grants R01 GM051836 and R01 GM073183. PHS found that the Respondent engaged in misconduct in science by falsifying and fabricating data that she included in grant applications 2 R01 GM051836-13 and 1 R01 GM073183-01.

PHS found that in grant application 2 R01 GM051836-13, Respondent knowingly and intentionally:

- Falsified Figures 5A and 5B by reusing figures from two of her earlier published papers and falsely labeling them to claim results that had not been achieved in her laboratory.

- Falsified Figure 7B by reusing a figure from one of her published papers and both relabeling it to claim she had detected the STAR-2 protein rather than the TRA-I protein actually detected and modifying the image in the application to disguise its origin.

- Falsified Figure 8C by using a figure produced by one of her students and relabeled it to show that RNAi treatment of C. elegans led to increased expression of the TRA-2 protein when this result had not been obtained by the student.

- Falsified the table on Page 20 of the application showing phenotypic frequencies of worms expressing star-2 (ok483) mutants by significantly overstating the level of aberrant phenotypes and fabricating certain categories of phenotypes not seen by the student conducting the research.

PHS finds that in grant application 1 R01 GM073183-01, Dr. Goodwin knowingly and intentionally:

- Falsified Figure 5 because she used the same two lanes in both Figure 5 and Figure 7, although they were flipped horizontally in one of the figures to disguise their reuse. In Figure 7, the lanes illustrated an effect on laf-1 during developmental stages of C. elegans, and in Figure 5, the same lanes purportedly illustrated an effect on laf-1 noncoding RNA. A witness testified that the result in Figure 5 had not been observed, while that in Figure 7 had, indicating that the claims for Figure 5 were falsified.

- Falsified Figure 8 by reusing photographs prepared by a student that identified the location of rRas-I expression in adult worms and claiming instead that the images illustrated the location of laf-1 mRNA. The images had been enlarged and cropped to disguise their location.

Figure 1.2. Cheaters are punished (http://ori.hhs.gov/content/case-summary-goodwin-elizabeth. Accessed March 21, 2011).

enabled to penalize defectors by refusing to play with them or by depriving defectors of winnings, noncheating players can effectively stop cheating.

A quick summary before moving ahead. Egoists should protect their interests by reporting wrongdoers only when so doing will advance their interests. If the egoist has perfect knowledge of all relevant factors, if the costs of squealing are high, if the chances of being caught are low, if the benefits of free-riding are palpable, and if the egoist is able to remain objective and unbiased throughout his calculations, then not reporting misconduct may be the right thing. But now the egoist must ask himself, Can I make these assumptions?

. . . and, furthermore, the community requires whistle-blowing

Here are two more factors to take into account. First, according to federal policy, the primary responsibility for reporting and investigating allegations of misconduct falls not on university law enforcement agencies or the foundation funding the research or the Office of Student Conduct but on the researchers themselves and their institutions. As a researcher, any student who does not report misconduct, therefore, may be breaking a federal law. Had Padilla not alerted someone about Goodwin's behavior, he would have become complicit in her misconduct. Ultimately, this consideration weighed heavily on his and his peers' minds as they came to their verdict about how to proceed.

Second, if we do not bring questionable research to light, the literature can become polluted with untrustworthy papers and unreliable results. Students citing shoddy papers in their literature searches or basing decisions for their own research on falsified data they find in the record will extend the bad consequences of the cheater's deeds into the indefinite future. Even whistle-blowing is no remedy, however, because papers that have been retracted continue to attract citations (Unger & Couzin 2006).

So the egoist should report misconduct because failure to do so will implicate her in the misconduct. What steps can she take to protect herself as she proceeds? All others things being equal, she should not make the allegation public until it has been fully investigated and confirmed. That said, if the misconduct has resulted in a situation in which public health or safety is endangered, then the whistle-blower should immediately let a public agency know about the threat. Authorities must also be notified if the misconduct involves the breaking of a civil law.

Gunsalus recommends that, if the situation is not dangerous, the potential whistle-blower should think through everything very carefully before acting (Gunsalus 1998). Once one has decided to move forward, one may protect oneself by rigorously Gunsalus's eight steps.

Step one	Review your concerns with someone you trust
Step two	Listen to what that person tells you
Step three	Get a second opinion and take that seriously, too
Step four	If you decide to initiate formal proceedings, seek strength in numbers
Step five	Find the right place to file charges; study the procedures
Step six	Report your concerns
Step seven	Ask questions; keep notes
Step eight	Cultivate patience!

Proceeding in this fashion might, might, allow you to come out ahead as a whistle-blower and, as Gunaslus puts it in her subtitle, "still have a career afterwards."

So, in situations of confusion and ambiguity, honesty seems the best policy – even for egoists

It is true that egoists have no principled reason not to cheat. Nor are they bound, in principle, to report misconduct. And yet we have begun to see that prudence may dictate that the egoist follow the rules of the research community. For egoists have their own internal fudge filters and have some investment in thinking of themselves as members in good standing with their chosen profession. Egoists, too, are surrounded by cheater detectors who not only disapprove of cheating but punish them. Egoists face laws that require whistle-blowing and have access to assistance from people who can help whistle-blowers have a career after they have done the right thing.

In the next three chapters we will encounter more reasons recommending rule-following. We'll ask, for example, whether any one researcher is really in a good position to see all of the data needed to make a wise assessment of the benefits and risks of cheating. How good are we at assessing the probabilities of various potential consequences?

Let us conclude with four points.

1. Excellent researchers are not necessarily ethical researchers

Some folks who engage in misconduct are cool calculators who are always weighing potential costs and benefits and trying to seize every opportunity to take advantage. But misconduct may also occur when otherwise good folks cut corners under stress and pressure.

2. Everyone is not doing it

We often hear that cheating is everywhere and this is what students told Ariely after he asked them to estimate the amount of cheating that they thought had occurred on a final exam. Their guess? Between 30 and 45% of their peers were cheating. But Ariely doubts that they are anywhere near being correct, "because less than 1% of students got a 90% or better (and the average got 70% correct)." He concludes that his "students' perception of cheating was much more exaggerated than the actual level" (Ariely 2011).

If large percentages of students are, in fact, not cheating, it is both false and counter-productive to perpetuate the meme that everyone cheats. Ariely observes that overestimating misconduct "can become an incredibly damaging social norm."

> The trouble [writes Ariely] with this kind of inflated perception is that when students think that all of their peers are cheating, they feel that it is socially acceptable to cheat and feel pressured to cheat in order to stay on top . . . . The bottom line is that if the perception of cheating is that it runs rampant, what are the chances that next year's students will not adopt even more lenient moral standards and live up to the perception of cheating among their peers? (Ariely 2011)

3. Faculty and administrators can do something about it

Faculty can help students by reminding them of the students' values. As Ariely found, students engage their own fudge filter if they are asked one simple question before taking a test (do you agree with the university honor code?). Faculty can provide advocates for students when students are thinking of blowing the whistle, preparing them ahead of time and counseling them about what to expect (McCabe *et al.* 2001).[4]

Faculty can make it more difficult for students to cheat than to do their own work. By giving a number of focused, variable assessments temporally distributed across the entire semester instructors can reduce the incentive to cheat that is presented in a single summative final exam. The answer McCabe heard most often from students was that faculty can communicate better and improve channels for dialog. After completing a survey of heads of laboratories Andrea Gawrylewski was led to recommend in "Fixing Fraud," (*The Scientist*, March 2009) that heads of labs take 12 steps to cultivate a fraud-free lab: hold weekly meetings; look at students' raw data; require detail in lab notebooks; set up a private data server; listen to your students; create open channels of communication; create a contract for new hires; follow the rules; know your limits; be fair and professional; get social; and get curious (Gawrylewski 2009).

Finally, faculty can create an atmosphere on campus by simply discussing research ethics on a regular basis in recurring forums. So let us note again the importance of being part of a vibrant research community. The University of Wisconsin students did not feel supported, felt they had no advocate, were up against powerful forces, and did not know to whom they could turn for assistance. Vibrant research communities deter cheating by encouraging whistle-blowing and protecting those who report falsification and plagiarism. To create such an atmosphere in a laboratory or at an institution is not difficult. The Graduate School Dean can introduce the topics with new students on Orientation Day and veteran students, faculty and administrative officials can follow up with conversations involving all students. Such steps create the kind of climate in which those who observe suspected misconduct feel safe enough to bring it to the light of day.

4. And students can do something about it

Students have a role as well. Since cheating has such bad consequences for them, poisoning the laboratory atmosphere and causing people to mistrust others' work, students have a stake in establishing a zero-tolerance attitude toward it. Cheating cheapens the value of an institution's degree and may have legal consequences for the cheater; the state of North Carolina, for example, regards cheating as a Class 2 misdemeanor. Students can do more; they can institute formal honor codes if their campuses lack them. They can argue for a policy of not using proctors during tests, even in huge lecture halls for, as it turns out, the campuses with the lowest incidence of cheating are campuses where students hold each other responsible.

Graduate students can work toward integrating their lab "horizontally" – that is, student to student – and "vertically," that is, with other faculty members, the director of graduate programs and the departmental chair. Multiple vertical relationships provide critical checks on situations in which students need advice but may not feel comfortable speaking with their supervisor. If departments are small, the chair has a professional obligation to fulfill this role.

---

[4] McCabe *et al.* (2001) recommend 12 steps to reduce cheating in the classroom. We've touched on most of them in this chapter, but here are two that seem to summarize the others: instructors should clearly communicate cheating policies to students, and should establish an atmosphere of respect and academic support with them.

Take home lessons

- To be considered misconduct, acts of falsifying, fabricating, or plagiarizing must have been committed intentionally, knowingly, or recklessly.
- Honest errors, differences of opinion, or insignificant departures from accepted practices are not research misconduct.
- Massaging data, omitting data, and excluding outliers may count as falsification.
- Grad students and postdocs found guilty of misconduct will most likely lose their positions; they may be dismissed from the university and declared ineligible for future federal funds, too.
- Understand clearly the expectations of your research group's leader.
- If you suspect misconduct, speak immediately with someone you trust, such as a faculty member, your department Chair, a member of an institutional ethics committee, or your university's ombudsperson.
- Do not make your allegation of misconduct public unless the misconduct clearly represents a threat to public health or safety.
- The primary responsibility for reporting and investigating allegations of misconduct lies with researchers and their institutions and not with the funders of research.
- The most important safeguard for whistle-blowers is protection from retaliation.
- Faculty should not take dissertation material and publish it without giving the student due credit.

Bibliography

Ariely, D. 2008a. *How Honest People Cheat.* Available at: http://blogs.harvardbusiness. org/cs/2008/01/how_honest_people_cheat. html [Accessed August 8, 2009].

Ariely, D. 2008b. *Predictably Irrational: The Hidden Forces That Shape Our Decisions,* 1st edn. New York: Harper.

Ariely, D. 2011. *Classroom Ethics 101.* Available at: http://danariely.com/2011/08/10/ classroom-ethics-101/#comments.

Bok, S. 1999. *Lying: Moral Choice in Public and Private Life Updated.* London: Vintage.

Cloward, D. 2005. Plagiarism: what's the big deal? *The Academic Standard,* **5**(1), 29–40.

Cosmides, L. & Tooby, J. 1992. *Cognitive Adaptations for Social Exchange.* New York: Oxford University Press, pp. 163–228.

Couzin-Frankel, J. 2010. Probation for biologist who admitted to misconduct. *ScienceInsider.* Available at: http://news.sciencemag.org/ scienceinsider/2010/09/probation-for- biologist-who-admitted.html [Accessed June 8, 2011].

Dennett, D.C. 1995. *Darwin's Dangerous Idea: Evolution and the Meanings of Life.* New York: Simon & Schuster.

Gawrylewski, A. 2009. Fixing fraud. *The Scientist,* **23**(3), 67–69.

Gert, B. 2001. Cheating. In L. Becker & C. Becker, eds. *The Routledge Encyclopedia of Ethics.* New York: Routledge.

Giles, J. 2005. Special Report: Taking on the cheats. *Nature,* **435**(7040), 258–259.

Gunsalus, C.K. 1998. How to blow the whistle and still have a career afterwards, or. . . how to conduct professional disputes professionally. *Science and Engineering Ethics,* **4**(1), 51–64.

Martinson, B.C., Anderson, M.S. & de Vries, R. 2005. Scientists behaving badly. *Nature,* **435** (7043), 737–738.

Mazar, N., Amir, O. & Ariely, D. 2008c. The dishonesty of honest people: a theory of self-concept maintenance. *Journal of Marketing Research,* **45**, 633–644.

Mazar, N. & Ariely, D. 2006. Dishonesty in everyday life and its policy implications, *Journal of Public Policy & Marketing,* **25**(1). Available at: at duke.edu/

~dandan/Papers/PI/dishonesty.pdf [Accessed June 20, 2011].

Mazar, N., Ariely, D. & On, A. 2005d. *(Dis) Honesty: a combination of internal and external rewards.* Working paper, Sloan School of Management, Massachusetts Institute of Technology, as referenced in Mazar and Ariely (2006).

McCabe, D., Trevino, L. & Butterfield, K. 2001. Cheating in academic institutions: a decade of research. *Ethics & Behavior,* **11**(3), 219–232.

McGinn, R. 2003. "Mind the gaps": an empirical approach to engineering ethics, 1997–2001. *Science and Engineering Ethics,* **9**, 517–542.

National Academies (U.S.), 2009. *On Being a Scientist: A Guide to Responsible Conduct in Research,* 3rd edn. Washington DC: National Academies Press.

Psychology Department, U. of C., Santa Barbara, n.d. *The Wason Selection Task.* Available at:

http://www.psych.ucsb.edu/research/cep/ socex/wason.htm.

Rhyne, B. 2008. Comment on Dan Ariely, "Why honest people cheat." Available at: http://blogs.hbr.org/cs/2008/01/ how_honest_people_cheat.html.

Ruhlen, R. 2006. What happens to the whistleblowers? (Letter to the editor). *Science,* **314**(5797), 251–252.

Unger, K. & Couzin, J. 2006. Even retracted papers endure. *Science,* **312**(5770), 40–41.

University of Wisconsin, College of Agricultural and Life Sciences. 2007. *College of Agricultural and Life Sciences Scientific Misconduct Policy for Graduate Students and Postdoctoral Research Associates.* Available at: http://www.cals.wisc.edu/research/ documents/compliance/resources/ CALS_Misconduct_Policy.pdf.

Max Weber noted years ago that the research world is nothing but a world of confusion and ambiguity. In such cloudy conditions, as we saw in the first chapter, honesty and whistle-blowing seem to be the best policy, especially for those looking out for themselves first and foremost. Now, it is also true, as we have seen, that most of us tolerate some amount of cheating and lying. Let's extend this analysis to the use of others' words in our speaking and writing.

Many of us do not object to so-called "white" lies (although even in this area there is much misunderstanding, a subject to which we shall return). But which lies are objectionable, and how much lying is too much? Wherever we draw the line in answer to that question, if we tolerate cheating beyond that line we reduce everyone's capacity to participate eagerly in the free flow of information. Since we cannot check every research result we use in our own research (indeed, we cannot check the vast majority of the results we use) we must trust in the truthfulness of others. But my willingness to trust others is diminished if I think others are plagiarizing. For I know how difficult it is to write up my research results and I know how upset I would be if I discovered someone else had gotten credit for an article that I had written. It is to an egoist's advantage when others properly acknowledge the egoist's written work. But does the egoist himself have any good reasons not to take unfair advantage of others' work?

Protect myself against charges of plagiarism

Let's begin by working our way toward a definition of plagiarism. When have I plagiarized someone else's text? An initial question we may ask is this: do I understand all of the sentences I have written? I have just strung a bunch of words together. What are the chances that I could have produced that particular string – or that particular sentence structure or paragraph arrangement – without having in front of me words written by others? The extent that I produced the string of words without removing my eyes from my computer screen may be the extent to which I can defend myself against a charge of plagiarism. The extent to which I could not have produced the string without looking at a source may be the extent to which I need to worry that I am plagiarizing (cf. Booth *et al.* 2008).

Here is a definition. Plagiarism is

"the deliberate or reckless representation of another's words, thoughts, or ideas as one's own without attribution in connection with submission of academic work, whether graded or otherwise."
(The University of North Carolina at Chapel Hill Instrument of Student Judicial Governance, Section II.B.1)

Research Ethics: A Philosophical Guide to the Responsible Conduct of Research. Gary Comstock.
Published by Cambridge University Press. © Cambridge University Press 2013.

What does "deliberate or reckless" mean? Consider the case of Frank Fischer (Figure 2.1). The paragraph on the left was written in 1980 by Alan Sheridan and published on pp. 139–140 in his book, *Michel Foucault* (Sheridan 1990). The paragraph on the right was written by Fischer in 2000 and published on pp. 26–27 of his book, *Citizens, Experts, and the Environment* (Fischer 2000).

But this power is exercised rather than possessed; it is not the "privilege" of a dominant class, which exercises it actively upon a passive, dominated class. It is rather exercised through and by the dominated. Indeed, it is perhaps unhelpful to think in terms of "classes" in this way, for power is not unitary and its exercise binary. Power in that sense does not exist: what exists is an infinitely complex network of "micro-powers", of power relations that permeate every aspect of social life. For that reason, "power" cannot be overthrown and acquired once for all by the destruction of institutions and seizure of the state apparatuses. Because "power" is multiple and ubiquitous, the struggle against it must be localized. Equally, however, because it is a network and not a collection of isolated points, each localized struggle induces effects on the entire network. Struggle cannot be totalized – a single, centralized hierarchized organisation setting out to seize a single, centralized, hierarchized power; but it can be serial, that is, in terms of horizontal links between one point of struggle and another.	Professional disciplines, operating outside of (but in conjunction with) the state, are thus seen to predefine the very worlds that they have made the objects of their studies (Sheridan, 1980). Because this power is exercised rather than possessed per se, it is not the privilege of a dominant elite class actively deploying it against a passive, dominated class. Disciplinary power in this sense does not exist in the sense of class power. Instead, it exists in an infinitely complex network of "micropowers" that permeate all aspects of social life. For this reason, modern power cannot be overthrown and acquired once and for all by the destruction of institutions and the seizure of the state apparatuses. Such power is "multiple" and "ubiquitous"; the struggle against it must be localized resistance designed to combat interventions into specific sites of civil society. Because such power is organized as a network rather than a collection of isolated points, each localized struggle induces effects on the entire network. Struggles cannot be totalized; there can be no single, centralized power. For this reason, argues Foucault, resistance can only be leveled against the horizontal links between one point of struggle and another (Foucault 1984).

Figure 2.1. Frank Fischer, plagiarism? The words in the right column in gray show apparent duplication, as alleged by Krešimir Petković and Alan Sokal (Bartlett 2010).

What is the lesson of the Fischer case? How many words could Fischer have copied in a row without being accused of "deliberate or reckless" copying? Students are understandably curious about the right answer to this question. But it is a bad question because it assumes that *counting words* is the correct way to avoid plagiarism. If this bad question had a good answer – which it doesn't – we might use the example above to suggest that the answer would not be as few as two or four words, even though Fischer has copied that number of words on at least four occasions. For we often see cases of good writing in which four words in a row appear in the original work and in another work. For example, a sense does not exist for a justifiable definition of plagiarism according to which one can be guilty of plagiarizing by taking four words in a row. And yet a sense does exist for a definition according to which plagiarism occurs whenever someone borrows 22 words in a row ("power cannot be overthrown and acquired once and for all by the destruction of institutions and the seizure of the state apparatuses"). Perhaps a good answer, then – assuming that there is a good answer – is that any time you find yourself wanting to borrow a half dozen or more words in a row you should pause to ask whether you are deliberately and recklessly copying.

But let us return to the point at which we began: the way to proceed here is not to try to count words. It is to ensure that you understand the author's ideas, that you are interpreting them accurately, and that you are expressing them in your own voice. Writing is a difficult skill to learn and it cannot be learned if we do not take the time to draft the article for ourselves, to revise and edit it in light of new findings and criticism, and to be ready to re-shape and re-work it again and again. Good arithmetic is not the answer here; good composition is.

When you write, think of yourself as entering a conversation. You must introduce yourself, find your own voice, acknowledge the contributions your colleagues have made, and add yours to theirs. To acknowledge theirs, cite and attribute.

First, cite. What is a citation? The Girl Scouts issue "citations" to members who have distinguished themselves in order to bring their achievements to the attention of others. Authors issue citations to other authors whose work they are quoting. In this context, citing is quoting, quoting is copying and pasting, and copying and pasting is permissible if we add quotation marks. No, common knowledge – information your audience already knows – does not need to be cited. How to cite? Single or double quotation marks? Before or after the attribution? Check the stylesheet of the journal to which you are submitting the article.

Second, attribute. To attribute is to give credit. For what do we give credit? Everything that is not common knowledge. Not just books and journals but ideas from informal conversations, movies, websites, and, yes, Wikipedia. If you reuse sentences or paragraphs of your own – ideas you have previously published elsewhere – be sure to attribute them to your prior publication, too. In this way you avoid self-plagiarism, which is publishing the same piece in two places. Careful attribution will also help you to avoid the temptation to publish the same paper in two very different places. For if you tried to hide from the editor of Journal #1 the fact that you were simultaneously offering the same paper to Journal #2, you would have a difficult time keeping up your ruse if you had to cite in Journal #2 all of the quotations you were using from your paper in Journal #1.

As my grandmother used to say, "Be sure your sin will find you out." I wonder whether Park *et al.* were prepared to be found out after they had submitted the results of their research to two journals, *Circulation* and *The New England Journal of Medicine*. After the NEJM found them out it published this editorial:

> In a subgroup of 81 patients described in the manuscript submitted by Park *et al.* to the
> *Journal*, intravascular ultrasound procedures were performed to evaluate the extent of restenosis.
> We later discovered that the intravascular ultrasound findings in these 81 patients had been

published in *Circulation* in February 2003 and that the two manuscripts had been under review simultaneously at the two journals. Park *et al.* had been explicitly informed about our policy against redundant publication, but they never told us about the existence of the other manuscript, even after it had been accepted for publication. Furthermore, their article in the *Journal* did not cite the article in *Circulation*.

As the International Committee of Medical Journal Editors points out, duplicate publication is contrary to "international copyright laws, ethical conduct, and cost-effective use of resources."

(Curfman *et al.* 2003)

It's also not a reliable way to build one's scholarly reputation.

Careful citation will also help you to avoid "salami" publications. When you're preparing a sandwich in the kitchen you want the sausage to go as far as possible. When you're preparing an article, however, you want your reader to be able to see the whole picture. If you slice and dice it into its LPUs – Least Publishable Units – you may pad your resume but you will also frustrate your reader. For readers are genuinely interested in knowing the whole story. Keeping coherent publishable units intact will attract readers; salami will drive them away.

Can I get away with it?

We plagiarize for many reasons. We don't have enough time to do the job right. We want a good grade on the paper. We can think of more fun ways to spend the weekend. Others are doing it, or so we believe. We just want to level the playing field.

A little copying here and pasting won't hurt me, will it? Who will ever know? Before you place much stock in your answer, google "plagiarism detection services." You'll get dozens of hits for companies like Turnitin.com, Article Checker, CopyTrackerOnline, Plagiarism-Detect.com, DOC Cop, SeeSources.com, Glatt, Dupli Checker, and PlagiarismChecker.com. If you're still not convinced that your odds of being caught are pretty high, try this exercise I learned from Charlotte Bronson. She has her graduate students select any six consecutive words from a journal article. She instructs them to put those words in quotation marks and enter them into Google.

In tests of dozens of strings of words, Bronson has witnessed only one case in which the search brought up more than one reference. She concludes that "six words in a row is usually enough to identify the source, and thus the six words in a row are likely due to plagiarism."[1] Admittedly, she adds, no senior researcher is going to accuse you of plagiarism if you happen to use the same half dozen words as someone else – assuming, of course, that you don't have a bunch of other copied phrases in your paper. However, the result should make you stop and think. If it's this easy to find the source of a six-word phrase, how difficult would it be for a reader to find the source you're pirating?

The 'half-dozen' rule captures two intuitions: first, that it is common to find two people using identical strings of words that are *shorter* than six words long, so these phrases are not likely to be plagiarized; second, that strings of words longer than seven or eight words, especially if they include technical terms, are likely to be plagiarized.

We are thinking about how likely it is that we will be caught in plagiarism. The issue raises a larger question about human nature and moral standards because we all know students who *have* gotten away with cheating. Would we hold ourselves to moral standards against cheating if we knew that *we* could get away with it? It's not a new question; the Greek philosopher Plato

---

[1] Charlotte Bronson, personal correspondence November 16, 2011, used with permission.

(d. 347 BC) discussed it in Book 2 of his *Republic* where a character named Glaucon ruminates about the mythical golden ring of Gyges. The piece of jewelry gives its owner the power to become invisible at will. (Yes, it's the same ring we see in Tolkien's *Lord of the Rings* and Rowling's *Harry Potter*.) Whenever Gyges wants anonymity, he simply slips it on and is free to go about doing whatever he wishes. So, Gyges can seduce the queen, murder the king, assume the throne, and never have anyone discover that he is the source of the evil. If one could go about one's dirty business with impunity, Plato has Glaucon wonder, what would be one's motive to act ethically? As no one could hold us responsible for our actions there would seem to be no reason to act morally. In many ways, "Why should I care about doing the right thing when I can get away with wrongdoing?" is the most basic question of the examined life.

The egoist's answer is straightforward. If I can get away with it I will. And I should. There is no objective moral standard apart from the one that tells me to pursue my own interests. But everything hinges on the conditional, "If I can . . . ." Can I get away with it? To answer the question I must carefully weigh all of the risks. And, as it turns out, the risks of getting caught are not insignificant, even though we all know of cheaters who have succeeded in their deception. But to what end? Their pay-off is almost always fairly minimal, they end up "cheating themselves" because they do not get the education they're paying for, and the risks are huge. If they are caught the professional damage to their reputations is potentially catastrophic. If that's true, there is almost never a good reason to plagiarize, even for the egoist. There's simply too much at stake and too little to gain.

Writing is very hard work and when you have done it well you deserve credit for accurate reporting, sensitive analysis, and nuanced judgment. This work cannot be done quickly and it cannot be borrowed from someone else. Egoists who want to be researchers should think twice before taking others' ideas or words. They should earn their credit, and they will earn it only if they do the work themselves.

To ensure that we can all accurately identify cases of plagiarism, work through the following exercise. In it you will have to figure out whether certain sentences are plagiarized from a publication in the plant sciences. (Versions of the exercise for other disciplines – physics, electrical engineering, plant pathology, physics education, public administration, and biochemistry – are available online at the OpenSeminar.[2])

Exercise: "Recognize plagiarism," by Charlotte Bronson and Gary Comstock[3]

1. Here is a paragraph quoted from a paper by G. S. Johal, S. H. Hulbert, and S. P. Briggs titled "Disease lesion mimics of maize: a model for cell death in plants" (Johal *et al.* 1995). Please read it carefully.

    A class of maize mutants, collectively known as disease lesion mimics, display discrete disease-like symptoms in the absence of pathogens. It is intriguing that a majority of these lesion mimics behave as dominant gain-of-function mutations. The production of lesions is strongly influenced by light, temperature, developmental state and genetic background. Presently, the biological significance of this lesion mimicry is not clear, although suggestions have been made that they may represent defects in the plants' recognition of, or response to, pathogens. . . . In this paper we argue that this might be the case. . .

[2] http://openseminar.org/ethics/courses/136/modules/3910/index/screen.do.
[3] Based on Charlotte Bronson, "What is Plagiarism?" *Bioethics in Brief* vol. 1, issue 2 (November 1999). Charlotte Bronson is professor of plant pathology and associate vice president for research, Iowa State University, cbronson@iastate.edu.

2. Which of the following sentences fail to give proper credit for the writing and/or ideas of the authors? Explain your answer.
   1. Currently, the biological significance of lesion mimicry in plants is not known, although suggestions have been made that they may represent defects in the plants' recognition of, or response to, pathogens.
   2. Currently, the biological significance of lesion mimicry in plants is not known, although suggestions have been made that they may represent defects in the plants' recognition of, or response to, pathogens (Johal *et al.* 1995).
   3. Currently, "the biological significance of lesion mimicry in plants is not known, although suggestions have been made that they may represent defects in the plants' recognition of, or response to, pathogens" (Johal *et al.* 1995).
   4. The biological significance of lesion mimicry in plants is currently not known, although some researchers believe that they may represent defects in the ability of plants to recognize or respond to pathogens.
   5. The biological significance of lesion mimicry in plants is currently not known, although some researchers believe that they may represent defects in the ability of plants to recognize or respond to pathogens (Johal *et al.* 1995).
   6. Lesion mimicry has been proposed to be due to mutations in genes controlling the ability of plants to detect and respond to pathogens.
   7. Lesion mimicry has been proposed to be due to mutations in genes controlling the ability of plants to detect and respond to pathogens (Johal *et al.* 1995).
   8. Disease-like lesions in plants may be due to mutations in genes controlling the ability of plants to defend themselves against pathogens (Johal *et al.* 1995).

Key

Instructor's note: The first sentence is blatant plagiarism in any discipline. Successive sentences become increasingly original, so that the last sentence is acceptable in any discipline. The opinions of students and professors diverge on the acceptability of the sentences in the middle of the list. Many students believe sentence number 5, for example, is acceptable whereas most professors believe it is plagiarism. This discrepancy demonstrates the need for better communication between students and faculty on this subject.

1. Currently, the biological significance of lesion mimicry in plants is not known, although suggestions have been made that they may represent defects in the plants' recognition of, or response to, pathogens.

   Almost everyone agrees that this is plagiarism because the wording is almost identical to that of Johal *et al.* and, in addition, there is no citation to give credit for the ideas.

2. Currently, the biological significance of lesion mimicry in plants is not known, although suggestions have been made that they may represent defects in the plants' recognition of, or response to, pathogens (Johal *et al.* 1995).

   Almost everyone agrees this is plagiarism because, even though the citation gives proper credit for the ideas, the wording is almost identical to that of Johal *et al.*

3. Currently, "the biological significance of lesion mimicry in plants is not known, although suggestions have been made that they may represent defects in the plants' recognition of, or response to, pathogens" (Johal *et al.* 1995).

   Almost everyone agrees that this is not plagiarism. However, it is improper quotation because the words in quotes are not identical to what Johal *et al.* wrote. Another point worth discussing is that quotes should only be used when the wording of the original author is so important that the information cannot be conveyed in the writer's own words. Quotations should not be used as a substitute for understanding.

4. The biological significance of lesion mimicry in plants is currently not known, although some researchers believe that they may represent defects in the ability of plants to recognize or respond to pathogens.

   Almost everyone agrees this is plagiarism because there is no citation to give credit for the ideas. Most readers also recognize that the wording is only a slight modification of that of Johal *et al*.

5. The biological significance of lesion mimicry in plants is currently not known, although some researchers believe that they may represent defects in the ability of plants to recognize or respond to pathogens (Johal *et al*. 1995).

   Most faculty consider such sentences plagiarism because, although a citation gives credit for the ideas, the wording is only a slight modification of that of Johal *et al*. This example is worth discussing at length because of the disagreement between students and faculty on whether it is plagiarism. Many students consider rearrangement and substitution of words, as in this example, to make a sentence their own. Note that it was not necessary to understand what Johal *et al*. wrote in order to write example 5.

6. Lesion mimicry has been proposed to be due to mutations in genes controlling the ability of plants to detect and respond to pathogens.

   It depends. Unless this information is already common knowledge, this sentence is plagiarism because no credit is given for the ideas.

7. Lesion mimicry has been proposed to be due to mutations in genes controlling the ability of plants to detect and respond to pathogens (Johal *et al*. 1995).

   This is not plagiarism. Note that, to write examples 6, 7 and 8, the writer had to first genuinely understand what Johal *et al*. had written.

8. Disease-like lesions in plants may be due to mutations in genes controlling the ability of plants to defend themselves against pathogens (Johal *et al*. 1995).

   This is not plagiarism; however, some readers astutely notice that there is more information in this sentence than in the paragraph by Johal *et al*. In fact, the writer had to read the entire paper to write this sentence.

Why words matter to the egoist

Let us return now to ethical theory. Can the egoist claim that plagiarism is wrong? Sure. Obviously, he will complain whenever someone takes his words; plagiarism is theft and the egoist is entitled to be angry when robbed. Theft diminishes the egoist, depriving him of something that is rightfully his. If I take his Harley Davidson Fat Boy, I hurt him. If I take his paragraph, I hurt him, too. It is obvious why egoists would object to others stealing their words. But can egoists give a reason why they should not take others' words? This is a more difficult question for the egoist to answer. Egoists have a response open to them, but it requires an elaboration of the social context in which the egoist operates.

The egoist researcher operates in a culture based on relationships of trust. This culture can survive occasional petty thefts and white lies told once in a blue moon. However, when individuals tell serious lies, and tell them again and again, the culture can quickly fail. For deception, exploitation, and widespread cheating does not only undermine the community.

It undermines each individual. For when the community tolerates such practices, it allows something subtle to be taken from the egoist – his ability to trust others.

Now, how much cheating and lying can the egoistic researcher allow before his ability to get what he wants is threatened? Where is the line between a few people telling a few little white lies in an otherwise just society and a corrupt society so full of pickpockets and slanderers that the corrupt structures barely hold together? There is no general answer. The answer depends on how the facts turn out – how widespread lying is and how much cheating is tolerated and how extensively such practices undermine the relationships of trust necessary for a functioning society. But there is no doubt that eventually a line can be crossed and a tipping point reached. At some point, widespread thievery undermines the ability of all professionals to trust each other. That is a cost to everyone, the egoist included.

When cultures tolerate lies they incur serious costs, and individuals – even if they are interested only in promoting their own self-interest – are harmed. Egoism can explain the wrongness of plagiarism for the egoist by pointing to the incremental and indirect way that such actions lead to social circumstances that may eventually impede the egoist from attaining her own goals. Indeed, egoists should generally not only not plagiarize, but they must be careful to protect themselves from being placed under any suspicion of having plagiarized for the suspicions may well come to hurt them.

It bears noting that discussions of research misconduct often begin by contemplating the theft of someone's words. Words matter because they convey our identity. It is possible that a precocious third grader, call him Little Mike, could see this sentence in a book and read it aloud "Disciplinary power in this sense does not exist in the sense of class power." But the string of words uttered by Little Mike would not mean the same thing as when it is uttered in a lecture by Michel Foucault himself. Arguably, the string of words on the youth's lips would not mean anything at all. On the one hand, he would not understand what they mean; on the other hand, his utterance would have a comic effect on his audience rather than the tutelary effect intended by Foucault. Sentences have the meaning they do only when they are spoken or written by someone who understands the words. To understand the words is to be able to wield them appropriately in other contexts. Foucault knows what Mike does not – what the words mean in other sentences, how people who understand the sentence are likely to react to it, and how to revise or amplify it so as to clarify its meaning. Competent users of a language know what incompetent users do not know: the semantic, syntactical, grammatical, and narrative rules that govern the combination of verbs and nouns. To know these rules enables one, too, to read audience's responses, anticipate misunderstandings, and re-focus their attention on one's actual intentions.

Furthermore, we must add one more fact to this story. We hone whatever linguistic skills are hard-wired into us with assistance from our parents and teachers. As children begin to deploy rules on their own, they begin to express themselves, in their own voices. Each one takes on her own identity as she enunciates words in her own individual cadence, her own accent, her own way of enhancing her meaning with a characteristic tempo, rhythm, and inflection. Each of us has acquired our idiosyncratic shorthands, our own favored metaphors, and nicknames for others. Our being, one is tempted to say, is inseparable from our speech.

That is why words matter to the egoist – as they matter to all of us – because they carry our personal identity. In this sense, when others steal an egoist's words they steal something of great value to the egoist. And when the egoist steals other's words, they similarly are guilty of psychological breaking and entering.

Can the same be said about our ideas? We have made the case that stealing words is plagiarism, but what about the thoughts that the words convey? Are they also wrapped up in our identity? Sure. If you read an article in Spanish or French or Chinese, translate the ideas into English and then include the English in your own article, you have taken someone else's intellectual property. True, you have not taken the person's (Spanish) words, but you have certainly taken their ideas, and the offense is the same.

Words are linguistic conventions. You can refer to a nation as a state, or *país*, or *peuple*, or 國. The token or word that you use is irrelevant when it comes to determining plagiarism. You plagiarize when you take someone's idea because the particular word used to express the idea is a convention. Because of their conventional nature, words can be changed and still refer to the same thing (state, people). To make this point clearer we might consider the conventions of card games. Spades are black in most card decks. But they could be gray, or even green. As long as the players all agreed that gray Spades are the same as black Spades they could get along just fine. What's important about a Spade in a game of Spades is not its color but its function; it can trump Hearts and Clubs. With words, it is the same. Stealing someone's words in their own language is plagiarism. So is stealing those ideas by simply changing the convention you are using to express their idea. This is a matter the research community cares about because we recognize that ideas as well as words carry an author's identity.

This is as true for egoists as for anyone. Words are critical to human beings because words are the vehicles by which we come to know who we are. How can an egoist know whether he is getting what he wants – how can he know what he wants – if he does not have words? "How do I know what I think," says Graham Wallas's 'little girl' (1926), "until I see what I say?"[4]

Conclusion

If you think you can get away with plagiarizing in a particular instance, rational egoism will not tell you it is always ethically wrong to do so. It will say that you are responsible for your actions, that if you want to get a graduate degree you must be perceived as following the rules of the game, and that the rules forbid cheating. How much plagiarism will the rational egoist tolerate in himself? The answer depends on the individual and the categorical interests he wants to achieve. If his goals are low, he may tolerate a lot of plagiarism. But acquiring an advanced degree is no mean feat, and it requires jumping some pretty tall hurdles. Egoists aspiring to be researchers, it would appear, cannot afford to tolerate much plagiarism in themselves.

How do we protect ourselves against plagiarism? Two words: write well. And three words: write by yourself. Read, re-read, and then set your sources aside before writing your first draft. Produce a "dirty" draft in which you just spew things out as they come into your head. Return to the texts for the next draft, quoting them carefully when quoting is necessary to clarify your point. Ensure that the words in your final paper are all in your voice. If the paper includes unusual phrases including technical terms, or sentences or significant parts of sentences of others, be sure to reference them. Check your usage against the conventions of your community whether you are writing an article, grant proposal,

---

[4] E. M. Forster also used the line in his *Aspects of the Novel* in 1927 (Forster 1956). As Davidson points out, however, Wallas was first into print with it (Davidson 1987).

essay, or progress report. Lean on your mentors; they can help you improve the draft. But don't let them lean too heavily on you. Professors should not be putting material from your dissertation into their published work without giving you appropriate credit. If you see that happening, a frank talk with the offending party should be in your future.

Take home lessons

- Attribute: use quotation marks to indicate the words you are copying from your source.
- Cite: use parentheses or footnotes to reference your source.
- Don't self-plagiarize by failing to cite yourself when reusing your published words; and don't publish salami or duplicate (redundant) papers.

Bibliography

Bartlett, T. 2010. Document sheds light on investigation at Harvard. *The Chronicle of Higher Education.* Available at: http://chronicle.com/article/Document-Sheds-Light-on/123988/ [Accessed August 30, 2010].

Booth, W.C., Colomb, G.G. & Williams, J.M. 2008. *The Craft of Research*, 3rd edn. Chicago: University of Chicago Press. Available at: http://www2.lib.ncsu.edu/catalog/record/NCSU2190397 [Accessed October 15, 2010].

Curfman, G.D., Morrissey, S. & Drazen, J. 2003. Editorial: notice of duplicate publication. *The New England Journal of Medicine*, **348**(2254). Available at: http://www.nejm.org/doi/full/10.1056/NEJMe038100.

Davidson, D. 1987. Knowing one's own mind. *Proceedings and Addresses of the American Philosophical Association*, **60**(3), 441–458.

Fischer, F. 2000. *Citizens, Experts, and the Environment: The Politics of Local Knowledge.* Duke University Press Books.

Forster, E.M. 1956. *Aspects of the Novel*, Harvest Books.

Johal, G.S., Hulbert, S.H. & Briggs, S.P. 1995. Disease lesion mimics of maize: a model for cell death in plants. *BioEssays*, **17**(8), 685–692.

Sheridan, A. 1990. *Michel Foucault: The Will to Truth*, new edn. Routledge.

Beware intuition

Egoism has much to recommend it. For one thing, it seems consistent with what biology suggests about the way the moral system might have evolved. Imagine our ancestors on the African plain competing for the attention of mates. Individuals who were indifferent about, unaware of, or insufficiently attentive to their own interests would be at a decided disadvantage. If individuals didn't look out for themselves, then who would look out for them? Those *Homo sapiens* skilled at getting what they wanted almost certainly had fitness advantages over individuals who were clueless, especially when it came to maximizing one's chances of finding a partner willing to have children with them. It seems, therefore, that egoists would win out over non-egoists, for they would outcompete whoever was not willing to scratch and claw to fulfill their needs.

Egoists must be conscious of observation bias

But things may not be so simple for the egoist. The reason is that many self-interested individuals have survived over time and, following this line of thought, many egoists must now exist. All of them, according to this story, must have exquisite means of reading, anticipating, and responding to others' behaviors, too. So if I'm an egoist today and I want to try to get away with slighting others in the contemporary research world, then, I will have my work cut out for me. In this chapter, we will explore the reasons that it's hard out there for an egoist.

Cheaters in the research community operate under unfavorable conditions. First, they must use their own perceptual equipment – which research shows is unreliable. Second, they are prone to overestimate their state of knowledge. Third, they are probably going to underestimate the influence of their own biases. And, fourth, they are most likely unaware of the extent to which their biases can mislead them into making bad decisions. Egoists, in sum, ought to be much more skeptical than they are about their ability to get away with cheating. Why should this be?

First, consider observation bias. It is very easy once one has acquired data that fits one's prejudices to seize upon these data as the final truth. Far harder to withhold judgment, to remain skeptical about one's hypotheses, to persevere in research and refrain from premature judgment (Kruger & Dunning 1999). As Ditto and Lopez showed, all of us have both conscious and unconscious ways to deceive ourselves. Individuals who are happy with the

Research Ethics: A Philosophical Guide to the Responsible Conduct of Research. Gary Comstock.
Published by Cambridge University Press. © Cambridge University Press 2013.

results of early information-gathering sorties can easily talk themselves into thinking that they have completed their mission. Data that are "consistent with a preferred conclusion is examined less critically than information inconsistent with a preferred conclusion and consequently, less information is required to reach the former than the latter" (Ditto & Lopez 1992). We are adept, in other words, at preventing ourselves from allowing unwelcome information to enter our consciousness. Von Hippel and Trivers provide an evolutionary explanation for why this trait is adaptive. Self-deception allows us to avoid relaying to others "the cues to conscious deception that might reveal deceptive intent" (von Hippel & Trivers 2011). Again we see the importance of a healthy dose of epistemic humility among those whose stated goal is to discover truths.

Second, our opinions rely heavily on the views we were taught to believe, and yet entrenched authorities cannot always be believed. The life of scholarship requires an extraordinary amount of courage, but everyone who thinks they can game the system must be especially vigilant about examining their hypotheses and particularly cognizant of how difficult it is to see things properly. As a species, humans are subject to biases, including the power of the answers – often mistaken – carried by tradition. We are subject to strong temptations simply to accept answers we have been taught. The research attitude of critical thinking, however, encourages us not to rest content with the commonplaces of alleged authorities.

One need not look beyond the history of the discovery of Saturn's rings for an example of observation bias, also known in the psychological literature as expectation bias. Today, using low-powered telescopes, school children can easily be taught to see the planet's rings. This was not always the case, however. After Galileo first reported, incorrectly as it turned out, that Saturn had two large moons – one moon on either side of the planet – observers thereafter consistently reported seeing moons, not rings. Albert Van Helden, a historian of science, has shown the power of our expectations. Inaccurate post-Galilean drawings of Saturn "came not from poor telescopes, but from the influence of Galileo's first reports on later observers" (Jeng 2006).

Third, it is easy to proceed in science by looking for the data we want. You adopt a strong theory and conduct experiments until the cows come home trying to prove it. Should any particular trial be inconclusive you ignore it, reasoning that it must have had design flaws. You publish only those trials that lend support to your hypothesis. You don't, in short, follow what Darwin called his golden rule:

> namely, that whenever a published fact, a new observation or thought came across me, which was opposed to my general results, to make a memorandum of it without fail and at once; for I had found by experience that such facts and thoughts were far more apt to escape from the memory than favourable ones.
>
> (Darwin & Barlow 1969)

. . . wary of misleading heuristics

Rhetoric – the way in which we frame a problem or word a question – has great power to lead us into errors of judgment. Our minds have shortcuts, what the cognitive psychologists Tversky and Kahneman call "heuristics," mental filters that may serve us well when we have to make snap judgments (Tversky & Kahneman 1974). But these same conceptual tools can often lead us not only to choose inconsistently but, most troublingly, to choose in ways that undercut progress toward our own goals. For example, if you tell me that a surgical procedure X offers an 85% chance of success, I will embrace it because it will get me what I want, an 85% chance of success. However, if you frame the issue differently, if you tell me that the same procedure offers a 15% chance of failure, I may well reject it – even though my choice will not get me what I want, an 85% chance of success.

This heuristic is known as the framing effect. Here is another example. Tversky and Kahneman told a group of research subjects that they could either choose to save 200 of 600 people afflicted with a deadly disease by choosing option A, or, by choosing option B, gain a 33% chance of saving all 600 while simultaneously risking a 66% chance of saving no one.[1] Given that choice, 72% chose option A, probably because it is less risky than option B and most humans are risk-averse. However, when Tversky and Kahneman gave a different group the same choice described in a different frame, the group reversed the decision. The alternate frame was this: you can choose option C with the result that 400 people die or option D that presents a 33% chance that no one will die and a 66% probability that everyone will die. Some 78% of the participants chose option D over C – even though D is equivalent to B and C is equivalent to A and the majority of us favor A over B. Are our responses really so malleable?

It seems so. Experimental evidence mounts in support of the idea that others can exercise significant control over my decisions simply by placing surreptitious anchors in my mind. Few MBA students know that Attila the Hun was defeated in the year 451. But if you want to lead them to guess a year that is lower than that figure, separate out those students who have phone numbers the last three digits of which are low (e.g., 008). Ask them to recall the last three digits of their phone number and write it down. If you then ask them when Attila the Hun was beaten they will guess numbers lower than 451 more often than chance would predict. (If you want to lead a group to guess a year higher than 451, segregate out those with high phone numbers and turn the same gears.[2]) Why should as mundane a mental activity as remembering my phone number affect my sense of when a critical historical event happened? Because the brain has a tendency to establish anchors, ideas that are readily accessible and not necessarily true or unbiased. We apparently search for anchors when looking for answers – and unconsciously fix on those we find, no matter how irrelevant or biased they may be. And never mind that they were placed there without our knowledge by others.

One might think these results are interesting but negligible since the examples come from peripheral areas of life (Attila the Hun and phone numbers?). But analogous results crop up in investigations of no less a significant domain of our lives than our moral character. Alice Isen and Paula Levin set out to determine whether they could persuade and dissuade people from acting charitably by manipulating their environment (Isen & Levin 1972). In 1972 they planted dimes in pay phones and then observed whether the folks who found the coins were more likely to help someone who had, as a confederate in the experimental protocol, dropped a sheaf of papers on the floor. The results were astonishing. Some 84% of shoppers would help if they had first found a dime – a dime! A mere 4% would help if they had not first discovered the change.

---

[1] Tversky & Kahneman 1981.
[2] Russo & Schoemaker 2002.

When interviewed, the helpful shoppers did not attribute their good nature to the fact that they had found a dime. Similarly, Princeton seminary students who stopped to help a man in need did not attribute their Good Samaritan behavior to the fact that they – unlike the majority of their peers who were in a rush – had plenty of time on their hands to stop and assist.[3] In both the dime in a phone and Good Samaritan cases, the cheery altruistic-minded subjects were quick to claim that their behaviors were consistent with their "character." They had good "habits," "traits." They were the sort of people that were naturally inclined to being virtuous. The evidence suggests that they are wrong. It seems that it is not our moral commitments that best predict our actions but, rather, the external environment.[4]

There is another reason egoists should be cautious when assessing their chances of getting away with something: their ability to understand themselves.

. . . and on guard against self-misunderstanding

How well do we understand ourselves? The so-called situationist literature provides reasons to doubt both that we know what makes us happy and that we exercise as much control over our decisions as we think we do. John Doris summarizes three of these reasons: the automaticity of many of our choices, source misattribution, and confabulation (J.M. Doris 2005).

Misunderstanding the causes of one's behavior is not confined to banal everyday activities such as finding a dime in a pay phone. Few choices are more consequential than our choice of a place to live. And yet even here unconscious influences work their magic on us. For example, consider my case. My name is Gary and my wife's name is Karen. Her father calls her Karey. When we decided to look for a house in North Carolina, we looked for almost a year before settling on one in Cary. It took us so long because we knew exactly what we wanted: transitional style under a certain price, wooded backyard, close to campus, etc. Between the two of us, we had a list of criteria as long as your arm. We would have found it amusing, and frankly demeaning, if you had told us that we settled on Cary because the town name sounds like ours. In fact, the similarity never even occurred to me until 8 years after we moved to Cary (indeed, as I was writing this paragraph).

Study after study suggests that nonconscious external causes play an unnervingly effective role in our decisions. One is more likely to move to a state that bears a resemblance to one's name (Georgia to Georgia, Virginia to Virginia) than chance would predict. Indeed, the rate is 36% higher for perfect matches. Similar studies show a similar influence of one's name on the profession one takes up. There is a higher than predicted number of Denises and Dennises in dentistry, and of Georges and Georgias in geoscience.[5] This is but a small sample of evidence suggesting that we make up stories to rationalize our judgments – sometimes of judgments we were never conscious of making in the first place. If offered a choice between two cards bearing pictures of different people and told to select the one we find most attractive, we will quickly make up a detailed

[3] Darley & Batson 1973.

[4] Doris 2005.

[5] Pelham, Mirenberg, and Jones, "Why Susie Sells Seashells by the Seashore: Implicit Egotism and Major Life Decisions."

reason why we chose the other person if through sleight of hand we are given the picture of the person we did not choose and asked to explain why we did choose her.[6] We are, it appears, inveterate rationalizers.

Accumulating data suggest that whereas we think we know immediately and intuitively who we are and why we are behaving in a certain fashion, it appears that we are often wrong about the actual causes of our behaviors. Consider the consequences for the rational egoist. If one makes decisions using automatic rather than reflective cognitive mechanisms and if one's assessments are subject to the powerful vagaries of automaticity, misattribution, and confabulation, then what chance do we have of accurately understanding our own interests? In these perilous psychological conditions, egoists have their work cut out for them. Their goal, remember, is to figure out what others are thinking so that they can cut corners without being caught. But what are their chances of success in this endeavor – deciphering what others are thinking about them – when all of the evidence suggests that it is difficult enough for them to figure out what they are thinking about themselves?

. . . not to mention probability ineptness

We are reviewing the challenges the egoist faces as he thinks of ways he might get away with cheating. Here is another hurdle, and probably the most formidable: the human tendency to over-estimate our skill in assessing probabilities. One might think evolution would have selected by now for ability to maximize chances to get what one wants. To the contrary, we lack advanced capacities for making choices critical to success in achieving our goals. The so-called Monty Hall phenomenon illustrates the point.

Case study: "Monty Hall," by Keith Devlin[7]

In the 1960s, there was a popular weekly US television quiz show called *Let's Make a Deal*. Each week, at a certain point in the program, the host, Monty Hall, would present the contestant with three doors. Behind one door was a substantial prize; behind the others there was nothing. Monty asked the contestant to pick a door. Clearly, the chance of the contestant choosing the door with the prize was 1 in 3. So far so good.

Now comes the twist. Instead of simply opening the chosen door to reveal what lay behind, Monty would open one of the two doors the contestant had not chosen, revealing that it did not hide the prize. (Since Monty knew where the prize was, he could always do this.) He then offered the contestant the opportunity of either sticking with their original choice of door, or else switching it for the other unopened door.

The question now is, does it make any difference to the contestant's chances of winning to switch, or might they just as well stick with the door they have already chosen?

---

[6] Johansson, "Failure to Detect Mismatches Between Intention and Outcome in a Simple Decision Task."

[7] Reprinted with permission of Keith Devlin from Mathematical Association of America Online 2010, Available at: http://www.maa.org/devlin/devlin_07_03.html. Keith Devlin is Executive Director, Human-Sciences and Technologies Advanced Research Institute, Stanford University. kdevlin@stanford.edu. Copyright the Mathematical Association of America 2010. All rights reserved.

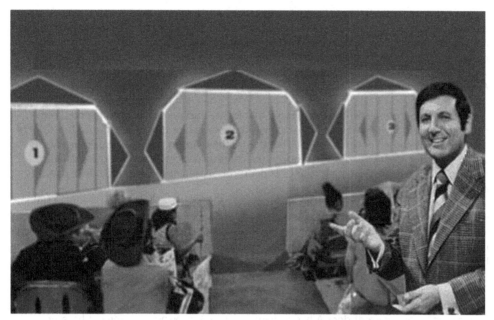

Figure 3.1. Let's Make a Deal.

When they first meet this problem, most people think that it makes no difference if they switch. They reason like this: "There are two unopened doors. The prize is behind one of them. The probability that it is behind the one I picked is 1/2, the probability that it is behind the one I didn't is also 1/2, so it makes no difference if I switch."

Surprising though it seems at first, this reasoning is wrong. Switching actually doubles the contestant's chance of winning. The odds go up from the original 1/3 for the chosen door, to 2/3 that the other unopened door hides the prize.

There are several ways to explain what is going on here. Here is what I think is the simplest account.

Suppose the doors are labeled A, B, and C. Let's assume the contestant initially picks door A. The probability that the prize is behind door A is 1/3. That means that the probability it is behind one of the other two doors (B or C) is 2/3. Monty now opens one of the doors B and C to reveal that there is no prize there. Let's suppose he opens door C. Notice that he can always do this because he knows where the prize is located. (This piece of information is crucial, and is the key to the entire puzzle.) The contestant now has two relevant pieces of information:

1. The probability that the prize is behind door B or C (i.e., not behind door A) is 2/3.
2. The prize is not behind door C.

Combining these two pieces of information yields the conclusion that the probability that the prize is behind door B is 2/3.

Hence the contestant would be wise to switch from the original choice of door A (probability of winning 1/3) to door B (probability 2/3).

Now, experience tells me that if you haven't come across this problem before, there is a probability of at most 1 in 3 that the above explanation convinces you. So let me say a bit more for the benefit of the remaining 2/3 who believe I am just one sandwich short of a picnic (as one NPR listener delightfully put it).

The instinct that compels people to reject the above explanation is, I think, a deep-rooted sense that probabilities are fixed. Since each door began with a 1/3 chance of hiding the prize, that does not change when Monty opens one door. But it is simply not true that events do not change probabilities. It is because the acquisition of information changes the probabilities associated with different choices that we often seek information prior to making an important decision. Acquiring more information about our options can reduce the number of possibilities and narrow the odds.

(Oddly enough, people who are convinced that Monty's action cannot change odds seem happy to go on to say that when it comes to making the switch or stick choice, the odds in favor of their previously chosen door are now 1/2, not the 1/3 they were at first. They usually justify this by saying that after Monty has opened his door, the contestant faces a new and quite different decision, independent of the initial choice of door. This reasoning is fallacious, but I'll pass on pursuing this inconsistency here.)

If Monty opened his door randomly, then indeed his action does not help the contestant, for whom it makes no difference to switch or to stick. But Monty's action is not random. He knows where the prize is, and acts on that knowledge. That injects a crucial piece of information into the situation. Information that the wise contestant can take advantage of to improve his or her odds of winning the grand prize. By opening his door, Monty is saying to the contestant "There are two doors you did not choose, and the probability that the prize is behind one of them is 2/3. I'll help you by using my knowledge of where the prize is to open one of those two doors to show you that it does not hide the prize. You can now take advantage of this additional information. Your choice of door A has a chance of 1 in 3 of being the winner. I have not changed that. But by eliminating door C, I have shown you that the probability that door B hides the prize is 2 in 3."

Still not convinced? Some people who have trouble with the above explanation find it gets clearer when the problem is generalized to 100 doors. You choose one door. You will agree, I think, that you are likely to lose. The chances are highly likely (in fact 99/100) that the prize is behind one of the 99 remaining doors. Monty now opens 98 of those and none of them hides the prize. There are now just two remaining possibilities: either your initial choice was right or else the prize is behind the remaining door that you did not choose and Monty did not open. Now, you began by being pretty sure you had little chance of being right – just 1/100 in fact. Are you now saying that Monty's action of opening 98 doors to reveal no prize (carefully avoiding opening the door that hides the prize, if it is behind one of those 99) has increased to 1/2 your odds of winning with your original choice? Surely not. In which case, the odds are high – 99/100 to be exact – that the prize lies behind that one unchosen door that Monty did not open. You should definitely switch. You'd be crazy not to!

Okay, one last attempt at an explanation. Back to the three-door version now. When Monty has opened one of the three doors and shown you there is no prize behind, and then offers you the opportunity to switch, he is in effect offering you a two-for-one switch. You originally picked door A. He is now saying "Would you like to swap door A for two doors, B and C . . . . . Oh, and by the way, before you make this two-for-one swap I'll open one of those two doors for you (one without a prize behind it)."

In effect, then, when Monty opens door C, the attractive 2/3 odds that the prize is behind door B or C are shifted to door B alone.

So much for the explanations. Far more fascinating than the mathematics, to my mind, is the psychology that goes along with the problem. Not only do many people get the wrong answer initially (believing that switching makes no difference), but a substantial proportion of them are unable to escape from their initial confusion and grasp any of the different explanations that are available (some of which I gave above).

On those occasions when I have entered into some correspondence with readers or listeners, I have always prefaced my explanations and comments by observing that this problem is notoriously problematic, that it has been used for years as a standard example in university probability courses to demonstrate how easily we can be misled about probabilities, and that it is important to pay attention to every aspect of the way Monty presents the challenge. Nevertheless, I regularly encounter people who are unable to break free of their initial conception of the problem, and thus unable to follow any of the explanations of the correct answer.

Indeed, some individuals I have encountered are so convinced that their (faulty) reasoning is correct that when you try to explain where they are going wrong, they become passionate, sometimes angry, and occasionally even abusive. Abusive over a math problem? Why is it that some people feel that their ability to compute a game show probability is something so important that they become passionately attached to their reasoning, and resist all attempts to explain what is going on? On a human level, what exactly is going on here?

First, it has to be said that the game scenario is a very cunning one, cleverly designed to lead the unsuspecting player astray. It gives the impression that, after Monty has opened one door, the contestant is being offered a choice between two doors, each of which is equally likely to lead to the prize. That would be the case if nothing had occurred to give the contestant new information. But Monty's opening of a door does yield new information. That new information is primarily about the two doors not chosen. Hence the two unopened doors that the contestant faces at the end are not equally likely. They have different histories. And those different histories lead to different probabilities.

That explains why very smart people, including many good mathematicians when they first encounter the problem, are misled. But why the passion with which many continue to hold on to their false conclusion? I have not encountered such a reaction when I have corrected students' mistakes in algebra or calculus.

I think the reason the Monty Hall problem raises people's ire is because a basic ability to estimate likelihoods of events is important in everyday life. We make (loose, and generally non-numeric) probability estimates all the time. Our ability to do this says something about our rationality – our capacity to live a successful life – and hence can become a matter of pride, something to be defended.

The human brain did not evolve to calculate mathematical probabilities, but it did evolve to ensure our survival. A highly successful survival strategy throughout human evolutionary history, and today, is to base decisions on the immediate past and on the evidence immediately to hand. If that movement in the undergrowth looks as though it might be caused by a hungry tiger, the smart move is to make a hasty retreat. Regardless of the fact that you haven't seen a tiger in that vicinity for several years, or that when you saw a similar rustle yesterday it turned out to be a gazelle. Again, if a certain company stock has been rising steadily for the past week, we may be tempted to buy, regardless of its stormy performance over the previous year. By presenting contestants with an actual situation in which a choice has to be made, Monty Hall tacitly encouraged people to use their everyday reasoning strategies, not the mathematical reasoning that in this case is required to get you to the right answer.

Monty Hall contestants are, therefore, likely to ignore the first part of the challenge and concentrate on the task facing them after Monty has opened the door. They see the task as choosing between two doors – period. And for choosing between two doors, with no additional circumstances, the probabilities are 1/2 for each. In the case of the Monty Hall problem, however, the outcome is that a normally successful human decision-making strategy leads you astray.

To safeguard judgments against prejudice and intuition, engage others

Most of us have a difficult time – a very difficult time – convincing ourselves that we ought to switch in the Monty Hall case. What does that tell us about the other armchair calculations that we make? Even in apparently simple decisions our guesses can be wrong – wildly wrong.[8]

There is a lesson here for researchers. While we must be ready to defend results in which we are confident, we must not succumb along the way to self-deception. How do we do that? The best antidote to self-deception is engagement with other researchers. John Stuart Mill (1806–1873) identified as one of the greatest qualities of the human mind that its "errors are corrigible" and that "[w]rong opinions and practices gradually yield to fact and argument." When we engage others in our reasoning, we open ourselves to criticism. This a desirable result for, as Mill notes, if "facts and arguments [are going] to produce any effect on the mind, [they] must be brought before it." Even when our immediate intuitions are

---

[8] For those still not convinced, see Keith Devlin, "Monty Hall Revisited," accessed, May 22, 2007, at Devlin's Angle, December 2005. You may also prove the point to yourself by playing the game here: The Let's Make a Deal Applet, accessed, May 22, 2007. Or, for the mathematically inclined, here's Devlin's proof:

> You select door A, and Monty opens door C to reveal that there is no prize there. So you now know that $p(C) = 0$. What are your new estimates for $p(A)$ and $p(B)$?
>
> We will apply Bayes' formula. Let E be the information that there is no prize behind door C, which you get when Monty opens that door. Then:
>
> $p(A|E) = p(A) \times p(E|A)/p(E)$
> $p(B|E) = p(B) \times p(E|B)/p(E).$
>
> We need to calculate the various probabilities on the right of these two formulas.
>
> $p(A) = p(B) = 1/3.$
> $p(E|A) = 1/2,$
>
> since if the prize is behind A, Monty may pick either of B, C to reveal that there is no prize there.
>
> $p(E|B) = 1,$
>
> since if the prize is behind B, Monty has no choice if he wants to open a door without a prize, he must open C.
>
> $p(E|C) = 0,$
>
> since if the prize is behind C, Monty cannot open it.
> Since A, B, C are mutually exclusive and exhaust all possibilities:
>
> $p(E) = p(A) \cdot p(E|A) + p(B) \cdot p(E|B) + p(C) \cdot p(E|C)$
> $= (1/3) \cdot (1/2) + (1/3) \cdot (1) + (1/3) \cdot 0$
> $= 1/2.$
>
> Hence, applying Bayes' formula:
>
> $p(A|E) = p(A) \times p(E|A)/p(E) = (1/3) \times (1/2)/(1/2) = 1/3$
> $p(B|E) = p(B) \times p(E|B)/p(E) = (1/3) \times (1)/(1/2) = 2/3.$
>
> Thus, based on what you know after Monty opened door C to show that there was no prize there, you estimate that the chance of winning if you stick is 1/3 and if you switch is 2/3. So you should switch (Devlin 2005).

true, we still must check them with others for, as Mill wrote, unless received opinion "is suffered to be, and actually is, vigorously contested, it will, by most of those who receive it, be held in the manner of a prejudice, with little comprehension of its rational grounds" (Mill 2004, ch. II, par 7).

To focus the community's attention on one's claims is not as easy as one might think. In his article, "It's Science, but Not Necessarily Right," Carl Zimmer shows how difficult it is to get studies published when they seek to confirm or disconfirm by replication previous studies (Zimmer 2011). Part of the blame for this situation lies with editors and reviewers who, if they are inclined not to publish papers that are based on well-designed experiments only because the papers have negative findings, may be complicit in publication bias. Bias skews the record and obscures the truth. So, to have beliefs in which one can have confidence, all must "keep their mind open to criticism of their opinions and conduct" (Mill 2004, p. 24). Rule of thumb: be your own worst critic, explicitly invite others to look for holes in your argument, look to colleagues for alternative interpretations of your results, and publish work even when it has disconfirming conclusions.

As egoists seek their own interests, they must be more attentive than others to the difficulty of assessing probabilities because they are not generally interested in the opinions of others. And yet, because the influence of heuristics and biases is both profound and hard to detect, egoists must be especially wary about the rationality of their decisions. Shared knowledge is knowledge possessed by several parties. This definition holds whether or not the parties know that others have the knowledge. Mutual knowledge differs from shared knowledge in that it brings the social power of knowing-that-others-know, too. Consider the parable of the emperor's new clothes. When only a few people admit to seeing his highness's unclothed state, their knowledge is shared but not mutual. Once everyone is in on the joke, however, the world changes. Power shifts from the emperor to all those who know that others know that he's naked.

The same is true in the Monty Hall case. Players who know how to assess probabilities have power over those who lack the knowledge. The lesson for misconduct is obvious. Ensure that you are in the know by discussing any questions you may have about responsible conduct with your mentors and colleagues. You not only want to understand how they understand the issues. You also want them to know that you know.

Take home lessons

- Don't trust your intuitions.
- Beware of observation bias and probability ineptness.
- Talk to your friends and advisors about the details of accepted research practices.
- Avoid being complicit in publication bias.
- Let your negative as well as positive findings be known.

Bibliography

Darley, J.M. & Batson, C.D. 1973. "From Jerusalem to Jericho": a study of situational and dispositional variables in helping behavior. *Journal of* *Personality and Social Psychology*, **27**(1), 100–108.

Darwin, C. & Barlow, N. 1969. *The Autobiography of Charles Darwin, 1809–1882: With Original Omissions*

Restored. Norton. Available at: http://darwin-online.org.uk/content/frameset?itemID=F1497&viewtype=text&pageseq=1.

Devlin, K. 2003. Monty Hall. *Mathematical Association of America.* Available at: http://www.maa.org/devlin/devlin_07_03.html.

Devlin, K. 2005. Monty Hall revisited. *Mathematical Association of America.* Available at: http://www.maa.org/devlin/devlin_12_05.html.

Ditto, P.H. & Lopez, D.F. 1992. Motivated skepticism: use of differential decision criteria for preferred and nonpreferred conclusions. *Journal of Personality and Social Psychology*, 63(4), 568–584.

Doris, J.M. 2005. *Lack of Character: Personality and Moral Behavior.* Cambridge University Press.

Jeng, M. 2006. A selected history of expectation bias in physics. *American Journal of Physics*, 74(7), 578–583.

Johansson, P. 2005. Failure to detect mismatches between intention and outcome in a simple decision task. *Science*, 310(5745), 116–119.

Kruger, J. & Dunning, D. 1999. Unskilled and unaware of it: how difficulties in recognizing one's own incompetence lead to inflated self-assessments. *Journal of Personality and Social Psychology*, 77(6), 1121–1134.

Mill, J.S. 2004. *On Liberty.* Agora Publications.

Pelham, B., Mirenberg, M. & Jones, J. 2002. Why Susie sells seashells by the seashore: implicit egotism and major life decisions. *Journal of Personality and Social Psychology*, 82(4), 469–487.

Russo, J.E. & Schoemaker, P.J.H. 2002. *Winning Decisions: Getting It Right the First Time.* Random House Digital.

Tversky, A & Kahneman, D. 1981. The framing of decisions and the psychology of choice. *Science*, 211(4481), 453–458.

Tversky, A. & Kahneman, D. 1974. Judgment under uncertainty: heuristics and biases. *Science*, 185(4157), 1124–1131.

von Hippel, W. & Trivers, R. 2011. The evolution and psychology of self-deception. *Behavioral and Brain Sciences*, 34(01), 1–16.

Zimmer, C. 2011. Why science struggles to correct its mistakes. *The New York Times.* Available at: http://www.nytimes.com/2011/06/26/opinion/sunday/26ideas.html [Accessed June 27, 2011].

Justify decisions

Give reasons to justify your decisions

One need not fabricate data or figures to be guilty of misconduct. "Significant departures" from "accepted practices of the scientific community" are also forbidden. When research- ers violate standards "intentionally, or knowingly, or recklessly," they are guilty of misconduct. What counts as a significant departure from accepted practice? Sometimes it is difficult to say. Consider the challenges of representing data through the use of images. Images are often easier to interpret than other formats and data may be more readily conceptualized if they are modified with image-enhancing software. Is using Photoshop to "clean up" or emphasize certain aspects of a digital image falsification? Is it a federal crime to add or change the colors of various structures in an image? Not necessarily. For if you can adequately justify your work to others, you will be on safe ground. To stay on safe ground, be sure to disclose what you have done – and read this chapter carefully.

Your being ready to provide reasons for your decisions is even more important in light of the fact that acceptable practices vary from field to field. Some rules even vary within a field, and some from lab to lab. It is not even unheard of for different students to receive different reprimands from the same professor for violating the same rule when the two students have different levels of experience. Nor do the complexities end there, for some- times rules change at the level of the professional organization – and without any formal notice. How can a junior member of the community expect to stay upright on such shifting ground? How can we keep up with nuanced changes or be expected to know how to behave in novel moral dilemmas for which there are, as yet, no accepted rules?

. . . especially in borderline cases

In almost no aspect of research are the lines between legitimate practices and illegitimate short-cuts more vague than in the digital presentation, enhancement, and manipulation of images. If one can make the salient features of one's work more visible by using advanced software to shape or crop, snip or flip, can one? Or are such acts always wrong? In areas as ambiguous as these, you must be prepared to answer challenges on the off chance – or perhaps not-so-off chance! – that other people question your method of presenting an

Research Ethics: A Philosophical Guide to the Responsible Conduct of Research. Gary Comstock.
Published by Cambridge University Press. © Cambridge University Press 2013.

image. You may have to explain, for example, why you added a dividing line between two groups of cells, or why you erased a band from your blot, or why you altered the contrast level in a particular fluorescence micrograph.

If you cannot provide plausible reasons for cropping this corner or outlining that cell, you may be guilty of a significant departure from an accepted practice, especially if you did so intentionally, knowingly, or recklessly. To protect yourself, know what you are doing, what the accepted practice is, and why your deviation from accepted practice is justifiable. Knowing which practices are acceptable helps you to avoid having to worry about constructing justifications for what you have done. And articulating to yourself and your colleagues why you are doing what you are doing will help you to defend yourself if you are called upon to do so.

What are acceptable practices in the area of cropping, recoloring, and manipulating images? Rossner and Yamada offer some valuable guidelines.

Case study: "What's in a picture? The temptation of image manipulation," by Mike Rossner and Kenneth M. Yamada[1]

It's all so easy with Photoshop.[2] In the days before imaging software became so widely available, making adjustments to image data in the darkroom required considerable effort and/or expertise. It is now very simple, and thus tempting, to adjust or modify digital image files. Many such manipulations, however, constitute inappropriate changes to your original data, and making such changes can be classified as scientific misconduct. Skilled editorial staff can spot such manipulations using features in the imaging software, so manipulation is also a risky proposition . . . .

The Journal of Cell Biology provides the following guidelines for its authors:

> No specific feature within an image may be enhanced, obscured, moved, removed, or introduced. The grouping of images from different parts of the same gel, or from different gels, fields, or exposures must be made explicit by the arrangement of the figure (e.g., using dividing lines) and in the text of the figure legend. Adjustments of brightness, contrast, or color balance are acceptable if they are applied to the whole image and as long as they do not obscure or eliminate any information present in the original. Nonlinear adjustments (e.g., changes to gamma settings) must be disclosed in the figure legend.

Because [this] set of guidelines is by far the most comprehensive we have found to date (full disclosure: we wrote them), we will continually refer back to them in the following discussions of the use and misuse of digital manipulations.

Blots and gels

Gross misrepresentation

The simplest examples of inappropriate manipulation are show in Figure 4.1. Deleting a band from a blot, even if you believe it to be an irrelevant background band, is a misrepresentation of your data (Figure 4.1A). Similarly, adding a band to a blot, even if you are only covering the

---

[1] Reprinted from *The Journal of Cell Biology* 166, no. 1 (July 6, 2004): 111–15. doi: 10.1083/jcb.200406019. Mike Rossner is Executive Director, Rockefeller University Press, rossner@rockefeller.edu. Kenneth M. Yamada is NIH Distinguished Investigator and Chief, Laboratory of Cell and Developmental Biology, National Institute of Dental and Craniofacial Research, National Institutes of Health. kenneth.yamada@nih.gov.
[2] The general principles presented here apply to the manipulation of images using any powerful image-processing software; however, because of the popularity of Photoshop, we refer to several specific functions in this application. Reprinted with permission from *The NIH Catalyst*.

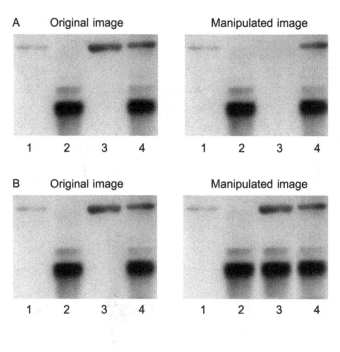

Figure 4.1. Gross manipulation of blots. (A) Example of a band deleted from the original data (lane 3). (B) Example of a band added to the original data (lane 3).

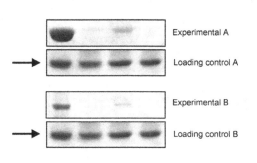

Figure 4.2. Gross manipulation of blots. Example of a duplicated panel (arrows).

fact that you loaded the wrong sample, and you know for sure that such a protein or DNA fragment or RNA is present in your sample, is a misrepresentation of your data. In the example shown in Figure 4.1B, the additional band in lane 3 has been generated by simply duplicating the band in lane 2.

Another example of using Photoshop inappropriately to create data is illustrated in Figure 4.2, in which a whole single panel has been replicated (arrows) and presented as the loading controls for two separate experiments.

More subtle manipulations

Brightness/contrast adjustments

Adjusting the intensity of a single band in a blot constitutes a violation of the widely accepted guideline that "No specific feature within an image may be enhanced, obscured, moved, removed, or introduced." In the manipulated image in Figure 4.3A, the arrow indicates a single

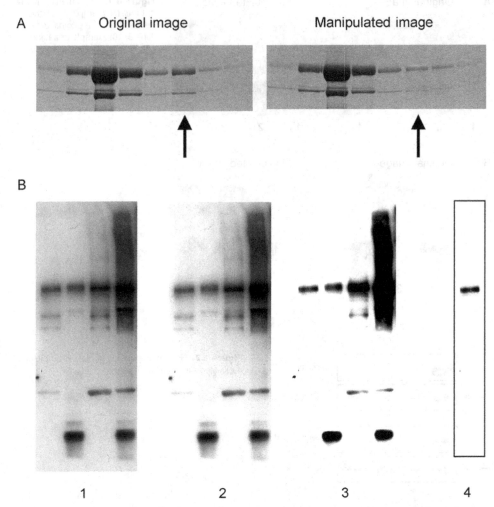

Figure 4.3. Manipulation of blots: brightness and contrast adjustments. (A) Adjusting the intensity of a single band (arrow). (B) Adjustments of contrast. Images 1, 2, and 3 show sequentially more severe adjustments of contrast. Although the adjustment from 1 to 2 is acceptable because it does not obscure any of the bands, the adjustment from 2 to 3 is unacceptable because several bands are eliminated. Cutting out a strip of a blot with the contrast adjusted provides the false impression of a very clean result (image 4 was derived from a heavily adjusted version of the left lane of image 1). For a more detailed discussion of "gel slicing and dicing," see *Nature Cell Biology* (2004) **6**:275 (editorial).

band whose intensity was reduced to produce an impression of more regular fractionation. Although this manipulation may not alter the overall interpretation of the data, it still constitutes misconduct.

While it is acceptable practice to adjust the overall brightness and contrast of a whole image, such adjustments should "not obscure or eliminate any information present in the original" (Figure 4.3B). When you scan a blot, no matter how strong the bands, there will invariably be some gray background. While it is technically within the guidelines to adjust the brightness and contrast of a whole image, if you overadjust the contrast so that the background completely drops out

Original
image

Manipulated
image

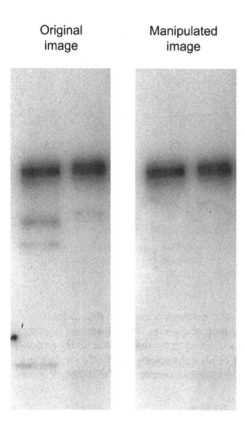

Figure 4.4. Manipulation of blots: cleaning up background. The Photoshop "Rubber Stamp" tool has been used in the manipulated image to clean up the background in the original data. Close inspection of the image reveals a repeating pattern in the left lane of the manipulated image, indicating that such a tool has been used.

(Figure 4.3B, part 2 vs. part 3), this should raise suspicions among reviewers and editors that other information (especially faint bands) may have dropped out as well.

It may be argued that this guideline is stricter than in the days before Photoshop, when multiple exposures could be used to perfect the presentation of the data. Perhaps it is, but this is just one of the advantages of the digital age to the reviewer and editor, who can now spot these manipulations when in the past an author would have taken the time to do another exposure. Think about this when you are doing the experiment and perform multiple exposures to get the bands at the density you want, without having to overadjust digitally the brightness and contrast of the scanned image.

Cleaning up background

It is very tempting to use the tool variously known as "Rubber Stamp" or "Clone Stamp" in Photoshop to clean up unwanted background in an image (Figure 4.4). Don't do it. This kind of manipulation can usually be detected by someone looking carefully at the image file because it leaves telltale signs. Moreover, what may seem to be a background band or contamination may actually be real and biologically important and could be recognized as such by another scientist.

Splicing lanes together

It is clearly inappropriate manipulation to take a band from one part of a gel and move it to another part, even if you do not change its size. But it is within usual guidelines to remove a complete lane from a gel and splice the remaining lanes together. This alteration should be clearly indicated, however, by leaving a thin white or black line between the gel pieces that have been

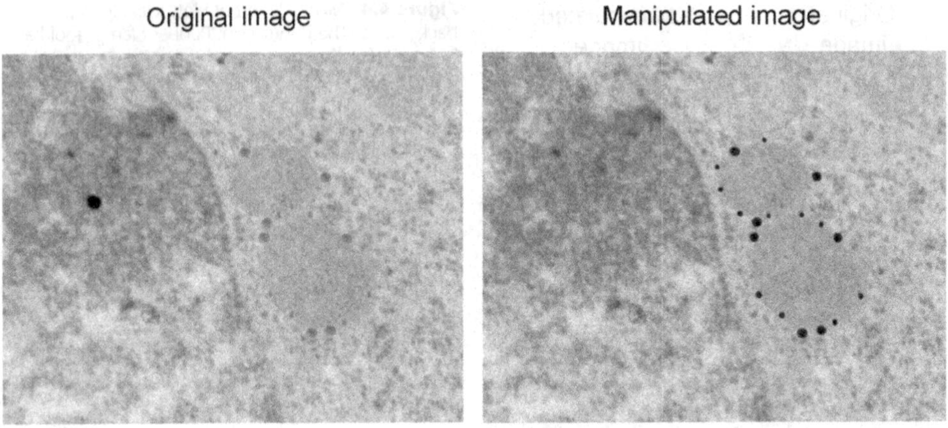

Original image

Manipulated image

Figure 4.5. Misrepresentation of immunogold data. The gold particles, which were actually present in the original (left), have been enhanced in the manipulated image (right). Note also that the background dot in the original data has been removed in the manipulated image.

juxtaposed. Again, it could be argued that this guideline is stricter than in the days before Photoshop when paper photographs of a gel were cut up and pieces were glued next to each other. This practice, however, usually left a black line indicating to the reader what had been done.

As it was with gel photographs, it is unacceptable to juxtapose pieces from different gels to compare the levels of proteins or nucleic acids. Rerun all of the samples on the same gel!

Micrographs

Enhancing a specific feature

An example of manipulation by enhancement is shown in Figure 4.5, in which the intensity of the gold particles has been enhanced by manually filling them in with black color using Photoshop. This type of manipulation misrepresents your original data and is thus misconduct. There are acceptable ways to highlight a feature such as gold particles, which include arrows or pseudocoloring. If pseudocoloring is done with the "Colorize" function of Photoshop, it does not alter the brightness of individual pixels, but pseudo-coloring should always be disclosed in the figure legend.

Other examples of misconduct include adjusting the brightness of only a specific part of an image or erasing spots. Using the "Brightness" adjustment in Photoshop is considered to be a linear alteration (see below), which must be made to the entire image.

Linear vs. nonlinear adjustments

Linear adjustments, such as those for "Brightness" or "Contrast" in Photoshop, are those in which the same change is made to each pixel according to a linear function. It is acceptable (within limits noted above) to apply linear adjustments to a whole image. There are other adjustments in Photoshop that can be applied to a whole image, but the same change is not made to each pixel. For example, adjustments of gamma output ("Color Settings" in Photoshop) alter the intensity of each pixel according to a nonlinear function. Adjustments of "Curves" or "Levels" in Photoshop alter the tonal range and color balance of an image by adjusting the brightness of only those pixels at particular intensities and colors. Such nonlinear changes are sometimes required to reveal important features of an image; however, the fact that they have been used should be disclosed in the figure legend.

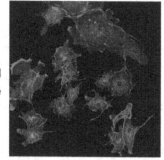

Manipulated
image

Figure 4.6. Misrepresentation of image data. Cells from various fields have been juxtaposed in a single image, giving the impression that they were present in the same microscope field. A manipulated panel is shown at the top. The same panel, with the contrast adjusted by us to reveal the manipulation, is shown at the bottom.

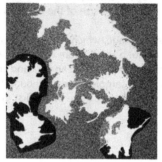

Manipulation
revealed
by contrast
adjustment

Digitally altering brightness or contrast levels can be misleading with fluorescence micrographs. Some authors mistakenly change the contrast of an experimental compared with a control photo, or change individual panels in a time course, or use different contrast levels when making merged images compared with the original images. All of these changes in individual pictures used for comparisons can be misrepresentations. On the other hand, certain adjustments such as background subtraction or using a filter or digital mask may be needed to extract information accurately from complex images. Reporting the details and logic of such manipulations that are applied to images as a whole should resolve concerns about their use. Standards and guidelines in the field will continue to evolve, but full disclosure will always be the safest course.

Misrepresentation of a microscope field

The reader assumes that a single micrograph presented in a figure represents a single microscope field. Combining images from separate microscope fields into a single micrograph constitutes a misrepresentation of your original data. In the manipulated image in Figure 4.6 (top panel), cells have been combined from several microscope fields into a single micrograph. This manipulation becomes visible when the contrast of the image is adjusted so that the inserted images become visible (bottom panel). You may want to combine images from several fields into a single micrograph to save space, but this assembly should be clearly indicated by thin lines between the pieces.

Resolution

A pixel is a square (or dot) of uniform color in an image. The size of a pixel can vary, and the resolution of an image is the number of pixels per unit area. Although resolution is defined by area, it is often described using a linear measurement – dots per inch (dpi). Thus, 300 dpi indicates a resolution of 300 pixels per inch by 300 pixels per inch, which equals 90,000 pixels per square inch (1).

High-resolution digital cameras (in 2004) can acquire an image that is 6 megapixels in size. This can generate an image of approximately 2400 × 2400 pixels, or 8 inches × 8 inches at 300 dpi. Note that, with the right settings in Photoshop, physical size and resolution can be traded off against each other without a gain or loss in the amount of information – that is, you can resize an image without altering the total number of pixels.

You should be aware of the resolution at which the image was acquired by the digital camera on your microscope. When that file is opened in Photoshop, you have the option of setting the size and resolution of the image. You should not set the total number of pixels to be greater than that in the original image; otherwise, the computer must create data for you that were not present in the original, and the resulting image is a misrepresentation of the original data – that is, the dpi of an image can only be increased if the size of the image is reduced proportionately.

It is acceptable to reduce the number of pixels in an image, which may be necessary if you have a large image at high resolution and want to create a small figure out of it. Reducing the resolution of an image is done in Photoshop by sampling the pixels in an area and creating a new pixel that is an average of the color and brightness of the sampled ones. Although this does alter your original data, you are not creating something that was not there in the first place; you are presenting an average.

Other data-management issues

It is crucially important to keep your original digital or analog data exactly as they were acquired and to record your instrument settings. This primary rule of good scientific practice will allow you or others to return to your original data to see whether any information was lost by the adjustments made to the images. In fact, some journal reviewers or editors request access to such primary data to ensure accuracy.

There are other important issues concerning data handling that we have not addressed by focusing on manipulations of existing data. Examples include selective acquisition of data by adjusting the settings on your microscope or imager, selecting and reporting a very unusual result as being representative of the data, or hiding negative results that may contradict your conclusions. Any type of misrepresentation of experimental data undermines scientific research and should be avoided.

Conclusion

Data must be reported directly, not through a filter based on what you think they "should" illustrate to your audience. For every adjustment that you make to a digital image, it is important to ask yourself, "Is the image that results from this adjustment still an accurate representation of the original data?" If the answer to this question is "no," your actions may be construed as misconduct.

Some adjustments are currently considered to be acceptable (such as pseudocoloring or changes to gamma settings) but should be disclosed to your audience. You should, however, always be able to justify these adjustments as necessary to reveal a feature already present in the original data.

We hope that by listing guidelines and publicizing examples of transgressions, all of us can become more vigilant, particularly in guiding junior colleagues and students away from the tempting dangers of digital manipulation. Just because the tools exist to clean up sloppy work digitally, that is no excuse to do sloppy work.

If you would have redone an experiment to generate a presentation-quality image in the days before the digital age, you should probably redo it now.

References for Rossner and Yamada

1. Rossner, M. and R. O'Donnell. 2004. The JCB will let your data shine in RGB. *J. Cell. Biol.* **164**:11.

2. 2004. Gel slicing and dicing: a recipe for disaster. *Nat. Cell Biol.* **6**:275.

Conclusion: some reservations about egoism

In this last part of the chapter we switch gears and return to theoretical matters introduced in Part A. The reason for this change of focus is that we are nearing the end of Part A and need to take stock of the adequacy of the theory that has guided us to this point.

Egoism, as we have seen, has several strengths. It recognizes that each of us has distinct motivations and goals; it allows us great freedom in choosing our own values; it is consistent with biological accounts of the evolution of our moral systems. Most notably, however, it provides a persuasive answer to the question: why be moral? I should be moral – meaning that I should comply with rules and regulations – because doing so is in my own interests.

But egoism also has two major strikes against it. It does not take seriously our need to justify our actions to each other, and it is not fair. Let us consider the second problem first because it is easier to summarize.

Egoism is arbitrary. It divides the world into two groups and always, unfairly, gives privileges to one of them. Just as the white racist sees only white people and black people, and always acts in ways that favor the first group, so the egoist has a metaphysics that divides the world into me and everyone else and an ethics that always serves to justify actions that favor the first group over the second. That's the very definition of unfair. Here's a hypothetical example. An egoist could decide to spread slanderous remarks on the internet about people they did not like. If doing so gave them even a little pleasure, and if they were computer savvy and could get away with it, say, by logging on anonymously, then they not only would fulfill their own desires by hurting others. They would be morally justified in doing so. But causing egregious harm to others for trivial benefits to oneself simply because others don't count seems wrong. Unless we can give some reason to prefer one group (or individual) over another, giving one privileges denied to others is nothing more than blatant prejudice. Egoism fails the fairness test.

And now we turn to the first problem, that egoism is not serious. At the end of Chapter 3, we noted that egoists who want to be researchers must do as we all do and become citizens of the community of question-askers. In this respect they are no different from anyone else who wants to be a professional researcher. The language we use in this community includes moral language; we say that one ought not to take others' ideas, that one should give credit where credit is due, that one must be able to explain why one is juxtaposing cells from various fields in a single image if they were not present in the same microscope field. We speak this way because we take other people seriously. Furthermore, taking them seriously means adopting a particular attitude about moral judgments. We do not merely give lip service to the moral judgments expressed in the language of ought and should; we actually believe that other people have interests that justify us in speaking that way. And we think that we should act in ways that respect others' interests.

Now, some egoists will have no problem adopting the attitudes required by this language. Some will want to take a sincere interest in the good of others. But if they adopt this stance, they will not have been required to adopt it by egoism. Egoists do not need to be serious about their moral obligations if they don't want to be. This is because their favored ethical theory tells them they are justified in disregarding the needs of others whenever it is in their interests to do so. An egoist need only train herself to talk the talk of research ethics; she need not commit to walking the walk. For nothing in egoism tells her that when she mouths the words "ought" and "should" she must mean what others mean when they use them. In sum, egoists need not use moral language in good faith. They may use it to trick other researchers into thinking that they speak the same language and use the same concepts – even if they have no intention of acting on them if they can get away with it.

You'll recall that, in the introduction, we said that ethical issues are difficult and emotional issues. They bother us. We have to think about them, sometimes for years at a stretch. But these issues need not bother the egoist, nor need the egoist give them a second thought. So long as the egoist can get away with acting as if they care about research ethics, then that is all he or she has to do. Egoists may very well mouth the words of morality in public while in the privacy of their own rooms they mock those who spend so much time and effort thinking through their obligations.

Here's another way to think about the problem. For egoists, ethical issues can be dissolved with a wave of their "I don't care" wand. If egoists can get away with stealing someone else's data, why shouldn't they? Why should the egoist care if others disapprove? The egoist does not disapprove and the egoist has no reason to pay attention to the complaints of others. Here is a second reason that egoism, even in its strongest form as rational egoism, satisfies few moral philosophers: it does not take ethical issues seriously.

There is a related point worth mentioning, one that may have occurred to you. Because egoism insists that one need not act on anyone's values except one's own, the following problem arises: what if one's categorical interests include harming others? Egoism has no way to condemn the successful researcher who discovers a truth by fabricating data or misleading proposal reviewers – much less by abusing patients if he or she can get away with it. For if one has freely chosen such ends as the ends one most wants to pursue, then egoism cannot explain why these ends are such objectionable ends.

Recall the conclusion to Chapter 3, namely that egoism cannot explain why some categorical interests are perverse. And yet some clearly are perverse. My wanting nothing more than to have the world's largest collection of toe nails does not require that I harm anyone in my pursuit of that goal. You may think my goal an odd one, but it is not wrong because I can happily pursue it without causing harm. But if I want nothing more than to be the world's greatest serial killer, I will have to harm others in pursuit of my goal. On what egoistic grounds could I be persuaded that what I was doing was wrong? According to egoism, as long as I act rationally and take the steps necessary to murder, say, as many young women as possible, I am acting morally. For as long as I am honest with myself (and do not, for example, lie to myself about the number of my victims) and am sincere and rigorous in disciplining my short-term urges so as to attain my long-term objective, I do not offend the egoist's requirement that I always act so as to attain my own long-range interests. And yet all of this is mad. To say someone acts morally simply because he is true to his ideals does not begin to capture our sense of what morality is.

The moral circle, we might say, seems unstable if we draw it only around ourselves. It is mere common sense that others have interests that I ought to take into account when deciding how to act. This is especially true for researchers, who have common interests by virtue of the fact that research is a social activity. And each of us is more than a researcher, of course. We are brothers, sisters, coaches, friends, confidants, judges, kindergarten teachers, accountants, musicians, auditors, consultants, CEOs, undertakers, and salespersons. Each of these roles is a social role, a role in which one's interests cannot be well described if one tries to restrict the description to oneself. As a friend, family member, or professional, I can only gain the satisfaction of my interests by helping others satisfy their interests. That is what it means to be a good teacher or a competent undertaker or an adept research assistant. My good is bound up with the good of those alongside whom I work, not to mention the good of those I love. And "bound up" is the right metaphor here. Our interests are literally tied to others' interests by promises and agreements, understandings implicit and explicit.

Every ethical theory – or at least every one that accords with commonsense – must take our social roles into account. Egoism, however, does not acknowledge that the reason we should explain ourselves to others is because others are reasonable people and that we owe it to them to provide reasons for our actions. Egoism does not recognize that other people matter. So much the worse for egoism for, as the prisoner's dilemma shows, if each agent pursues her own interests exclusively, all agents – including herself – will be worse off. That is why the moral circle cannot encompass us alone. It must include others in it or it will collapse entirely.

We can now state the obvious: egoism seems like an odd place to start a discussion of ethics.[3] And it is. Most of us were raised to think that morality is a way of thinking about our obligations "unto others." And the logic of the concepts we use in thinking about morality are decidedly anti-egoistic (e.g., we tend to believe that "no one should count for more than anyone else," and "don't use one standard for this person and a different standard for another person"). Egoists can deny this logic or flaunt the concepts. They can't, however, insist that their theory makes them take seriously our talk about helping others, respecting rights, and trying to make the world a better place for all.

These reservations about egoism force us to turn to a more familiar idea, the notion that we ought, at a minimum, to keep our promises. This brings us full circle, because this was the point with which we opened this chapter. Don't we owe it to others to honor the agreements we make with them? If we find that we cannot do so, shouldn't we provide them with the reasons that we let them down? Our second theory, contractualism, is based on this line of thought.

Take home lessons
- Disclose alterations you've made and explain why you made them.
- Don't delete bands from blots even if you're sure they're irrelevant.

---

[3] For the view that all rational justifications of the moral life must be prudential, see Plato's *Republic* (Plato *et al.* 1992). For a contrary view – that it is impossible to show that living morally always coincides with prudence – see Prichard (1912).

- Don't delete outliers from statistical plots even if you're sure they are mistakes.
- Don't enhance, obscure, move, remove, or introduce specific features into images.
- When in doubt, consult with your mentor.
- Don't rest content with egoism as an ethical theory.

Bibliography

Plato, Grube, G.M.A. & Reeve, C.D.C. 1992. *Plato: Republic*, 2nd edn. Hackett.

Prichard, H.A. 1912. Does moral philosophy rest on a mistake? *Mind*, 21(81), 21–37.

Rossner, M. & Yamada, K.M. 2004. What's in a picture? The temptation of image manipulation. *The Journal of Cell Biology*, 166(1), 11–15.

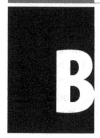

Part

Promote our interests

I once heard a postdoctoral fellow refer to researchers as pack animals. It's true, even the most hardened and self-absorbed of egoists at the university must cooperate with others. Every graduate student has his or her committee; every faculty member has his or her task force; and every department chair consults with others, publicly in seminars and privately in the hall. But why, we might ask, would an egoist care about the pack? Why wouldn't egoists simply find out what their professional codes say about some issue, decide whether it serves their own interests – obey it if it does, ignore it if it doesn't – and move on?

It is an important question for the egoist because in research we find ourselves constantly having to explain our decisions to others. If an egoist decides that it is against her interests to abide by her professional code, she cannot let the matter lie there, much as she might wish to do. She will have to offer those researchers who are affected by her decision some justification or other for her behavior.

Now, on occasion, a code might contain confusing advice or have two rules that contradict each other. Most codes, for example, tell professionals that their education and training entitle them to autonomy. That is, they have the right to use discretion about professional matters – as, for example, when a professor decides to deal with a disruptive student in class by having a private conversation with that student. However, the same code may also require that the professor report all disruptions to the dean. How can the professor both report and not report a class disruption? It's a puzzle. Is the professor entitled to legislate for herself in this matter, or must she defer to an authority? To protect themselves, egoists must be prepared to say why they've not conformed to professional codes – if that's what they've done – and know how to handle potential conflicts while working within the requirements of their professional codes. They must know how to give reasons for the rules in the code.

Egoistic researchers must not only know what their codes say, but they must also understand how others are going to react to the egoist's decision not to live by the code if that's what the egoist decides to do. Notice that egoism has suddenly become an unstable position. Any egoist who sincerely wants to become a researcher must look at the world from the perspective of her colleagues. Now, egoists can agree with this point and yet insist that they are taking another person's point of view only because they must do so in order to promote their own interests. But egoists cannot stop there. For once egoists sincerely and honestly take another's perspective, they cannot help but see that the other's interests matter to them. It is a hardened heart indeed that, having taken the first step, will not take the second, and begin to empathize with the other person. For the mere step of seeing the world

---

Research Ethics: A Philosophical Guide to the Responsible Conduct of Research. Gary Comstock.
Published by Cambridge University Press. © Cambridge University Press 2013.

from another's point of view is impossible to take without also realizing that the other person's goals and desires make a difference to his or her welfare. And if that's true, then the egoist has now stepped into a bigger and brighter world, and a terrain that is much more familiar, ethically speaking. For every moral theory, every theory other than egoism that is, begins and ends with the moral significance of others. Am I my brother's keeper? Yes – or, at least, that is our usual answer. And that answer is the gateway to ethics as commonly understood.

How should we treat others? This is a difficult and complex question. Let's begin by exploring one issue that will be relevant to your developing career – promise keeping – and a second moral framework from which to consider it, contractualism. As we'll see, contractualists hold that we should keep our promises because other people are like us in their ability to understand human actions as behaviors guided by reasons.

Graduate students sign diverse contracts

When you accepted the invitation to become a graduate student at your university, you agreed to adhere to the institution's policies in return for a degree upon your completion of academic requirements. They are agreements in which at least two parties state the expectations each has of the other. They may also explain enforcement mechanisms and penalties in the event that one party breaks the agreement. When a university accepts funds from the US government, it agrees to abide by the granting agency's regulations. When principal investigators apply for grants, they consent to observe rules pertaining to, among other things, responsible fiscal conduct, the disposal of hazardous materials, and the export of intellectual property. In turn, they receive money to conduct their research.

Let us call the doctrine that our behavior should be bound by the terms of the contracts we sign narrow contractualism.

Narrow contractualism: One should always act in accord with the terms of contracts he or she signs.

Note that narrow contractualism is not logically inconsistent with rational egoism; it simply recognizes the fact that we sometimes enter into agreements. (If a contract requires an egoist to do something that does not best satisfy the egoist's categorical interests, the two theories will conflict, but this issue need not concern us here.)

What contracts have you signed? Recall the "Graduate Student Contract" for the Department of Food Science and Technology at Virginia Tech University from Part A. This 21-page document begins with these clauses.

1. All graduate assistants are expected to adhere to the Graduate School's expectations of graduate study available at http://www.grads.vt.edu/academics/expectations/index.html.
2. All graduate assistants are expected to conduct themselves in a mature, professional, courteous manner toward students, staff and faculty regardless of their race, gender, religion, sexual orientation, or national origin. Graduate assistants should act in accordance with the standards outlined by the Virginia Tech Principles of Community (http://www.multicultural.vt.edu/pdf/Virginia_Tech_Principles_of_Community.pdf), (http://ghs.grads.vt.edu/) and the Graduate Honor code.
3. All graduate assistants are expected to take primary responsibility to inform themselves about specific regulations and policies governing their graduate studies at the department and Graduate School levels, including ensuring that they meet departmental and graduate school deadlines.

4. All graduate assistants are expected to manage time effectively for maximum professional development as well as personal health and well being, balance competing demands such as being a student, a graduate assistant, a parent, a spouse, a caregiver, etc. (Department of Food Science and Technology, Virginia Tech University n.d.).

The department requires each student, along with a faculty member, to sign the document. By signing, students agree that they have been given an opportunity to discuss the terms with their faculty members. Their signatures also indicate promises to meet each of these conditions:

i. Maintain at least a 3.0 grade point average.
ii. Satisfy enrollment requirements (9–12 hours) during the academic year.
iii. Make satisfactory progress toward degree as defined by academic department and graduate school.
iv. Have "regular" admission status.
v. Meet regularly with major professor. All meetings should be scheduled and every effort maintained to keep the appointment.
vi. Attend all laboratory and FST graduate student meetings as designated by your major professor. You must be excused from meetings in advance; only one excuse per semester will be allowed, regardless of situation.
vii. All students on assistantship are expected to spend at least 10 or 20 hours a week on laboratory duties or focused on extension work.

   20 hours = full assistantship
   10 hours = partial assistantship.

Those who disobey the rules will likely pay: the document goes on to stipulate that students whose GPAs drop below 3.0 are in trouble, while those who take less than 9 credit hours may lose their assistantships.

Contracts like this one vary from institution to institution. The University of Hawai'i may require a lower minimum number of hours; Purdue may have a different rule about minimum GPAs; North Carolina State may have different expectations about student participation in open departmental meetings. The Department of Anthropology at the University of Montana requires all PhD candidates in cultural heritage studies to maintain a portfolio that includes a curriculum vitae, all papers written for courses, and "the results of all work performed for internships" (Department of Anthropology, University of Montana n.d.). Your department surely encourages you to have a portfolio, but may not require you to keep one, and if it does require it, may not require you to have all of your course papers in it.

Yet all are part of one contractual community

When researchers pursue their work as a business, they compete not only for grant funds, intellectual property rights, jobs, and promotions, but also for prestige and honors. Because competition strains cooperative relationships, researchers have explicit agreements that detail the rules – and exceptions – that govern collaborations. But since research is also a vocation, we rely on a vast number of implicit, unwritten rules, too. You will want to ask around to find out exactly what these unspoken expectations are, but universities usually assume that graduate students agree to get sufficient sleep, eat reasonably well, exercise regularly, and keep themselves in the mental, physical, and emotional state necessary to meet the requirements of the explicit contracts they signed.

The central point concerning implicit agreements is this: we must give reasons for our actions. The practice of giving reasons is required at the interpersonal level, as when explaining one's absence from a lab meeting. And when it comes to explanations, some are better than others. "I was sick" will do, but "I don't know why I have to go to these things" won't. Giving reasons is also binding at the policy level. Suppose your university's faculty handbook claims that grad students are not entitled to grievance hearings against faculty members unless they first put their complaints in writing to the faculty member in question. Suppose the graduate council, however, has no such policy. Which policy applies? Perhaps one thinks the faculty document applies, because it sets out the terms by which faculty are governed. Perhaps one thinks the graduate council policy applies, because it sets out the terms by which graduate students are governed. However the issue is decided, it will have to be decided on the basis of good reasons. But what constitutes a good reason? This is a question contractualism can help us to answer.

Few of us have ever signed a document in which we promise to give reasons for the actions we take in our research – and yet we all assume that we all will do so. For example, most university and college policies don't include a written rule requiring instructors to distribute syllabi. But what would happen to an instructor who did not provide students with one? He'd probably be reprimanded for having violated a fundamental norm of transparency in the educational process. If the instructor, when asked by his department chair to justify his practice, said, "Why should I?" he might lose his job on the spot.

And for good reason. When a student's grade is left to the mercy of a professor's word – as it is when students have no course syllabi – the teacher acquires more power over students than is proper. Instructors who change their minds midcourse about how much weight to give to each assignment or about how to determine the grade of end-of-year group presentations leave students open to abuse and exploitation. Instructors have numerous reasons for providing syllabi, all of them pertaining to the power relationship between teachers and students. The syllabus, in sum, provides a contract about the determination of grades and gives students a basis to complain when they encounter deceptive professorial practices.

These reasons are likely not stated in any university contract. Yet they refer to conditions essential to the proper functioning of a university. This fact highlights a glaring deficiency of narrow contractualism. For narrow contractualism does not acknowledge the importance of unwritten agreements; in fact, it says nothing about them. What if we never put our agreement in writing? What if we just gave our word over the phone or simply shook hands? We must understand implicit agreements and honor them, even if we have not signed written documents.

Narrow contractualism faces another difficulty. What if you signed a contract, but did so under duress? Or without really understanding its terms? Or subsequently signed a second contract making it impossible to keep the terms of the first contract? How are our obligations to be decided when contracts conflict?

Consider the terms of the contract established by the US Public Health Service (PHS) Syphilis Study. Begun in 1932 in Tuskegee, Alabama, to determine the causes of, and possible treatments for, syphilis, the experiment enrolled 399 rural African American men with the disease. The medical community could offer no treatment for syphilis in the 1930s, so PHS agreed to give the men regular checkups, hot meals, free transportation to their exams, and burial plots. By 1943, penicillin had become widely available as an effective treatment, but the men enrolled in the study did not receive this medicine until the study ended in 1972. By then, over 100 men had died, dozens of their wives had become infected, and several children had been born with the disease.

In 1969, several of the scientists were asked to justify the study. Suppose they explained the reasons for their actions this way: withholding penicillin gives researchers the unusual opportunity to advance science by following the disease's natural course from beginning to end; and after all, the men signed contracts, the terms of which did not include treatment with penicillin.[1] Furthermore, if the men, most of them poor sharecroppers, were not in the study, they would not receive any healthcare at all. By enrolling, participants agreed to allow researchers to study the natural course of their disease in the hope that the knowledge gained would save many more lives, lives that would be lost if the study did not continue. In exchange, the patients receive checkups and so on, but not treatment with any new therapies. In defending the study, the scientists might well have expressed regret that some men would suffer and some would die. But more men would suffer and die, they might argue, without the study. The contract was justified because it served a greater cause: the progress of science and the prevention of syphilis in future generations.

Notice how counterintuitive the conclusion is. Medical researchers should not callously, knowingly, and willfully send patients to their deaths in the course of their research, even if subjects voluntarily sign documents essentially agreeing to it. But the Public Health Service syphilis study points to the problem with narrow contractualism, for narrow contractualism provides an ethical justification for abusing the research subjects enrolled in the study. And this offensive consequence points to the weakness of the theory.

Do contractualists have an alternative? Yes, one that claims we should observe all agreements, written or unwritten, so long as free and equal people would consider the agreements reasonable. No fair-minded, competent person would find an agreement reasonable if it stated that experimental syphilitic subjects should not receive penicillin unless they have specifically contracted to receive it. Certainly the Tuskegee men would not have agreed to such a contract, a contract which would have been an affront both to the specific norms of the medical profession and to conscience generally. That is why the Public Health Service Syphilis "experiments" have become a textbook example of how not to conduct research.

In the end, researchers – the askers of questions – are also rightly the givers of reasons. And the community of which they are a part insists that their moral as well as scientific reasoning stand up to public scrutiny.

. . . in which giving reasons comes naturally

Giving reasons comes as second nature to us. If accused of wrongdoing, a child is quick to provide an explanation. It is a fact of human psychology that, when challenged, we can and want to justify ourselves. And when challenged this way, we do our level best to defend ourselves, not by resorting to weapons but by arming ourselves with reasons. This process

---

[1] After penicillin had become widely available and used to treat syphilis, the Public Health Service convened an Ad Hoc Committee "to examine data from the Tuskegee Study and offer advice on continuance of this study. Participants of the February 6, 1969 meeting included: ... Dr. Sidney Olansky, Professor of Medicine, Emory University Clinic." www.gwu.edu/~nsarchiv/radiation/dir/mstreet/commeet/meet1/brief1/br1i.txt Accessed 3/7/06. According to Stephen Thomas, Olansky defended the syphilis trials as late as 1979. www.kaisernetwork.org/health_cast/uploaded_files/Tanscript_Thomas.pdf. Accessed 3/7/06.

of justification through giving reasons is not simply a strategy for the contractualist. It is a strategy for every human being embedded in a community. For other humans are potent forces in our lives; they have the power to affect us in many ways. If we care about their opinions and they come to resent us for something we have done or said, we want to make amends, repair the relationship. Other agents are powerful, even in the egoist's life, because the egoist's own well-being can be undermined (or promoted) by others.

We've all experienced resentment, guilt, and shame. As these emotions make clear to us, we are vulnerable to others' words and attitudes. If we were not, if we were invulnerable, we would never be moved by others' attempts to embarrass or harass us. Few of us have been so lucky; almost all of us have been hurt at some point in our lives by jokes made at our expense or muttered words intended to ridicule us. We cannot afford to be unaware of social slights, for the welfare of those we love, as well as our own psychological health, depends on how we are perceived by others. If we were impotent and invulnerable with respect to each other, we would have no need to try to strike mutually advantageous bargains or to pay for protection. However, the fact that others are potent in this way, and that we are vulnerable, provides each of us with a motive to contract with each other. Here, perhaps, is the reason that the ring of Gyges – the ring that confers invisibility and with it the power to act anonymously – so appeals to us. What wouldn't we give to be invulnerable to the power others have over us?

Without a magic ring, adults try to protect themselves by making and securing agreements. Agreements are reached through negotiations wherein each party offers reasons for the words it wants in the contract. If a contract is signed and then broken, we engage in complicated verbal maneuvering to try to explain ourselves. When two contractors have an argument about terms, they are not necessarily involved in a verbal fight. Arguments, in this sense, are a series of statements in which one party is trying to convince another party of the soundness of some conclusion.

Let's look at an example of an argument. A student is accused of plagiarism. He responds with this explanation:

> Most people from my ethnic background think that my action does not qualify as plagiarism.

Implicit is the idea that his actions would be widely accepted within his community. The conclusion that he hopes his accuser will draw from his explanation is this:

> Therefore, you (my teaching assistant) should not report me.

Is this a good argument? Clearly not. It's missing a key premise:

> If most people from my ethnic background think that my action is not plagiarism, then it is not plagiarism and you (my instructor) should not report it.

Here is a reconstruction of the full argument:

1. Most people from my ethnic background think that my action was not plagiarism.
2. If most people from my ethnic background think my action was not plagiarism, then it is not plagiarism and you (my instructor) should not report it.
3. Therefore, you (my teaching assistant) should not report it.

Now the question is: do the premises justify the conclusion? Is the argument valid? To assess validity, we assume all of the premises are true and then ask whether they entail the conclusion. That is, the conclusion of a valid argument must be true if all of the premises are true and no mistakes have been made in reasoning. In this case, if 1 and 2 are true, 3 follows logically and must also be true. The argument is valid.

Valid arguments are better than invalid ones, but valid arguments are not necessarily sound. An argument is sound if it is both valid and all of its premises are true. So, are the premises of the argument given by the student true?

Let us grant that the first premise, 1, is true – that the arguer is correct about the view held by most people in his ethnic group. So far, so good. But is the second premise true? That is, is it the case that whatever standard one's ethnic community holds about plagiarism is the correct standard? Obviously not, because plagiarism is a kind of misconduct defined by the relevant scholarly community, not one's familial community. Because the arguer mistakenly thinks the standards of his culture apply in a research context, his second premise is false. And if an argument has a false premise in it, then the argument is not sound. And an unsound argument, even if it's valid, is not a good argument. Note that the conclusion may be still be true (there may be other reasons that the teaching assistant should not report the incident), but the argument given does not provide a good reason to believe the conclusion.

We have been exploring the characteristics of moral reasoning. Moral reasoning is only possible, however, because we have two other skills, language and moral emotions.

. . . because we are emotional, social animals

Social animals naturally affiliate with others of their kind and especially with the others who treat them in the ways they wish to be treated. From the time we are infants, we not only lean in close to our mothers who care for us but we also wave goodbye to strangers we do not recognize. Early on we learn to synchronize our activities and to play with others. We are the kinds of beings who instinctively cooperate. We share these prosocial tendencies with other primates, species that are also inclined to aid others of their kind. And so we find ourselves hanging around in groups; seeking emotional support from our loved ones, and in turn wanting to provide the same to them. Like the chimpanzees studied by Frans de Waal, we are mutual animals willing to assume short-term costs to gain longer-term rewards.[2] Our desire to live in peaceful and productive communities strengthens the group and satisfies our need for companionship.

Interacting with others brings emotional risks and benefits. We are all familiar with anger, disgust, fear, shame, joy, sadness and surprise – the six emotions Paul Ekman identifies as common to every culture (Ekman 1982). Of these six, the simple emotions (e.g., joy, anger, sadness) do not require the ability to take another person's point of view. For example, when a 7-year-old gasps in delight at a fireworks display, her expression is spontaneous, not deliberated, and not dependent upon her understanding someone else's view of her.

But the moral emotions require that we have the capacity to imagine how our behavior is affecting another person's opinion of us. For example, suppose you are trying to cheat in an exam. You feel your heart rate accelerate and your palms begin to sweat. You are experiencing simple fear and anxiety. However, if you now notice the instructor looking at you, your automatic physiological fear response is displaced by another emotion, a moral

---

[2] F. B. M. de Waal, *Good Natured: The Origins of Right and Wrong in Humans and Other Animals* (Cambridge, MA: Harvard University Press, 1996).

emotion. For as you become conscious of the image of you forming in the instructor's mind, the basic biological state of heightened arousal gives way to shame, a socially constructed emotion that involves the understanding of another person's opinion of you.

The so-called moral emotions – e.g., regret, embarrassment, shame, guilt, pride – are responses in which we impute to others perceptions of our own social transgressions. The result is that we have a negative feeling about where we stand with relation to the other person. We may have positive feelings, too, if we are convinced we have accomplished something others have not. Consider pride, the positive feeling that accompanies the belief that my standing in the group hierarchy is rising. These feelings, positive and negative, are social emotions insofar as they require me to read others' minds and register how their mental states are affecting me in the group.

If moral emotions motivate us to give reasons for our actions, language provides us with the conceptual tools we need to express those reasons. Readers who understand this book use a common grammatical system; no one who understands these words comes to understand them by using their own private language. Consider this last sentence. It is an English sentence that I wrote to express a fact of human psychology. The sentence is only one among many I could have composed to convey the fact that you, the reader, are now entertaining multiple interpretations of what I have written, evaluating them to settle on one that makes sense to you, connecting the sentence in question to the sentences that come before and after it. You are engaged in constant, active debate with yourself as you read, and you debate in a way with me as you assess the meaning and significance of what I've written.

Language, like the moral emotions, is a capacity given to us by nature and developed by us with the assistance of our parents and teachers. The sort of interchange in which we are engaged, mediated by the text in your hands (or on your computer screen), is complex, extensive and learned. Philosopher Noam Chomsky once wrote that language is so complex that no 2-year-old could learn it unless he or she was hard-wired to acquire it. But even if he's right that our brains are programmed to learn language, the fact remains that we would not have it were it not for our parents and siblings and friends teaching us our mother tongue. The inability of so-called feral children to learn to understand spoken language underscores the point (Rymer 1994; Curtiss *et al.* 1974).

From an early age, under the steady hand of a caring adult, children can begin to imagine themselves in others' shoes because language allows them to express their wonderment about causality and character. "Why did Sarah hit me, Mommy?" Children can represent to themselves the proposition that others have interests different from their own because they can recognize, appreciate, and learn how to respect the interests of others. And their caregivers can explain the moral world to them – "Sarah just wants her toy back; it is hers, you know."

None of this interchange would be possible if we were not linguistic creatures. That includes egoists. Without language, the egoist cannot understand her past, much less work on shaping her future. The community, we may say truthfully, is part of our identity – and part of the egoist's identity – because our categorical interests are linguistic representations of the futures we desire for ourselves. All linguistic representations are public in that they are constructed of elements that are socially created. Babies do not create their own words, syntax, or semantics. To communicate, they use tools that exist before them and independently of them.

This point, so problematic for egoism, bears emphasis. Egoists seem blind to the facts of our social nature when they construe their identity as something they created and for which they can claim credit. They thus ignore the conditions in which they have come to exist, conditions in which others have cared for them, educated them, and helped them to mature. We live in houses we did not build, as we are reminded by the biblical author of *Joshua*. We reap from fields we did not sow. The proper emotional response to the fact of our existence is gratitude. Gratitude expresses itself in sincerity, honesty, and a resolve to keep the promises we make. For our very identity is something we make using gifts brought to us by our cultures, communities extended through time.

Contractualism begins where egoism ends, with the fact that our identities are social identities constructed on the bases of shared emotional, linguistic, and rational capacities. In conflicts of interest cases, therefore, the contractualist cannot and does not assume that his interests automatically take precedence. The contractualist recognizes that to think egoistically – to presume that my vision of the good life is primary and others' visions must always take a backseat to it – is not only ungrateful. It is ignorant. For egoism fails to acknowledge the fact that we did not create ourselves or the linguistic, emotional, and moral systems that constitute us.

Contractualism understands that we are able to form long-term categorical interests only because we are affiliative creatures. So, contractualists ask first not how can I arrange matters to get what I want, but how can we arrange matters to get what we want? This is a difficult question to answer because we are creatures who forever cause problems for each other. Let's briefly note some of these problems.

. . . and yet the community is constantly threatened by unreasonable decisions

The good of any community is based on reciprocity; you groom Elias, Elias grooms you. If you groom Elias and then he refuses to cooperate, having only feigned a cooperative spirit and then reneging on his promise, you will not trust him and may organize your friends to ostracize him from the ordinary workings of the group. When someone does not collaborate, he makes it difficult for others to want to take his point of view. Not only are defectors a disappointment to those counting on them, defectors are a threat to the entire community.

For we are not always on the lookout for the good of others. Each of us is handicapped to some extent by slothfulness and fatigue, if not by antisocial tendencies. We are prone to forgetfulness and are easily tired, weak willed, and deceptive. Our failings elicit negative emotions in others: anger, envy, spitefulness. And we are inclined to cut corners ourselves when we learn that others have cut corners.

Recall Professor Goodwin, not the first researcher to take unreasonable risks with her career and others' careers. Other examples abound; if you need convincing that the research community is constantly under threat from within – from researchers putting their own and others' interests in jeopardy – pay another visit to the Office of Research Integrity website. Alas, you will probably see new cases posted every few months.

One final point about the moral emotions before moving ahead. The emotional bonds that tie us together compel us to want to give reasons for our moral transgressions. The reason we want to explain ourselves when accused of, say, falsifying an image in a grant application or plagiarism in our dissertation is that we are aware of how this charge makes us look. Negative social emotions are not under our control and are not welcome; we do whatever we can to avoid them. But since they are inevitable, we have created mechanisms to help us discharge them. For example, we require those making accusations to give reasons for their charges. If their reasons are not persuasive, we ask them to withdraw their accusations. If their charges are groundless and yet they refuse to admit their error, we might take more aggressive actions, such as trying to shame them to give up their attacks – or finally even ostracize them from the group if they continue to be disruptive.

Reason-giving contractualism is the view that a person should always act in accord with principles that no free and equal person could reasonably reject

As we've noted, narrow contractualism fails to take account of our unwritten contracts. It is not capable, then, of accounting for the gratitude we ought to feel to those who have given us the ability to give reasons for our actions.

A theory that recognizes our explicit and implicit agreements is reason-giving contractualism:

> Reason-giving conctractualism: one should always act in accord with principles that no free and equal person could reasonably reject.

Reason-giving contractualism is not just the view that we should be ready to provide reasons whenever we decide what to do. It is the view that the principles guiding our decisions must be principles that are interpersonally persuasive. How the world looks from another's perspective is the key here. If your decision makes sense to you, but places another person at a grave disadvantage or at risk of loss, then that person need not accept the principle. If a person who is free, informed, and in control of her faculties objects to the principle on which you plan to act and does so on grounds that are reasonable, then reason-giving contractualism requires you not to adopt the principle you are considering.[3]

For contractualists of this sort, morality consists in the rules that free and equal persons would agree to be bound by if they knew that their colleagues would also be bound by them. In this way, morality consists of the larger good of all rather than the narrower good of individuals. To put it another way, this version of contractualism holds that actions are right if and only if they are permitted by rules that free, equal, and rational persons would agree to live by, assuming that all other moral agents must obey the rules, too. Actions are wrong if and only if they are not allowed by the rules. Suppose Goodwin had asked Mary Allen to spend the first 3 months of her year writing Padilla's literature search, the next 3 months finishing Ly's experiments, the next 3 months replicating the procedures of the lab's postdoc, and the next 3 months preparing the galleys for Goodwin's forthcoming textbook. Suppose further that none of these four outcomes would be possible without Mary Allen's help. By sacrificing 1 year of Allen's time, Padilla, Ly, a postdoc, and Goodwin would all advance their careers. The scenario depicts a case in which the overall goodness of outcomes is maximized and would be morally acceptable on egoist grounds – if Goodwin could get away with it.

---

[3] It should be noted that it does not follow that the reason-giving contractor may not perform the act being considered, as there may be another principle that no free and equal person could reasonably reject with which the act is in accordance. The mere fact that you are acting from an unacceptable principle doesn't mean that the act is not licensed by this form of contractualism. Thanks to Rob Streiffer for encouraging me to clarify this point.

According to reason-giving contractualism, however, the scenario would only be morally justifiable if Goodwin could justify her actions on grounds that everyone involved could not reasonably reject. It is hard to imagine how this would be possible. Allowing the head of the lab to exploit Mary Allen is obviously unacceptable to Allen. It will cost her a year of her time, is not part of the bargain to which she agreed, and would be a clear violation of a mentor's prerogatives. The harm to Allen is considerable, even when – as we have stipulated – the aggregated consequences for all involved are positive. Mary Allen is perfectly reasonable to reject Goodwin's attempt to use her in this way.

If, on the other hand, Goodwin had asked Allen to perform these actions in exchange for each of the involved parties donating 3 months of their time to Allen's project, and if everyone involved agreed that the arrangement would be to their mutual advantage, then contractualism would deem the action morally permissible. For if all involved are fully informed and genuinely agree to the proposal, then no reasonable person could object.

Here is another example to illustrate the importance of being able to justify our actions to reasonable people. Suppose you promised Jane that you will complete the literature search for an article you are coauthoring by Thursday. If something comes up and you can't do it, you'll owe Jane a reason. Let's suppose something does come up: your sister gets in an accident on Wednesday and you have to visit her in the hospital, postponing your ability to fulfill your promise until Saturday. This reason, unlike, say your deciding to tan at the beach for the next few days, is not just any reason. It's a morally good one, one that other reasonable people would acknowledge as weighty.

In essence, contractualism, a well developed and widely held view among contemporary, English-speaking moral philosophers, is based on the idea that insofar as we make promises to each other, we owe it to each other to keep our word – or come up with very good reasons to justify ourselves if we must break our word. Broken promises elicit hard feelings. But even a significant transgression ("You haven't finished the lit search? Really?") can be wiped clean with a good reason ("Your sister lost her arm? Really?").

The view that society is based on the nature of humans as givers of reasons to friends and foes alike is aligned with what's called the social contract tradition in moral philosophy, a tradition associated with political theorist Thomas Hobbes (d. 1679) and philosophers John Locke (d. 1704) and Immanuel Kant (d. 1804). Each of these thinkers explained this view differently. But each believed that the morally right action would always be the action that could be justified to the people affected by the action. Their common insight is that we should observe the terms of our contracts insofar as they are socially beneficial and because we have entered them voluntarily.

Contractualism's central theme, then, is this: conventional rules governing social activities in complex organizations must be justifiable on the basis of reasons that other reasonable people can accept. If someone accuses you of acting negligently or irresponsibly, you will want to know what rule you've broken. You may then want to know what makes the rule valid. When group rules – be they for the lab, studio, family, pickup basketball game, or carpool – can be explained to each member in such a way that no member can reasonably object to them, then the rules are moral rules, according to contractualism. Rules, which may be implicit or explicit, maintain group cohesion and identity. But they are only the right rules, ethically speaking, when no free and equal person can reasonably object to them.

Contractualism does not aim to bring about the most good for the most people. In this respect it is similar to egoism because both theories maintain that a decision leading to a large number of trivial benefits for a large number of people should not outweigh one person's complaint that the decision would bring her insufferable and unmerited harm. For egoists, only one person's complaint matters: me. For rational contractors, on the other hand, the complaints of all persons who are free and reasonable matter. For, according to this view, acts are morally wrong when any individual has stronger reasons for accepting a principle according to which the act is wrong than the individual has for accepting a principle according to which the act is right. Individuals can only object to decisions or rules, in other words, on their own behalf; they need not appeal to their group's interests to make their case.

Consider again the Virginia Tech rules. Can they be justified? The document doesn't address this question, but we can answer it without too much difficulty. What about the rule that students must attend all lab meetings? It can be justified by pointing out that when some lab members are above the rules and consistently miss meetings, the consequences for group morale can be disastrous. And how is *that* claim justified? On the basis of experience; delinquents do not learn about new developments in the lab, are unaware of problems that arise, and are incapable of helping the group to solve problems. When students are not up-to-date on information the entire culture of the lab suffers, since those members are unable to assist others with lab tasks. There is a reason for the Virginia Tech rules, and when we ask questions about the rules, we can provide answers, answers that others in the research and university community cannot reject as unreasonable.

On the other hand, the policy as stated may still be rejected as unreasonable because it allows such limited exceptions. If the policy requires, for example, attendance at lab meetings even when one is seriously injured and in the hospital then it would seem to be unreasonable. Faculty can work with students to find creative ways to keep students involved and informed even when students cannot be physically present for extended periods. To be fully defensible, the Virginia Tech rule about lab meeting attendance would have to be responsive to these kinds of nuances.

Let us review. Egoism surrenders to contractualism in the face of the human condition. We are beings without identities unless we have social interaction, moral emotions, language, and reason. None of these capacities are our own inventions. I cannot claim credit for possessing any of them; the capacities are presents I received from those who nurtured me. Contractualists are grateful for what they have been given. Contractualists, recognizing the role others have played in the formation of their character, want in turn to figure out what is in *their group's* interests. They want, in turn, to figure out what they can do individually to promote the achievement of the group's interests.

How to proceed as a contractualist

Remind yourself of the contracts you have signed. Pull out the copies you were given at orientation and read the fine print. Then study the professional codes that govern conduct in your field. Ask yourself if the rules are ones that no free and equal person could reasonably reject and hence can be justified on the basis of interpersonally persuasive reasons. If the rules pass that test, observe them. If they do not pass that test, raise questions about them and encourage your profession either to provide the justifications necessary – or change the rule. Unreasonable attendance policies, for example, may be criticized and modified in light of moral principles and practical considerations. This is work junior and senior researchers may do together.

Bibliography

Curtiss, S. *et al.* 1974. The linguistic development of Genie. *Language,* **50**(3), 528–554.

Department of Anthropology, *University of Montana, Cultural Heritage Studies.* Available at: http://www.cas.umt.edu/anthro/documents/graduate/phd_contract_example.pdf [Accessed June 23, 2011].

Department of Food Science and Technology, *Virginia Tech University, Graduate Student Contract.* Available at: www.fst.vt.edu/graduate/handbook/graduatehandbook.pdf [Accessed June 23, 2011].

Ekman, 1982. *Emotion in the Human Face,* 2nd edn. Paris: Cambridge University Press.

Rymer, R. 1994. *Genie: A Scientific Tragedy.* Harper Paperbacks.

Waal, F.B.M. de. 1996. *Good Natured: The Origins of Right and Wrong in Humans and Other Animals.* Cambridge, MAs: Harvard University Press.

Chapter 5

Articulate reasons

Researchers are professionals, people who have earned positions in groups with social obligations and special privileges. Those who professed constituted the first profession – the clergy – and the clergy was followed eventually by two other professions: medicine and the law. Modernity knows of many professions, all of which share three characteristics: members have special knowledge resulting from advanced education; a solemn charge to advance the good of society; and the privilege of policing themselves.

If professionals do not conduct themselves in ways that inspire public trust, society may respond by imposing regulations. To fulfill its mission and retain its freedoms, a professional society develops a code of conduct. Many of the rules address situations commonly faced by members; these rules are developed by drawing on the collective wisdom of the group. Other rules address questions not commonly faced by members; sometimes these situations require special task forces to study the issue and issue a recommendation.

Ethical questions that commonly arise should generally be answered in the same way by all members. Should a doctor or lawyer give a newspaper reporter personal information about their patient or client? No. Should an elementary teacher discuss a student's mental health problems on a blog? No. Should researchers mislabel photos or plagiarize manuscripts? No. Such issues are settled. However, if a given professional does not know how to behave in such familiar circumstances, they will probably be able to find the appropriate response articulated in the code. For while the ethical issues professionals face are not ethical issues the rest of society faces, they are issues that other members of their group have faced. And these familiar problems have given rise to common rules that members should internalize.

However, professionals may also find themselves having to deal with difficult cases in which members disagree about how a given issue should be resolved. An example of such a case in medicine is the so-called "duty to warn" case, in which a doctor must decide whether to break patient confidentiality in order to warn a family member about a possible danger from the patient. And novel questions arise in the professions, questions that have not been settled or, perhaps, even previously encountered. Should a researcher in ecology, for example, uproot endangered plants and secretly transport them across a national boundary knowing full well that doing so is against the law if they are convinced that doing so is the only way to preserve the species? Should a statistician who is only a consultant on a research project intervene if a mentor in another department gives questionable statistical advice to a graduate student? Should a graduate student report another graduate student for dropping an outlying data point? Even accomplished researchers will disagree about the correct answers to such questions.

Research Ethics: A Philosophical Guide to the Responsible Conduct of Research. Gary Comstock. Published by Cambridge University Press. © Cambridge University Press 2013.

The answers to such questions will probably not be found in any formal codes of conduct. In such cases, professionals must be able to rely on their specialized training and personal judgment to find the right answer. For society expects professionals to be able to make the right decision when no one else knows what the right decision is.

In answering questions of either kind, common or novel, professionals must be able to make wise choices under pressure and, eventually, to articulate their reasons for their choices. For that is the special responsibility of the group, to be able to explain their actions to others. In commonly encountered cases, as we have noted, the correct decision will usually be found in the profession's code. If a doctor or lawyer has acted to protect a patient's or client's confidentiality and her action is subsequently questioned, she can defend herself by explaining that her action was consistent with her group's rules. Most moral decisions faced by professionals are, almost by definition, "common" in the sense that others in the group have previously faced the same issue, found the appropriate response, and codified the rule. Professionals need not think up reasons for following the rule on each occasion. Generally, they need only appeal to the rule articulated in the code.

When facing truly novel dilemmas, however, professionals may have to discover by themselves both the right final decision and the reasons for it. What sort of response must the professional's response be? For contractualists, it must be the sort of response that a fair-minded person would accept. Let us explore this matter further.

Professional codes articulate two types of rules

As we say, some issues in research ethics are garden-variety issues and should be addressed with rules that are second nature to members of the profession; do not lie, do not cheat, do not steal. Communities of research support their youngest members by keeping rules simple and resorting to expert advice in the difficult cases. An atmosphere of collegiality is easily formed and maintained when the lab director and institutional officials openly and frequently discuss these issues. When the climate is transparent, when the door to the senior member of the group is open, and when senior members are helping junior members to understand and articulate reasons for their actions, researchers will prosper.

Other issues, however, require extensive discussion and investigation, e.g., should ecologists value the property rights of peasant farmers more than the continued existence of rare plant species? To resolve these questions we cannot rely on the automatic application of intuitive rules. We need professional expertise and judgment. While we should train ourselves to act without thinking on the common rules, we must regularly discuss the novel questions with an eye to refining our professional responses as new knowledge comes to light.

Common rules that members should internalize

As we have said, most codes contain routine duties and expectations. Do not make statements known to be false, obey the law, be honest in all dealings, respect the integrity and reputation of colleagues, protect the safety of the public, and so on. For example, the National Society of Professional Engineers' Code of Ethics states that engineers "shall be objective and truthful," "avoid deceptive acts," and "conduct themselves honorably, responsibly, ethically, and lawfully in their reports" (National Society of Professional Engineers n.d.). The International Association of Assessing Officers requires an "ongoing commitment to the core values of integrity, honesty, fairness, openness, respect and responsibility" (International Association of Assessing Officers 2005).

Why are the codes replete with admonishments not to depart from expected norms of the community? One reason is that contemporary professions exist in large, complex, and competitive societies. To succeed in this milieu, the members of a profession must be able to trust each other. If I doubt the reliability of the information you're telling me I won't be able to do my job. If professionals disobey rules, they won't be able to trust each other. So, by internalizing these common injunctions – habituating oneself to observe the basic rules – each member contributes to the health and productivity of the group. Occasionally the common rules warrant critical scrutiny, especially if they do not reflect tenets of our common morality or if circumstances have changed since the rule was first formulated. Usually, however, we can and should trust the common rules, particularly to the extent that they reflect hypernorms – norms that are necessary in any conceivable human society.

Specific rules that members should examine critically

If some rules are generic, well-established and relatively uncontroversial, others may be quite specific, more recent and, occasionally, problematic.[1] For when novel situations arise, professionals may find that the usual rules do not tell them how to behave. In such situations we must think for ourselves, reason to the right conclusion and, occasionally, ask whether the received rule is a good one. Professionals must also think for themselves in another situation: when two or more common rules conflict with each other. Here's an example. Suppose a mechanical engineer comes to think that a bridge they have had a hand in designing has a structural flaw. The engineer begins to worry that the bridge may eventually shift in a dangerous way, or even collapse. But there is no certainty here, only probabilities and percentages. In such a case, how should one decide when to blow the whistle on oneself?

The engineer will look in vain for an answer to this thorny question in any professional code, much less the code of the National Society of Professional Engineers. For the NSPE code contains injunctions that may yield conflicting judgments in particular cases. For example, the first line of the NSPE document explicitly requires that all engineers "hold paramount the safety . . . of the public." That seems clear enough; we should blow the whistle at the earliest sign of anything wrong. However, later on in the code we read that engineers must observe their obligations to those who hire them, and that they must "act for each employer or client as faithful agents or trustees." How can one be a faithful agent for one's employer if one blows the whistle on oneself with the result that the employer loses millions of dollars when they have to reconstruct the bridge? Although it seems obvious that the public's safety should come first, the code seems to leave the point open for discussion.

Suppose, to take another engineering example, that your company asks you to certify the safety of a process in which a plant is pumping radioactive material into a waterway. You investigate and determine that there is a 10% risk of an environmental disaster. A small risk, perhaps, but your supervisor does not want it reported. He removes your finding from the final report (cf. Inez Austin's actions, Online Ethics Center for Engineering and Research 1998). Should you protest? Again, is your primary obligation to protect the public's safety?

---

[1] I don't mean to imply that one should only question new or specific rules and never old or general rules. It's an open question whether a new rule will be controversial, as it's possible that a common rule ought not to be obeyed in a particular case. There are occasions when one ought to think critically about both sorts of rules.

Or is it to act as a "faithful agent" for your employer? And, if a 10% risk of disaster is not sufficient for you to blow the whistle, what level of risk is sufficient?

. . . and be able to justify

Professionals sometimes must make difficult decisions. These decisions are not always justifiable on the basis of any of the official codes that govern one's career. In such situations, we must be able to marshal our thoughts, identify our options, make the best decision, and defend our line of reasoning with data and sound argument. To protect yourself, then, take a moment now to locate and carefully read your professional code. Examine it for the reasons it offers, if any, in defense of each rule or policy. Watch for two types of policies, generic policies likely to be shared with other professions, and specific rules not likely to be shared by other professions.

Not all policies are acceptable and some may impose unacceptable costs on those who must abide by them. How do you know when a cost is unacceptable? Ask yourself whether you would consider yourself fair-minded if you had to be on the receiving end of your decision. If a policy is in accord with agreements you have made, or with agreements your profession might reasonably be expected to make in light of its explicit and implicit social contracts, you are probably doing the right thing.

To illustrate the procedure of trying to justify a code's claims, read these paragraphs of the Ecological Society of America's code.

Case study: The Ecological Society of America Code of Ethics[2]

Preamble: This code provides guiding principles of conduct for all members of the Ecological Society of America and all ecologists certified by the Society. It is the desire and purpose of the Society to support and encourage ecological research and education, and to facilitate the application of ecological science in the management of ecological systems. Towards these ends, this Code is intended to further ecological understanding through the open and honest communication of research; to assure appropriate accessibility of accurate and reliable ecological information to employers, policy-makers, and the public; and to encourage effective education and training in the disciplines of ecological science. Individuals aware of breaches of this Code are encouraged to refer to the Society's procedures for addressing violations of the Code, and to communicate with the Society's Executive Director who will explain the code and process.

General: All members of the Ecological Society of America and all ecologists certified by the Society should observe the following principles in the conduct of their professional affairs.

a. Ecologists will offer professional advice and guidance only on those subjects in which they are informed and qualified through professional training or experience. They will strive to accurately represent ecological understanding and knowledge and to avoid and discourage dissemination of erroneous, biased, or exaggerated statements about ecology.

b. Ecologists will not represent themselves as spokespersons for the Society without express authorization by the President of ESA.

c. Ecologists will cooperate with other researchers whenever possible and appropriate to assure rapid interchange and dissemination of ecological knowledge.

d. Ecologists will not plagiarize in verbal or written communication, but will give full and proper credit to the works and ideas of others, and make every effort to avoid misrepresentation.

---

[2] Reprinted from Ecological Society of America, http://www.esa.org/aboutesa/codeethics.php [Accessed June 20, 2011].

e. Ecologists will not fabricate, falsify, or suppress results, deliberately misrepresent research findings, or otherwise commit scientific fraud.

f. Ecologists will conduct their research so as to avoid or minimize adverse environmental effects of their presence and activities, and in compliance with legal requirements for protection of researchers, human subjects, or research organisms and systems.

g. Ecologists will not discriminate against others, in the course of their work on the basis of gender, sexual orientation, marital status, creed, religion, race, color, national origin, age, economic status, disability, or organizational affiliation.

h. Ecologists will not practice or condone harassment in any form in any professional context.

i. In communications, ecologists should clearly differentiate facts, opinions, and hypotheses.

j. Ecologists will not seek employment, grants, or gain, nor attempt to injure the reputation or professional opportunities of another scientist by false, biased, or undocumented claims, by offers of gifts or favors, or by any other malicious action.

Certified Ecologists: Ecologists certified by the Ecological Society of America are expected to adhere to all sections of the Code; the following principles apply particularly to such individuals.

a. Certified ecologists will present evidence of their qualifications, including professional training, publications, and experience, when requested in connection with their work as a certified ecologist.

b. Certified ecologists will inform a prospective or current employer or client of any professional or personal interests which may impair the objectivity of their work, and, upon request, provide clients and employers with this Code.

c. Certified ecologists will respect requests for confidentiality from their employers or clients, provided that such confidentiality does not require violation of this Code or of legal statutes. Should conflicts arise between maintenance of confidentiality and legal or ethical standards, certified ecologists should advise clients or employers of the conflict in writing.

d. In seeking employment through bids, certified ecologists will describe salaries and fees and the extent and kinds of service to be rendered as accurately and fully as possible.

e. Certified ecologists should use resources available to them through institutional employment, in performance of work contracted independently of their employing institution, only with the full knowledge and consent of the employing institution. Inappropriate use of access to institutional resources should be avoided; the appropriateness of particular uses of institutional resources should be addressed by the employing institution.

f. Certified ecologists will accept compensation for a particular service or report from one source only, except with the full knowledge and consent of all concerned parties.

g. Certified ecologists will utilize, or recommend utilization of appropriate experts whenever such action is essential to solving a problem.

h. Certified ecologists will not knowingly associate professionally with, or allow the use of their names, reports, maps, or other technical materials by any enterprise known to be illegal or fraudulent.

i. Certified ecologists may advertise their services, but may not use misleading, false, or deceptive advertising. If Society certification is noted in advertisement, the level of certification must be included.

Common rules in this code encourage understanding, open and honest communication, and "effective education and training" – the sorts of things we'd expect to find in all codes. The directives not to represent oneself as a spokesperson of the Ecological Society of America or to allow suspect parties to use one's maps, however, are exhortations not likely to be in the codes for the American Physical Society or the Society for Developmental Biology.

Suppose a member of the Ecological Society were asked to justify General rule i., that ecologists should clearly differentiate facts from opinions. Suppose an ecologist challenged the rule on philosophical grounds, claiming that ecologists cannot do what the code requires because facts are value-laden, because opinions can be soundly based on facts, and because the rule seems to rely on a distinction between facts and values that does not exist. How would an ESA member go about justifying the rule?

They might turn to contractualism and argue that this rule is justified because it is consistent with the implicit contractual agreement between ecologists and society. If it is true that ecologists and members of the general public have implicitly agreed to separate facts and opinions and to allow ecologists only to report facts, then the requirement that ecologists should only report facts may be a rule that all reasonable persons would agree to be bound by, assuming that all other persons agreed to be bound by it, too. Reasoning in this way would be to offer a justification of the rule on contractualist grounds.

Or an ecologist might turn to egoism and argue that the rule is justified because it is consistent with that ecologist's categorical interests. Or an ecologist might turn to rights theories or utilitarianism – two theories we will explore in more detail in Parts C and D – and argue that the rule is consistent with respect for persons or because observing the rule will lead to maximizing aggregate good consequences.

In this chapter's Background essay, Gary Varner draws on all four ethical theories (if somewhat indirectly) to address the question. While his title emphasizes the utilitarian roots of his view, the particular kind of utilitarianism he defends is consistent with the contractualist emphases of this chapter. In the course of exploring the justification of the ESA code's rules regarding the proper treatment of animals, Varner compares the ESA statement with the code of the American Veterinary Medical Association and notes that the two codes contain different emphases in this area.

Varner draws heavily upon utilitarianism, providing us with an opportunity to look ahead to Part D with a few words of introduction about that theory. Varner's preferred version of utiliarianism is two-level utilitarianism. As we mentioned in the Introduction to the book, two-level utilitarianism is based on the work of R. M. Hare. According to the theory, ordinary citizens engage in, and ought to engage in, two very different kinds of moral thinking. In ordinary circumstances, we should think and act as contractualists and routinely do what we have agreed to do. At the first level, then, professionals need not reason about whether they should observe the rules of their professional codes; they should automatically and unreflectively keep them. These rules are an instance of what Varner calls Intuitive Level System (ILS) rules – rules we ought to follow because habituating ourselves to follow them will counteract unwelcome tendencies to act selfishly and unreasonably.

As we saw in Part A, we are prone to spin the facts in our favor, rationalize our behaviors, and fool ourselves into thinking that we're acting for others' benefit when we are actually just trying to get what we want. The common contractual understandings found in most professional codes – fulfill promises, seek understanding, be honest, etc. – require that professionals not act egoistically in most circumstances. The idea here is that if all professionals follow the code, they will collectively and unreflectively produce better overall results than if each one acts only on his or her personal desires.

The second level of moral thinking, on the other hand, applies to unusual cases, those rare instances when the professional is facing a novel conundrum. Perhaps a new dilemma has arisen in the law practice, or a particularly vexing issue in the chemistry lab. When one's code does not address an issue, or when there are two or more conflicting rules in the code, agents must employ critical thinking. In critical thinking we discover which of the actions open to us will lead to the best overall results. The best overall results may include obeying one's promises, being fair to others, and respecting individual rights. One of the purposes of thinking critically, however, is to ask whether unusual situations can arise in which we are justified in acting contrary to an otherwise reliable ILS rule. In sum, Hare's two-level utilitarianism requires that we respect the strengths of egoism and contractualism while denying that either theory is sufficient by itself. For Hare denies that moral decisions can be made on the basis of self-interest or contractualist agreements alone. It is appropriate at this juncture in the book, therefore, to consider Varner's use of two-level utilitarianism in examining the code we have just read. For Varner explains the importance of two points. First, Varner emphasizes the importance of thinking and acting most of the time as a contractualist thinks and acts – that is, as someone who observes intuitive level system rules almost all of the time. Second, Varner emphasizes the importance of thinking critically when moral conflicts arise. And he makes both points in the context of examining the particular code, the code of the Ecological Society of America, that we have just read.

Background essay: "Utilitarianism and the evolution of ecological ethics," by Gary Varner [3]

. . . [R. M.] Hare's theory [1, 2, 3] provides closely related answers to two . . . questions . . .: (1) what explains the existence of codes of professional ethics? and (2) what justifies the tenets of a code of professional ethics? Intuitive Level System (ILS) rules in general are designed to guide human beings, who are incapable of perfect archangelic thinking, in the kinds of situations they normally encounter. A code of professional ethics is a set of ILS rules designed with a specific population in mind. What defines the population is that they normally encounter certain kinds of ethically charged situations that the population at large does not normally encounter. If Hare's theory is correct, what explains the existence of codes of professional ethics is the fact that members of different professions normally encounter situations that members of the general public do not. What justifies the tenets of a code is the fact (if it is one) that professionals will tend to do a better job of maximizing aggregate happiness when they encounter those kinds of situations if they have internalized those tenets. If the authors of the code have done a good job of critical thinking that will indeed be a fact.

. . .

Specifying the contents of a code

As anyone who has reviewed various codes of professional ethics will realize, there is much overlap among them. From a Harean perspective, it is obvious why this should be so: a wide range of professionals normally encounter the same kinds of ethically charged situations that members of the laity do not. For instance, a wide range of professionals engage in research and publication, and for this reason many codes of professional ethics discuss things like plagiarism, co-authorship, and so on. Similarly, codes of closely related professions, e.g. those of doctors and nurses, will share provisions that are not found in unrelated professions.

On the other hand, some professions are such that their members normally encounter ethically charged situations of a unique kind, and this is reflected in the fact that their codes of ethics include rules that are found in few or no other professions' codes. For instance, police officers' codes might contain provisions about high-speed chases, and codes of military ethics should contain provisions about targeting non-combatants. Such provisions are found in no other

---

[3] Reprinted from *Science and Engineering Ethics*, 2008, 14(4), pp.551–573. Gary Varner is professor of philosophy, Texas A&M University; gary@philosophy.tamu.edu.

professions' codes, and they reflect the fact that members of these professions will, in the normal course of their work, encounter situations that members of other professions never encounter in the normal course of their work. Including related provisions in their codes of ethics ensures that properly socialized members of these professions will have developed strong dispositions to behave in certain ways in these situations.

This emphasis on instilling dispositions comports with the view that a code of professional ethics must somehow be informed by virtue theory . . . . The Harean approach incorporates virtue theory directly into the way ILS rules are "internalized." To properly internalize an ILS rule is to develop a disposition to behave accordingly and to judge accordingly. This is why a moral agent feels compunction after breaking an ILS rule, even if she has been led to do so by clear critical thinking. Internalizing an ILS rule requires more than being able to recite it, it requires developing a disposition to act and judge accordingly, and that disposition remains in place when one acts "out of character." A good scientist is not just able to recite the provisions of his profession's code; a good scientist is one who has internalized these provisions in a way that gives him certain traits of character. If the provisions are well crafted, then developing these character traits will contribute to the leading of a morally responsible scientist's life. This is how, on the Harean view, to internalize the provisions of a code of professional ethics is to acquire certain virtues.

. . .

The Code of Ethics of the ESA

The current Code of Ethics of the ESA [4] discusses authorship standards, proprietary data, and simultaneous submission to multiple journals (principles a.–e. under "Publication"), and it prohibits plagiarism and fabrication of data (principles d. and e. under "General"). As noted in the preceding section, such provisions are appropriate in any profession whose members actively engage in research and publication. Ecologists also contract out their services and employ staff, and the ESA code also includes provisions found in many business and professional codes, concerning discrimination, harassment, and confidentiality (principles g. and h. under "General," and c. under "Certified Ecologists").

It makes sense that the ESA code includes such provisions, but from the Harean perspective it also makes sense to ask whether ecologists normally encounter ethically charged situations that members of other professions and the general public rarely if ever encounter. The preamble of the ESA Code does say that "this Code is intended to further ecological understanding," but aside from stating the obvious (that what ecologists are concerned with understanding is ecology), is there anything that distinguishes ecology as a profession? Is there nothing unique or special about the kinds of situations that members of this profession normally encounter that calls for any principles that would not be found in the codes of other professions whose members sell their services and publish their research?

As an illustration of this point, consider side-by-side the codes of the American Society of Civil Engineers (ASCE) [5] and the Association for Computing Machinery (ACM) [6]. The ASCE Code requires members to "hold paramount the safety, health and welfare of the public and shall strive to comply with the principles of sustainable development in the performance of their professional duties" (Fundamental Canon #1). The ACM code includes, under "General Moral Imperatives," a provision mentioning the public's "health and welfare" and "potential damage to the local or global environment" (Imperative 1.1), but there is no mention of sustainable development.[4] There is, however, an imperative to "Access computing and

---

[4] The ASCE follows the Brundtland Commission, defining "sustainable development" as "the challenge of meeting human needs for natural resources, industrial products, energy, food, transportation, shelter, and effective waste management while conserving and protecting

communication resources only when authorized to do so" (#2.8). Thus the two codes address (if somewhat obliquely) the question of what special kinds of situations members of their professions normally encounter that members of other professions do not. For while civil engineers use computers, they do not, like computer engineers, routinely find themselves in a position to access large amounts of securely stored information which only other people are supposed to access. And for their part, concern for sustainable development is a natural reflection of civil engineering's history . . ..

A Harean perspective on professional ethics suggests that, when revising its code, the ESA should attend to the question of what, if anything, makes ecology unique as a science, and the ESA should craft principles that reflect what they decide that is.

One possible route would be to do something analogous to what conservation biologists have done, by asserting that being an ecologist means being committed to certain specific values or management goals. In a famous article from over 20 years ago, Michael Soulé described conservation biology as being committed to various "normative postulates," including that *"Biodiversity has intrinsic value*, irrespective of its instrumental or utilitarian value" [8, p. 731 – italics in original]. More generally, conservation biologists commonly describe their science as both "mission-oriented" and "crisis-oriented" [9]. Its mission is to provide society with knowledge and techniques necessary to further the general goal of preserving biodiversity. This implicitly describes the kind of problems conservation biologists focus on: preserving the natural variety of species and functioning ecosystems. Preservation projects commonly require social engineering, however, so conservation biology is conceived of as highly interdisciplinary, involving not only field observations and laboratory experiments, but also "adaptive ecosystem management," which is an experimental and community-involving approach to managing sustainable development [10]. Conservation biology is "crisis-oriented" because species and habitats are being lost at an unprecedented rate, and this has made many conservation biologists comfortable with a level of advocacy that scientists are usually taught to shy away from. Soulé even says that "In crisis disciplines, one must act before knowing all the facts; crisis disciplines are thus a mixture of science and art, and their pursuit requires intuition as well as information" [9, p. 727].

Two provisions of the current ESA code suggest that, by contrast, the ESA expects its members to shy away from making claims about ethics or values and from advocacy. Consider, for instance, general principle i:

> i. In communications, ecologists should clearly differentiate facts, opinions, and hypotheses.

No guidance is given for distinguishing "facts" from "opinion," but in scientific circles, moral judgments and statements about values are generally classified as "opinion, not fact." General principle a. has a similar implication:

> a. Ecologists will offer professional advice and guidance only on those subjects in which they are informed and qualified through professional training or experience. They will strive to accurately represent ecological understanding and knowledge and to avoid and discourage dissemination of erroneous, biased, or exaggerated statements about ecology.

While it does not explicitly rule out communicating one's intuitions or hunches, it would certainly be in the spirit of this principle to label them as such, since an intuition or hunch is generally regarded as a step down the epistemological ladder from a hypothesis. Also, ecologists do not receive "professional training" in ethics, and values are not open to "experience" in the sense that was presumably intended in general principle a. So adherence to the current ESA Code

---

environmental quality and the natural resource base essential for future development" (ASCE Code, footnote #3).

of Ethics would seem to make it impossible for members to "offer professional advice and guidance" on ethical questions that are not explicitly addressed in the Code itself.

General principles a. and i. thus suggest that the ESA will not want to follow conservation biology's lead by committing its members to a specific view about what has intrinsic value or any specific management goals. However, general principle f. could be taken to express, rather indirectly, two kinds of value commitments:

> f. Ecologists will conduct their research so as to avoid or minimize adverse environmental effects of their presence and activities, and in compliance with legal requirements for protection of researchers, human subjects, or research organisms and systems.

One kind of value commitment is suggested by the command to "avoid or minimize adverse environmental effects of their presence and activities." Unfortunately, this general principle provides no guidance on what would count as an "adverse" environmental effect. Without such guidance, one is left wondering whether all such effects can be understood in terms of the instrumental value of ecosystem functioning, or whether there can be, according to the ESA's Code of Ethics, effects that are "adverse" for the environment itself, even if there is no effect whatsoever on human interests.

That ecologists should have some concern for animal welfare is also expressed in general principle f., although the principle does not explicitly mention animals and it implicitly prioritizes the value of animal welfare vis-à-vis avoiding "adverse environmental effects." Animal welfare is included by the reference to "legal requirements for protection of . . . research organisms," for these legal requirements include federal and state animal welfare statutes governing animals used in laboratory research, as well as standards imposed by wildlife agencies when granting permission for various kinds of field research. This concern for animal welfare is implicitly prioritized, however, because the same principle instructs ecologists to "avoid or minimize adverse environmental effects" whether or not the law requires it. The current ESA code thus says, in effect, that ecologists should take "environmental effects" more seriously than effects on animal welfare.

From a Harean perspective, any profession whose members' activities routinely impact the interests of sentient animals should embody in its code of ethics some form of respect for those animals.[5] This is true even though morality, in Hare's view, is a construct of human language. Plants have no moral standing in Hare's view, because it is impossible to imagine experiencing the effects of actions on them. For any sentient[6] being, however, this is possible. Thus both mentally incompetent human beings (who may lack language and the ability to make moral judgments) and sentient nonhuman animals have morally significant interests from a Harean perspective. Put informally: the Golden Rule requires one to judge as if one had to "stand in everyone's shoes, not just our own"; but many nonhuman animals are sentient[7] and thus "have shoes"; so all sentient animals count, morally speaking.

So from a Harean perspective, it would be appropriate to amend the ESA code so that it does not tie concern for animal welfare to existing legal requirements. At the same time, however, it is true that from the Harean perspective, it would be appropriate to embody concern for animal welfare differently in different professions' codes. To see why, compare the

---

[5] This may be an over-simplification: Harean ethics makes what is appropriate to a society sensitive to background ecological and economic conditions, so perhaps it is more accurate to say that in modern societies, any such profession should embody concern for animal welfare in its code of ethics.

[6] Here "sentient" is intended in the standard sense it takes in the literature on animal rights and animal welfare, where it means "capable of conscious suffering and/or enjoyment."

[7] The question of which animals are sentient is a large and complicated one, but the best answer seems to be that probably all vertebrates are capable of suffering (at least from physical pain) while invertebrates (with the exception of cephalopods) probably are not. For a detailed treatment of the issue, see [11, Chap. 5]

situations of an ecologist studying predator–prey relations and a veterinarian practicing in a small animal clinic. The American Veterinary Medical Association (AVMA) [12] code of ethics states that "Veterinarians should first consider the needs of the patient: to relieve disease, suffering, or disability while minimizing pain or fear."[8] From the Harean perspective, one profession's code of ethics should differ from another's if the members of that profession encounter, in the course of their normal work, ethically charged situations that members of other professions do not. Studying predator–prey relationships is a perfectly normal activity for an ecologist, but it requires "letting nature take its course" in ways that result in significant amounts of preventable disease, suffering, disability, pain, and fear. The veterinarian in clinical practice, by contrast, does not normally study predator–prey relationships and is generally committed to thwarting the natural course of diseases and injuries. So while it is true that, from a Harean perspective, any profession whose members' activities routinely impact the welfare of animals should embody a concern for animal welfare in its code of ethics, the ESA Code should do this in a different way than the AVMA Code. Prioritizing concerns about animal welfare and "adverse environmental effects" in the way the ESA Code currently does may be an appropriate way of doing this. In effect, general principle f directs ecologists to follow current legal requirements regarding animal welfare, whatever those may be, while allowing ecologists to bracket any more stringent requirements that might be appropriate in other professions' codes of ethics.

Another approach would be to amend the ESA Code to include a stand-alone principle that articulates an appropriate attitude of respect for conscious animals. Such a principle could mention any practices that are both (a) likely to be suggested in the course of ecological research, and (b) likely to cause suffering to animals. An appropriate principle would not rule out these practices, but it would call for minimizing such practices as far as possible, consistent with good experimental design and sound management. Including this kind of principle might subtly but importantly improve the ESA Code from a Harean perspective because, as indicated in the preceding section, part of the function of ILS rules is to instill virtues; properly internalizing an ILS rule produces dispositions to judge and act accordingly. Allowing or causing animal suffering may be a "necessary" part of ecological research, so producing in ecologists a disposition to avoid causing "unnecessary" suffering and a corresponding disposition to condemn it in others would certainly be a good thing. Some second-guessing of conventional field research methods and experimental designs might also result, and this could lead to improvements from an animal welfare perspective. In this way, building concern for animal welfare directly into its Code rather than incorporating it by reference to existing legal standards would have the effect of making compassion a virtue of ecologists.[9]

. . .

---

[8] In the context of Hare's theory, note that the AVMA Code also states that the basis of its principles is the Golden Rule.

[9] Another point about general principle f that bears mentioning from a Harean perspective is that, as emphasized previously, ILS rules often have a decidedly non-utilitarian "flavor." From the perspective of Harean critical thinking, nothing has intrinsic value except the conscious experiences of sentient beings, because critical thinking is explicitly utilitarian. Nevertheless, one could argue that ILS rules for ecologists should inspire some kind of non-utilitarian love or respect for ecosystems. The rationale would be that an ecologist who thinks of ecosystems as more than "mere" resources, that they (or their functioning) are intrinsically valuable, will love or respect them in a way that someone who thinks that only conscious beings have intrinsic value will not, and will, as a result, be more likely to avoid indirectly harming people and other sentient animals. Bryan Norton has argued [10, 13] that the implications of environmental holism and "enlightened" anthropocentrism will converge in practice. This "convergence hypothesis" is plausible in a general way [14, 15], so it is questionable whether ecologists will do a better job if they believe that ecosystems have intrinsic value. Surely an air conditioner repairman would not do a better job if he stopped thinking of air

Conclusion

R.M. Hare's two-level utilitarianism suggests that codes of professional ethics arise because members of various professions encounter, in the normal conduct of their jobs, ethically charged situations that members of the lay public only encounter in unusual situations. While it is to be expected that a code of professional ethics for ecological scientists will have many provisions that overlap with those for other scientists, from the Harean perspective two issues arise for ecologists.

First, from a Harean perspective, it makes sense to ask if there is anything about the normal activities of ecological scientists that sets their enterprise apart. It may be that there is not, but if there is, that should be taken up explicitly when the ESA next revises its code.

Second, from a Harean perspective, any profession that routinely impacts the welfare of nonhuman animals should address this in its code. The current ESA code does this by directing ecologists to conform to existing legal requirements concerning animal welfare, and, given the kinds of research that ecologist normally perform, this may be appropriate. On the other hand, amending its Code to explicitly endorse the view that the lives of all sentient animals have intrinsic value would, from a Harean perspective, further the goal of instilling important virtues like compassion.

. . .

It is worth noting that Hare's theory mirrors the complexities, uncertainties, and hazards of the moral life as it is encountered. It is simultaneously prescriptive and descriptive and it does not give clear-cut answers in complicated cases. Yet while humans are not archangels (who could decide such hard cases in a snap), neither are they proles (who are incapable of dealing with any case in which ILS rules conflict or give inadequate guidance); the reality is that humans are something in between, and while there is good reason to be diffident when engaging in critical thinking, hard cases . . . call out the courage to engage in critical thinking in the face of uncertainty.

The rules written down in a code of professional ethics will never give complete guidance on the truly hard cases. The rules will highlight various salient aspects of such cases, but if the cases are really difficult ones then the code, taken by itself, will not resolve them. From the Harean perspective, it is in dealing with such cases that we must try to think like archangels, knowing all the while that we are, at best, highly fallible at it. The really hard cases thus transcend what is provided in a code of professional ethics, but if the code is well formulated its rules will at least highlight some of the salient features of the case from which our heroic attempt at critical thinking must begin.[10]

References for Varner

1. Hare, R. M. (1993). *Essays on Bioethics.* New York: Oxford University Press.

2. Hare, R. M. (1973). Critical study: Rawls' theory of justice—I and II. *Philosophical Quarterly*, 23, 144–155, 241–252.

Reprinted in Norman Daniels (Ed.), *Reading Rawls* (1975). Oxford: Blackwell.

3. Hare, R. M. (1981). *Moral Thinking: Its Levels, Method, and Point.* New York: Oxford University Press.

4. Ecological Society of America. Code of Ethics. http://www.esa.org/

---

conditioning as having merely instrumental value to the residents of the house, but maybe that is the case with regard to very complex systems. Perhaps it inspires a healthy dose of humility.

[10] Research for this paper was supported in part by National Science Foundation (NSF) grant #0620808, but the opinions expressed herein are the author's and do not necessarily reflect the views of NSF. Jonathan Newman, Ed Harris, and Gary Comstock provided feedback on an early draft of this essay. An anonymous reviewer for this journal also provided particularly focused criticisms that goaded me into shoring up the argument and analysis at various points.

aboutesa/codeethics.php. Accessed 25 Sept. 2008.

5. American Society of Civil Engineers (ASCE) Code of Ethics. (2008). http://www.asce.org/inside/codeofethics.cfm. Accessed 25 Sept. 2008.

6. Association for Computing Machinery (ACM). (2008). http://www.acm.org/constitution/code.html. Accessed 25 Sept. 2008.

7. Harper, R. F. (1904). *The Code of Hammurabi*. Chicago, IL: University of Chicago Press.

8. Soulé, M. E. (1985). What is conservation biology? *BioScience*, **35**, 727–734.

9. Van Dyke, F. (2003). *Conservation Biology: Foundations, Concepts, Applications*. Boston: McGraw-Hill.

10. Norton, B. (2005). *Sustainability: A Philosophy of Adaptive Ecosystem Management*. Chicago, IL: University of Chicago Press.

11. Varner, G. 2012. *Personhood, Ethics, and Animal Cognition: Situating Animals in Hare's Two-Level Utilitarianism*. Oxford University Press.

12. American Veterinary Medical Association (AVMA). (2008). http://www.avma.org/issues/policy/ethics.asp. Accessed 25 Sept. 2008.

13. Norton, B. (1991). *Toward Unity Among Environmentalists*. New York: Oxford University Press.

14. Varner, G. (1998). *In Nature's Interests? Interests, Animal Rights and Environmental Ethics*. New York: Oxford University Press.

15. Varner, G. (2007). Review of Bryan Norton, sustainability: a philosophy of adaptive ecosystem management. *Environmental Ethics*, **29**, 307–312.

Conclusion

Study your profession's code and watch for common rules, rules likely to be found in other codes, and discipline-specific rules, rules not likely to be found in another code. Watch, too, for the ways in which both kinds of rules are justified. The defense of common rules will bring into focus moral truisms and values shared by all research fields. The defense of discipline-specific rules will clarify the particular practices and special competencies of the different fields. Ask yourself whether your code does a good job of giving reasons for its rules. If your professional society is considering whether to revise its code, encourage it to answer Varner's questions: what makes your field unique, what intuitive level rules reflect this uniqueness, and is it the case that aggregate happiness is more likely to be maximized if members internalize those rules? Those charged with writing or revising a code might reasonably aim at providing not a complete guide with answers for every specific question, but a general and coherent statement of the fundamental values to which the profession is committed.

Bibliography

Ecological Society of America, Code of Ethics. Available at: http://www.esa.org/aboutesa/codeethics.php [Accessed June 20, 2011].

International Association of Assessing Officers. 2005. *Code of Ethics and Standards of Professional Conduct*. Available at: http://www.iaao.org/sitePages.cfm?Page=70 [Accessed June 18, 2011].

National Society of Professional Engineers, NSPE Code of Ethics for Engineers. Available at: http://www.nspe.org/Ethics/CodeofEthics/index.html [Accessed June 18, 2011].

Online Ethics Center for Engineering and Research, 1998. *Inez Austin-Protecting the Public Safety at the Hanford Nuclear Reservation*. Available at: http://www.onlineethics.org/Topics/ProfPractice/Exemplars/BehavingWell/austinindex.aspx [Accessed June 18, 2011].

Varner, G. 2008. Utilitarianism and the Evolution of Ecological Ethics. *Science and Engineering Ethics*, **14**(4), 551–573.

Write cooperatively

6

Co-authors are colleagues with whom we implicitly contract to publish articles. Few activities are as important as publishing to launch a young researcher's career. For good or ill the old saw, "publish or perish," remains as true today as it ever was. To keep yourself moving forward professionally your name must appear regularly in the author line of journal articles. In some disciplines (philosophy, literary criticism) single-authored publications are the norm. However, in many fields today research is collaborative, a fact that gives rise to thorny questions about who is entitled to be an author. When has a junior member of a team done enough work to qualify? May the lead author exclude someone who has made significant intellectual contributions but not done any of the writing? Do authors differ from contributors? Whose names should be placed in the acknowledgments? In what order should names appear in the byline? How often may I publish my own work; may I publish the same paper simultaneously in a conference proceedings and in a refereed journal? And, who should make such decisions? The background essay answers these questions and provides a foundation for the issues raised in the case study.

Background essay: "Responsible authorship," by James R. Wilson, Lonnie Balaban and Gary Comstock[1]

As researchers, we must communicate our results with others. We are expected to write up our findings and share them, both in informal lab meetings and departmental seminars, and in more formal settings, such as conference proceedings and refereed journals.

---

[1] This article is itself a study in authorship. It is based on Wilson's February 2002 paper, "Responsible authorship and peer review" at http://www.ncsu.edu/grad/preparing-future-leaders/rcr/modules/module_2.doc [accessed July 19, 2011], a modified form of which appears as Wilson, J. R. 2002. Responsible authorship and peer review. *Science and Engineering Ethics* 8 (2): 155–174. Available at http://www.ise.ncsu.edu/jwilson/files/wilson02see.pdf [accessed July 19, 2011]. Comstock and Balaban are primary authors of the section called *Authorship is complicated* and Wilson is primary author of the section called *Acknowledging coauthors*. Wilson's article appears with the following Acknowledgment:

This work was supported by NSF Grant SES-9818359. Special thanks go to Tom Regan, Rebecca Rufty, Margaret King, and Nell Kriesberg (North Carolina State University) for many enlightening conversations on reasearch ethics. Thanks also go to Stephanie Bird (MIT), Frank Davidoff (Executive Editor, Institute for Healthcare Improvement; Editor Emeritus, *Annals of Inernal Medicine*), and the anonymous referees for numerous suggestions that substantially improved this

---

Authorship documents one's contributions to the advance of knowledge and is critical to the advancement of one's career. If we have not published, we cannot provide hard evidence of our ability to write well. The overworked slogan "publish or perish" suggests that authorship is the most respected form of expressing results; researchers of all ages rely on publications to advance their careers. If we fail to write up and publish our work then our colleagues will not know about what we have done – and we might as well have done nothing in the first place. Being able to communicate one's work effectively is essential to one's job prospects and it requires that we know the rules and conventions of authorship, an arena in which matters are not always straightforward.

Authorship is complicated

In past centuries, articles were mostly written by single researchers acting on their own. Deciding who was entitled to be an author was less of a problem and it was easier to give proper credit to everyone involved. Unfortunately, as research becomes more complex and interdisciplinary, the answer becomes increasingly complicated. Hollywood's image of the lone scientist bent over a workbench late at night is anachronistic. In fact, scores of individuals often cooperate to produce twenty-first-century research. While the size of research teams varies from discipline to discipline – some fields in the humanities continue to work on the single-researcher model and many articles in philosophy and history continue to be single-author works – research in most fields of science and engineering typically involves more than one person and discipline. In recent years, there has been a rapid proliferation of large, interdisciplinary research teams writing articles with tens or even hundreds of potential authors; in high-energy physics it is not unusual to find articles with dozens of authors. "A High Statistics Study of the Decay $\tau \rightarrow \pi - \pi^0 \, v_\tau$" lists more than 250 authors.[2]

But today, authorship is a much more complex issue. Should someone be listed because he/she supplied equipment or a strain of bacteria for experiments? (One is reminded of the lauded DNA discovers Francis Crick and James Watson, who downplayed the contributions of Rosalind Franklin in their famous *Nature* article, even though Franklin's photographs of the double helix launched their success. She didn't rate a byline, but was rather cordially thanked.) Should the director of the lab – whose only contribution was to secure funding for the project – be added to the list? What about other senior figures whose names would add prestige? Should undergraduates who have contributed to the work but may not fully understand its results be added as "honorary" authors? No, to all of these questions. Honorary authorship is – or should be – a thing of the past. If a Big Name has gotten funding for the work, or if colleagues and staff have gone out of their way to assist with the project, their contributions can be recognized in the acknowledgement section. We should also get rid of salami science (using the same opening and closing paragraphs in different articles while simply switching out the data in the middle) and fragmentary publishing (dividing a single set of data into two publications only to multiply lines on one's vita).

Just who is entitled to be an author? More than ever, we need explicit answers to this question. Blaise Cronin (2005) writes in *The Hand of Science: Academic Writing and its Rewards*, "Historically authorship implied writing. Today, the concept of authorship has expanded to accommodate a diverse array of contributions and inputs, some of which may require little or no engagement with the text qua text" (p. 55).

---

paper. James R. Wilson is professor of industrial engineering, North Carolina State University, jwilson@eos.ncsu.edu. Lonnie Balaban is a freelance writer and editor, Cary, NC, lonnie. balaban@gmail.com. Gary Comstock is professor of philosophy, North Carolina State University, gcomstock@ncsu.edu.
[2] http://www.arxiv.org/PS_cache/hep-ex/pdf/0512/0512071.pdf.

With large complicated science projects come many individuals performing large or small contributions to the whole. It is not surprising that authorship disputes are occurring more frequently [1,2]. So, who is responsible for the work, and exactly who should get the credit? Can you be an author without writing a word?

Common sense holds that anyone who makes a significant contribution to the work being reported deserves to be an author. But what does "significant contribution" mean? Common sense does not provide a clear answer this question. And yet providing an answer is critical to the continued success of a research team. Consider the consequences of not doing so.

One of the most famous researchers of the last two decades is Ian Wilmut, creator of the first cloned sheep. Dolly, whose birth appeared in the media all over the world, was described in a seminal 1997 paper in *Nature*. Almost 10 years after Dolly's birth, however, Wilmut's team was embroiled in controversy over the order of authors of the paper [3]. Wilmut's name appears as first author, a position that carries great weight in many fields, conveying the idea that this person was primarily responsible for the work. However, Wilmut himself admits that he did not do the majority of the work. What follows are comments by Wilmut, fellow scientists and technicians.

In an unrelated employment dispute in Edinburgh, Scotland, Wilmut responded to a lawyer's question by admitting that Professor Keith Campbell, an expert on the biology of cell cycles, deserved 66% of the credit for Dolly [3]. Doctoral candidate Angelika Schnieke, the researcher who earned the second spot on the *Nature* paper byline, was a graduate student at the Roslin Institute in Edinburgh at the time. She said Wilmut should not have been named first author and he should have given more credit to all the people involved. While Schnieke admitted that the co-authors agreed that Wilmut should be named first author, she also said that Wilmut wanted to be first author [4].

Meanwhile, a technician on the project, Bill Ritchie, has been quoted saying that he and another technician were responsible for most of the arduous laboratory work leading to Dolly's creation. He said that his and Mycock's names appear in the acknowledgement section of the paper, but that they should have appeared on the list of authors [3].

One might conclude from this public quarrel that the animal cloning scientific community is agreed that the lead scientist did not properly acknowledge his team in this case. To draw that conclusion, however, would be premature. Eckhard Wolf from the Institute for Molecular Animal Breeding at the University of Munich in Germany said, "If the basis of the (Dolly) research was (Wilmut's) idea, then there is no reason why he should not be first author" [4]. And Miodrag Stojkovic, a scientist in Spain, said that while Wilmut may have taken too much credit, this is common practice in scientific publishing [4].

In another recent incident Hwang Woo Suk, named the 2005 *Scientific American's* Research Leader of the Year, committed research fraud by falsely claiming he cloned a human embryo using far fewer donor eggs than expected, and in a later report claimed he created Snuppy, the first cloned dog. The findings of this extraordinary work were published in the prestigious journals *Science* and *Nature* (www. thelancet.com, January 7, 2006). The results were faked. After being exposed by a whistle-blower in his own lab, Hwang expressed remorse, but explained his behavior a result of stress and the expectations of others for him to succeed. While Hwang's case is scientific fraud it reveals issues in the scientific community's authorship conventions. Hwang invited well-known American researchers to be co-authors on his articles, hoping to add credibility to the work. The sole American researcher, Gerald Schatten, a professor from the University of Pittsburgh's School of Medicine, who was listed as senior author on the 2005 *Science* paper, "had little to do with the research" (www.thelancet.com, v.36, January 7, 2006; *Washington Post* December 30, 2005, p. 1; *NYT* December 25, 2006, p.1). According to a January 2006 *Lancet* editorial Schatten is now also the target of a formal university investigation.

Authorship disputes can be costly, consuming time and energy that could be better spent on more productive activities. In the next section you will read a case that vividly displays these costs. Should you become involved in a similar episode, one that drags on and on, the consequences could be debilitating professionally and personally. Before we turn to the case, however, let us introduce two models of authorship.

Acknowledging coauthors

Understanding the potential pitfalls of authorship should encourage you to discuss with your mentor the criteria used in your laboratory and discipline. Criteria for authorship vary not only among disciplines, but even between faculty members within the same discipline. The more you know about how your discipline and working group view authorship, the better off you will be. Our first piece of advice, therefore, is to discuss this issue with your mentor. Knowing how your mentor views the subject will help you to work with them to fend off potential problems.

Nearly everyone agrees that authorship requires contributing significantly to the intellectual content of the article. But what is a "significant contribution?" Answers differ from field to field, so we encourage you to begin with your mentor. As a beginning point for discussion, however, we describe three different models.

According to the first model, which we will call the traditional model, each principal investigator (PI) is individually responsible to decide authorship issues. The PI assesses the contributions of each person involved in the work and then uses criteria implicit in the accepted practices of the discipline to decide whether to include someone. Obviously, this model gives the PI a great deal of power, for the lead author is not only capable of adding a marginal figure to the authorship list but that person is also free to exclude a major contributor from the list. The fact that the traditional model delegates so much power to the senior person is one reason that it has been called into question. This is true in part because research teams get larger and larger and the number of authors submitting papers expands, too. Consequently, a second model is emerging in place of the received view.

According to the second – which we will call the democratic – model, selection of authors (or contributors) for a paper is jointly agreed by all collaborators. As soon as the group has decided on the assignment of responsibilities and workload for each member of the group, the group decides together who will be an author and in what place of authorship each person's name will be found. This idea, articulated first, perhaps, by the International Committee of Medical Journal Editors,[3] and largely adopted by the IEEE,[4] was motivated by the recognition that failure to achieve such consensus at the outset can have serious repercussions later. Perhaps the most extreme example of such a failure is the original paper on cold fusion [7], which Fleischmann and Pons prepared in such haste that they inadvertently omitted their co-author Marvin Hawkins – even though Fleischmann and Hawkins had done the bulk of the work in the months prior to the submission of the paper [8]; and there is some evidence that Hawkins heavily pressured his collaborators to be included as a coauthor in the list of errata [9] that soon followed [10].

Let us explore the democratic model before describing the third option.

ICMJE recommends that authorship credit be given if and only if a person has performed each of the following tasks:

(1) substantial contributions to conception and design, or acquisition of data, or analysis and interpretation of data;

(2) drafting the article or revising it critically for important intellectual content;

(3) final approval of the version to be published.

---

[3] ICMJE adopted guidelines in 1977 and a summary of the guidelines below represents the 2005 updated version available on their website http://www.icmje.org/index.html. Apparently, over 500 journals have adopted the ICMJE guidelines [5,6].

[4] For IEEE, authorship requires a "substantial intellectual contribution." Revisions to Section 8.2.1.A – Authorship, of IEEE PSPB Operations Manual, Amended 23 June 2006, require the review and approval of the IEEE Board of Directors. http://www.ieee.org/portal/cms_docs_iportals/iportals/publications/PSPB/opsmanual.pdf.

In the first category is scientific leadership and original ideas. Who came up with the original idea for the work? Who framed the hypothesis and designed the methods? Who organized and oversaw the progress of the research, ensuring that adequate equipment, space, time and personnel were provided? Who collected, processed, stored, organized, and interpreted the data? Who analyzed and made sense of the results?

Merely securing funding for a project or having a recognizable name in the field is not sufficient to be an author; one must be involved in a "hands-on" way. A substantial contribution includes providing leadership, designing an approved protocol, collecting and analyzing data, reviewing literature, and making sure that deadlines and objectives are met.

In the second category is writing: drafting, rewriting, revising, and reviewing the manuscript. ICMJE believes that participating in this process is necessary, not optional, for authorship. Who produced the first "dirty" draft? Who reworked and reorganized the material for coherence and precision. Who revised the piece for ease of readability?

In the third category is the responsibility for, and the right to, approve the final draft. As revisions are made, the claims made in manuscripts can change in subtle but significant ways. Every author must be given the opportunity to read the final version carefully, should ask probing questions about any discrepancies or new materials introduced to that version, and be prepared to defend that version in public. If coauthors do not perform these tasks, they may find themselves in the position Bertram Batlogg found himself in when his coauthor, Jan Hendrik Schon, was accused of fabricating data in a paper they had published in *Nature*. Without Batlogg realizing what had happened, Schon had inserted, on at least 16 occasions in various papers, reused data sets, mislabeled figures, and graphs produced on the basis of mathematical functions rather than, as advertised, with experimental data. What was Batlogg's responsibility in this case? The committee that reviewed the case said in its report that Schon and Batlogg were making extraordinary claims in their papers and asked whether Batlogg should not have "insisted on an *exceptional* degree of validation of the data in anticipation of the scrutiny that a senior scientist knows such *extraordinary* results would surely receive" (as quoted in Brumfiel 2002 [11]).

So, authors must meet 1, 2, and 3. Each author must have participated sufficiently in the work to take public responsibility for appropriate portions of the work. These guidelines suggest that every person listed as an author must have participated in the research by providing intellectual input, writing, and review of the manuscript.

When research involves large groups of individuals and centers, the group itself should take responsibility for identifying authors. The same criteria apply; only individuals meeting all three criteria – including willingness to accept direct responsibility for the manuscript – should be listed.

ICMJE recommends that the order of authors be a joint decision of all co-authors, and that the group be prepared to explain the order.[5]

Contributors who do not meet all three criteria for authorship should be listed in an acknowledgement section. This category can acknowledge those who provided technical help, writing assistance, individuals such as department chairs who provided general support, and other individuals, institutions, or agencies contributing financial or material support. The function played by each person may be specified, such as "clinical or participating investigator," "served as scientific advisor," "critically reviewed the study proposal," "collected data," or "provided and cared for study patients."

From a larger perspective, an even more serious problem in such situations is the lack of a clear-cut assignment of responsibility among all the potential authors for ensuring the integrity of the entire article and for answering any questions about the article that may arise after publication. These issues have led many scientists and scientific editors to propose alternatives to the traditional model for authorship outlined above. In particular, Rennie, Yank, and Emanuel [1] proposed

---

[5] Visit http://www.icmje.org/ for the latest updates to these requirements.

replacing the concept of an author with the concept of a contributor, whose role in the work is precisely specified in a footnote to the published paper; moreover in the same footnote at least one contributor (usually a co-investigator) is designated as a guarantor for the integrity of the article as a whole. Davidoff [2] asserts that full disclosure of the contributions of each collaborator merely ensures that the same high standards for accurately reporting the scientific information in the article are also applied in the assignment of credit and accountability for the work.

To follow up a 1996 conference held in England, "Is it time for a new approach to authorship?," the Council of Science Editors (CSE) convened a *Task Force on Authorship*, where a paper written by Paul J. Friedman [12] suggested researchers provide a modified copyright form which would be filled out an signed by all the authors. "A new standard for authorship" proposed a check-off list. Friedman, an MD from the University of California, suggested that contributions of the individuals associated with a manuscript be published to document the byline. Authors would check off the contribution categories and sign the form. The form lists relevant activities: concept, design, supervision, resources, material, data collection/processing, analysis/interpretation, literature search, writing, critical review, and other. CSE reports that several journals have implemented the contributorship plan in slightly different form and are collecting information about how well the system works (www.councilscience editors.org/authorship.cfm).

The selection of authors for a paper should be jointly agreed by all of the collaborators on a project as soon as the group has decided on the assignment of responsibilities and workload for all members of the group. Considerations of the division of labor naturally lead to the question of who shall be the primary or lead author.

The primary author is the author listed first in the article's byline. That person must have demonstrated the ability and willingness to exert intellectual leadership of the project so as to (a) assume responsibility for a major professional aspect of the work, and (b) ensure that all the project objectives are met. Thus the primary author of a paper is generally chosen based on an evaluation of that individual's contributions to the conception, planning, and execution of the study. Selection of the primary author often occurs after the experimental work has been performed but just before the paper is written. If two or more authors have contributed equally to the project, then the primary author should be the one who by mutual consent actually coordinates the overall writing of the paper. According to Houk and Thacker [13], individuals who satisfy one or more of the following criteria should be considered as candidates for primary authorship:

- Originality of contribution – the primary author made an original theoretical or methodological contribution that proved to be a highly important basis for the paper.
- Major intellectual input – throughout the study, the primary author generated ideas on the study design and modifications, on ensuring availability and use of appropriate experimental subjects or material, on productively conducting the study, on solving measurement problems, on analyzing and interpreting data in a particular way, and on preparing reports.
- Major feature of the manuscript – the primary author originated and developed the feature of the paper that is of central importance.
- Greatest overall contribution – the primary author did the most work, made the study succeed, provided intellectual leadership, and analyzed and interpreted the data.

No one is entitled to primary authorship solely because of administrative position or expertise in a particular subject or discipline. Selection of the primary author should reflect a consensus of the paper's coauthors on the most deserving individual.

Note that other designations such as first author, senior author, corresponding author, and last author are sometimes used to show different divisions of responsibility than were described above for the primary author [14]. For example, the senior author may be a faculty adviser (mentor) who coordinated the overall writing of a paper on a student's doctoral dissertation research, with the student listed as the first author, followed by any other members of the student's supervisory committee who played a significant role in the work, and with the senior author listed last. The term primary author is used in this paper to simplify the discussion.

We come now to a third option, the contributorship model. According to Rennie, Yank, and Emanuel [1] and Davidoff [2], all authors should arrive at mutually agreed-upon descriptions of their individual contributions to the paper, a mutually agreed-upon ranking of the relative importance of those contributions; and determination of the order of contributors in the byline based on the ranking; and explicit indication of each contribution in the article. The difference between the contributorship model and the democratic model is that the contributorship model specifies the work that each person has done. Here is an example taken from Hackam and Redelmeier [15]:

> **Author Contributions**: Dr Hackam had full access to all the data in the study and takes responsibility for the integrity of the data and the accuracy of the data analysis.
> *Study concept and design*: Hackam, Redelmeier.
> *Acquisition of data*: Hackam.
> *Analysis and interpretation of data*: Hackam, Redelmeier.
> *Drafting of the manuscript*: Hackam, Redelmeier.
> *Critical revision of the manuscript for important intellectual content*: Hackam, Redelmeier.
> *Statistical analysis*: Hackam, Redelmeier.
> *Obtained funding*: Redelmeier.
> *Administrative, technical, or material support*: Redelmeier.
> *Study supervision*: Redelmeier.
> *Literature retrieval*: Hackam.

Whichever of the three models you adopt, the primary author should coordinate the contributions of all the coauthors, who are responsible for both the style and content of their respective sections of the paper.

§§§

The following case is based on a real incident; names have been changed to protect the participants' confidentiality.

Case study: "Authorship: new faculty," by James R. Wilson, Daniel J. Robison and Gary Comstock[6]

Steven Plim was a tenure-track assistant professor of microbiology at Eagle River State University (hereafter "ERSU"). During the second year of a three-year contract he was undergoing the typical probationary review to determine whether the university would offer him a second three-year contract, during which time he would be considered for tenure.

---

[6] James R. Wilson is professor of industrial engineering, North Carolina State University, jwilson@eos. ncsu.edu. Daniel J. Robison is professor of forestry and associate dean for research, college of natural resources, North Carolina State University, robison@ncsu.edu.

For a case study involving a professor preparing to publish without acknowledging the contributions of his graduate student, see C. K. Gunsalus, M. C. Loui, and their students, "Responsible Conduct of Research Role-Plays: Authorship," http://nationalethicscenter.org/resources/126 [accessed October 25, 2011]. We gratefully acknowledge Gunsalus and Loui for inspiring us to write up our case. Their paper also contains pedagogical materials we have used to great benefit in the classroom.

Plim completed his PhD in Microbiology at Southeastern State University (hereafter "SSU") working under the direction of Associate Professor David Ryerson. There, Plim published several papers with Ryerson in journals such as *Microbial Products Abstracts* (hereafter, "MPA"), solid journals if not the top two or three in the field. Plim found working with Ryerson difficult because Ryerson did not seem to return papers promptly and Plim believed he was underpaid. Ryerson in turn found Plim minimally competent, vain, and unresponsive to his teaching methods. Nonetheless, the two were able to write a half dozen articles together and publish them in conference proceedings and similar venues.

Plim worked in Ryerson's lab for 5 years, but was continually frustrated by his inability to land a job despite getting interviews at prestigious universities. He began to think Ryerson was not supporting him and began to harbor resentments against his mentor. He was irritated that Ryerson would take weeks or even months to respond to drafts of manuscripts. Ryerson was in turn irritated that Plim did not work hard enough and did not have "good hands" in the lab. Nonetheless, Ryerson was instrumental in getting Plim his first position as a temporary Research Assistant Professor at SSU and then the tenure-track job at ERSU.

During his first year at ERSU, Plim published another paper based on data collected while at SSU. His department chair had told him that a single-authored paper counted more for building his resume for tenure. Plim figured that Ryerson – already a full professor and director of a research institute – neither needed nor wanted the credit. Working on those assumptions and knowing Ryerson's track record in returning manuscripts to him, Plim decided not to list Ryerson as a coauthor.

In August of his second year at ERSU, Plim found the following email in his inbox from Ryerson, his former mentor at SSU.

From: David Ryerson
Sent: Friday, August 20

To: Steven Plim
Subject: MPA (2007) 189, pp. 72–81

Hello Steven,
The paper I reference in the subject line above, is one I just discovered. Typically I scan the MPA contents of every issue, but somehow missed this one until just now. This paper is of course, 'Microbial response to stress in a sugar substrate' by you, Steven.

This is work we did together here at SSU, under my research direction, with my budget, from which we published a preliminary paper (Plim and Ryerson 2006) in the edited book by Short, Roberts and Strevens 2006 ("SRS"), which I helped to write and am a coauthor on, and which includes a full list of helpers in the acknowledgments section. And as coauthors you and I again published another piece of the work from this same research effort in *The Sugar Substrate* Vol 1 ("TSS"), which you cite in the MPA paper. The analytical work reported in MPA paper was done with equipment loaned to us from another scientist at SSU, who you do not acknowledge in MPA.

As you know, and participated in while you were here, the practice in the SSU lab under my direction is to be fully inclusive in coauthorship, as is the common and appropriate practice in every research group I have familiarity with.

The genesis for the work reported in these publications was the result of my thinking and the research direction I was steering our group. You were most certainly a collaborator and lead scientist on the actual effort, but you were not alone in this work in any fashion. I was to this effort far more in many ways than you indicate in the acknowledgments to your MPA article, "Dr. David J. Ryerson was involved in discussions of this work."

In all the work you did here, and for the data which you took with you to your new job to finish, I was integrally involved, and director of the research. On all other papers from your work here that I am aware of, we are coauthors. In fact I have been very flexible in giving you lead credit.

When we discussed how to construct the oral presentation and then paper for the 2006 SRS paper, we specifically decided to limit the extent of the data we would report, so that we would have the bulk of the data available for a peer-review journal. We discussed how the experiment was going and additional samples/data we might collect from the experiment, in order to fully utilize the experimental setup, and use it to develop an excellent peer-reviewed paper, such as in MPA. Soon after the SRS paper, when you were already at your new position, you put together the paper for TSS, and again we worked as coauthors, as was appropriate. This paper dealt with another dimension of the same study. Then out of the blue came the MPA paper with you as a sole author.

This is a serious professional ethical lapse. I am very disappointed to discover this. Publishing collaborative work without appropriate authorship is wrong. The sentences you used in MPA that are word for word from SRS and perhaps also from TSS, were words that I helped to write, have coauthorship of, and proper attribution of someone else's words, even when written collaboratively, is required.

If you felt like I should not have been a coauthor on the MPA paper, about work done within my own research program, you should have engaged me in a discussion. You did not. I cannot even begin to imagine an acceptable explanation for your decision to proceed as you did.

Publishing this way gives a false impression to the editors and readers of scientific journals, and is a disservice to direct collaborators. In addition, publishing this way may cause concern among those who funded the work and have been familiar with its development, fails to give proper credit to the scientists and the institutions that deserve credit, and it misrepresents the manner in which you have worked. In the manuscripts which remain to be completed from our collaborative work, I will be sure to include you as a coauthor as it is the proper thing to do. I will expect you to do the same. I cannot help but wonder if there are other papers you have written as a sole author which should have included other scientists as coauthors. Please tell me if you have published or are preparing to publish any other work from your efforts here at SSU without sharing authorship. Even one such paper is a serious matter.

- David

David J. Ryerson, Ph.D.
Associate Professor, Director – Microbial Products Research Institute
Southeastern State University

A week later, Plim responded as follows.

Date: Fri, 27 Aug
From: Steve

To: David Ryerson

Dear David,
I appreciate your communication, but wish you did not have those opinions. I believe that I used solid decision-making in determining that the MPA manuscript should be single author. I could explain my reasoning, but will spare you the detail. I am very much involved in my work here, this issue is behind me, and should be for you as well. I do wish I had done a better job on the Acknowledgements section of the MPA paper, especially about the people who helped me. Sorry about that.

There are indeed additional manuscripts to work on. I'll not exclude you from any that you perceive you worked on, when I complete them.

My very best,
Steve

Plim sent the message hoping he would not hear back from Ryerson. He was not so lucky. Ryerson contacted two colleagues at SSU, one an expert on research ethics and one a journal editor and the author of a paper on ethics and authorship issues. Ryerson also found in his files an early version of the MPA paper, a PowerPoint presentation listing Ryerson as first author and Plim as second author. Between the two previous papers and the PowerPoint, and general practices of authorship, Ryerson concluded there was no reason for Plim to exclude him as an author.

A half dozen emails ensued between Ryerson and his two SSU colleagues. They met face-to-face for several hours to discuss the situation. After this extensive consultation and careful consideration of the issue, Ryerson decided not to let the issue drop.

Steve,

I am pursuing the question of coauthorship I raised with you. This issue is not resolved and from your response it does not appear you fully appreciate what you have done or its implications. You should not have, 1) published MPA as a sole author, 2) used my words in a paper without attribution, 3) failed to acknowledge the people and institution where the work was conducted, and 4) implied in your acknowledgments section in the MPA paper that I was aware of this manuscript. I would not have agreed that you would be sole author on this work – as that would not be truthful – you did not work alone.

I notice the following in the MPA Guide for Authors available on the web:

Submission of an article implies that the work described is approved by all authors and tacitly or explicitly by the responsible authorities where the work was carried out.

Your acknowledgment to me in the MPA paper could reasonably be construed to affirm my tacit approval of the submission of the paper. Since I was not even aware of the existence of this paper at the time it was submitted, however, your acknowledgment of me amounts to a misrepresentation of the truth.

You need to contact the MPA journal and request that an erratum be published indicating that I am a coauthor. Before you do this you need to, 1) indicate to me that you will do this and when, 2) provide me a copy of the erratum verbiage before you submit it and allow me to approve its final wording, 3) copy me on all written correspondence with the journal in this regard, and 4) provide me an opportunity to carefully read the revised MPA paper and include in the errata any corrections I may have about the paper since I never had a chance to work on the manuscript previously.

In your email response of 20 August, you state, "There are indeed additional manuscripts to work on. I'll not exclude you from any that you perceive you worked on, when I complete them." I do not understand what you mean by "...that you perceive you worked on..." You should be aware that any work you did here with my budget and under my research direction – – is work that I was directly involved in. Such work belongs to me and SSU, as well as you. Sharing of authorship of such work is the full expectation.

This is a very serious issue.

Sincerely,

David Ryerson

Plim, piqued by Ryerson's response, wrote back as follows.

Hello David –
The following are my responses to the items you continue to raise.

Your letter of August 20th was so difficult to follow that I could not be expected to understand what you think I did that was incorrect. Perhaps you are right, that, "it does not appear you (me) fully appreciate what you have done and its implications." But then it is your role here to explain these things in a way that makes sense.

I was a new research "appointment" professor when this work was done, on your paid staff, but you were already a well established tenured professor. I collected the data concerns and did the real work. While you may assume authorship for information developed by graduate students and postdoctoral scientists under your guidance and working with your support, you cannot do this with a research professor.

The work done for the MPA manuscript was mostly done by me. It was my idea, my experimental design, my physical work, and I wrote the paper. Your effort was minimal and involved approval of my plan, and providing contacts. These are the contributions I mentioned in the Acknowledgements. I think you looked in on the work a couple times – I even remember one visit. Not much more. Did you do more on this effort? I suppose you did guide me on some challenges, however mostly I did the research work.

It seems to me that you got credit on all the papers from the lab regardless of how much you did on each. This is not something I ever protested. There were others in the group though who did complain to me. There was even one paper in JOMB that I should have been listed as first author and you later, but I gave the first position to you.

My big issue is that I always waited longer than I wanted to get comments back from you on draft papers. Seems it once took more than a couple years to get comments. And thus I could not publish as much as I wanted and this caused me to be overlooked for jobs that I was being interviewed for. You need to realize the impact of your behavior on people who work around you. On the paper in TSS I never did get any comments from you.

With regard to your assertion that in the MPA work I used your words without permission; I should say that those words were my words too and why would I need permission to use my own words?

I do not agree at all with your contention that I presented a false impression to the journal reader of your involvement in this work. You'll recall (and you'll see if you look at the document) that I wrote that you were "involved in discussions of this work."

We have had some problems in the past, and I hope you'll keep those in confidence. I have stories that could be problematic for you if I told them. I suppose you intend to do that to me. We can have that kind of interaction if you want.

I might be willing to do an erratum for MPA, if you want, but I caution you that I too will make inquiries of the editor about you. I feel you are wrong on the authorship issue, but we can continue to communicate about it.

Regards,
Steven

Ryerson and Plim continued emailing back and forth intermittently for several months. At one point, Plim agreed to publish an erratum in the journal not only listing Ryerson as coauthor but also acknowledging, at Ryerson's insistence, someone who had contributed the analytical apparatus and support staff who had provided training. After Plim agreed, Ryerson told his authorship ethics expert colleague that he believed they were on the path to a low-stress resolution.

When the time came to submit the joint letter to the journal, however, Plim changed his mind. He wrote to Ryerson as follows.

David – After speaking with people here and considering the issue I have decided that it will be bad for both you and me to publish an erratum. You'll recall that in the preliminary version of the erratum that you drafted and provided to me, it did not indicate why an additional author was being added, only that it was. Surely we'd need to explain "why" to the editor.

Given that the MPA paper is already in print, no one would ever see you name anyway on the paper or in reference searches. So it would be a waste to do this, and besides, you did not do anything on this research.

There are other and better ways to help each other and get past this problem. Should you be willing to drop your request that we do an erratum, then I think you should submit the outstanding paper that you have on your desk now, and as a sole author. I can even help you edit it. That way we'll be equal with single author papers.

No matter what, even if you insist on the erratum, I will not do so without putting my own reasoning into it. And, further, my understanding of this entire episode was explained to you in my earliest response to you.

This is my position.

– Steven

The end of the story can be quickly summarized. When Ryerson's colleague who had written about ethics and authorship did not hear from Ryerson for a year, he emailed Ryerson to ask whether the issue had been resolved. Ryerson said no, responding that he had done nothing further. His concluding thoughts were these:

I am still a pillar of indecision on this.
Do I care? Sure.
Does it matter to me? Only in a "fairness" way.
Do I want to nail this guy? Strangely enough, no.
Would I like to compel him to do the right thing? Yes.
Do I want to open the can of worms and take this to the editor and/or his dept head? Not sure.
Do I have an ethical obligation to take this further, even if I decide it's not important to me? Not sure.
If I take this further, it will cost me more time, and do I want to spend any more time on this? No.
Will I always feel like I let him get away with this? Yes.
Do I have any satisfaction out of the sweat I have caused him thus far? Some, if it means he'll clean up his act in the future.
If I send this on to the editor, does it also make sense to send it to his dept head at the same time? Not sure.
Do I send the whole thing unedited to the editor/dept head, or would I need to first write a summary, etc.? Probably for it to be useful and fair to these other people a summary is required.
Do I want to spend the time to write a summary and organize the emails? No.
Should I do this? Perhaps yes.
After I send the stuff on, I will surely have to answer questions from these people, and no doubt be made to reply to Steven's various counter arguments. What a drag.
If I go through this whole affair, then what? No satisfaction there either I am sure.
When I see his dept head this summer, do I say anything? Probably shouldn't, but maybe it's a good venue to do so, not sure.
What to do???
Am I grateful to the time and energy you have put into this? SO VERY GRATEFUL TO BE SURE – THANKS. Now what. . ..?

And that is where the matter rests to this day.

To avoid wasting time by becoming involved in an authorship dispute, ask questions early and often whenever you believe you may be entitled to be a coauthor of some work. Here are a few recommendations consistent with the spirit of both authorship models discussed above.

- Discuss authorship at the very beginning of a project. If your mentor does not bring it up, you bring it up.
- Do not add a friend's name as a quid pro quo.
- Do not ask a friend to run some standard statistical procedures to justify putting their name on the paper.

- Do not put a senior faculty member's name on a paper because they generally supervise the lab or secured the funding.
- An author may be responsible for only one part of a paper, but that author must have performed intellectual and compositional work for that part.
- Disagreements? Pick up the phone. Do not email. Email is not suited to discussion of sensitive matters that require each party to hear inflections of voice. Unlike email, phone conversations communicate verbal and nonverbal cues such as silences, allowing us to anticipate and head off misunderstandings.

Here are some practical questions and answers.

Guidelines: "Publication ethics: a common sense guide," by Wesley E. Snyder[7]

Should I acknowledge my sponsor in a publication?

Unless, for some special reason, your sponsor does not want their support acknowledged, your paper should include an acknowledgement, usually including the program and grant number.

Can I publish the same paper in two different places, for example in an electrical engineering conference and a mechanical engineering conference?

Yes you can, provided that in whichever is published second, you state something like "this is a copy of a paper originally published in the International Conference on Eggplant Engineering". And, provided the editor of the second publication is aware of this and approves it.

Can I submit a paper to two journals at once?

Normally no, this is considered an ethical violation, if for no other reason than the amount of work you are putting reviewers to. I recently heard of a reviewer who received the same paper to review simultaneously from four journals. It was declined by all. An exception could be made if both editors are made aware of the situation and approve (which they will not do).

What can I quote in a paper without citation?

Nothing.

What about figures?

If I use a figure which is trivially simple, can I simply photocopy it from another paper and use it without citation? If it is genuinely generic, e.g. a block diagram of a PID controller, you have two choices: you can redraw it or photocopy it. If you copy, you MUST gain permission. If you redraw it, no citation is necessary.

What about using my own previously published work?

That depends on where the work was previously published, and who the copyright holder is. If you simply copy some segment of work you previously did, you should state where it is copied from. For instance, "in our earlier work published in the Journal of Unverifiable Experiments, we said 'Cold Fusion is Hot' [Snyder, 98]." For more extensive quotes, over a page, or a figure, you should gain permission of the copyright holder. The IEEE policy on this topic states that an author may use his/her work again, provided it is cited.

---

[7] Wesley E. Snyder, "Publication Ethics: A Common Sense Guide" originally published in the June 2004 issue of *IEEE Robotics and Automation Magazine*. © 2004 Institute of Electrical and Electronics Engineers, Inc. http://www.ncsu.edu/IEEE-RAS/RAS/RASnews/041107PubEthicsGuide.htm. Sections reprinted here with permission of copyright holder. Wesley E. Snyder is professor of electrical and computer engineering, North Carolina State University, wes@ncsu.edu.

What about publications by authors who work for the US federal government?
In general, such publications may not by copyrighted, and you may copy, for example, a figure from such a publication without requesting permission. However, you still need to say "from the IEEE Transactions on Eggplant Engineering," – you don't just have to add "used with permission." Any time government employees publish a paper, they are supposed to include a disclaimer which says that copyrights are not owned by the publisher. Some other governments may have similar policies – I have not been able to sample every country; however, my colleagues from Europe and Japan tell me that the US seems to be unique in this aspect. In most other countries at least, copyrights are owned by the publication and/or the author, and not by the government.

What about web publications?
The problem with web publications is that the authors usually do not identify whether or not the publication is copyrighted. The author may have taken a figure from his/her publication in a journal (which is copyrighted) and put it on the web page. You should make every effort to track down the actual copyright holder. It is not always easy to do that (I once encountered a case where the copyright holder had died, and I had to contact the family), but you need to try very hard.

Finally, in the spirit of being explicit about the relative extent of each author's contributions, note that some authors are now providing estimates of the relative work each has done. Sripada and Stich recently declared in their first footnote: "Our best estimate of the relative contributions of the authors is: Sripada 80%, Stich 20%."[8] The more specific the information the better when authors are crediting their relative contributions.

Take home lessons

- Authors should contribute to the intellectual labor of designing or acquiring or analyzing data, and to the composition labor of drafting or revising the article, and should give final approval of the version to be published.
- Inexperienced assistant professors still learning the ropes may need guidance about authorship, and should be willing to accept such guidance.
- Senior professors should diplomatically provide guidance and work to arrive at mutually acceptable expectations with less experienced counterparts.
- Even if you have done most of the work on a project, you are not entitled to exclude others from authorship.
- Authorship issues are serious; do not take a cavalier attitude toward them.
- Research collaboration does not end with publication; each author has a responsibility to defend the paper.
- If your method or analysis deviates from generally accepted practices, describe why you chose the unconventional approach, its limits, and the ways in which it differs from common procedures.
- If an institution discovers falsification or fabrication of data or plagiarism in an article published by one of its faculty it must consider asking the journal to retract the paper.

---

[8] Chandra Sripada and Stephen Stich, "A Framework for the Psychology of Norms," to appear in P. Carruthers, S. Laurance and S. Stich, eds., *Innateness and the Structure of the Mind*, Vol. II. http://www.rci.rutgers.edu/~stich/Publications/Papers/Framework_for_the_Psychology_of_Norms_7-23-05.pdf.

- The corresponding author is also responsible if falsification or fabrication of data or plagiarism is found in the publication.
- Avoid honorary authorship, salami science, fragmentary publication, and quid pro quo arrangements.

References for Wilson, Balaban and Comstock

1. Rennie, D., Yank, V. & Emanuel, L. (1997) When authorship fails: A proposal to make contributors accountable. *Journal of the American Medical Association* **278**: 579–585.

2. Davidoff, F. (2000) Who's the author: problems with biomedical authorship, and some possible solutions. *Science Editor* **23**: 111–119.

3. Sample, I. (2006) Scientists dispute credit for Dolly. *The Guardian*, 10 March 2006. Available at: http://www.guardian.co.uk/science/2006/mar/11/genetics.highereducation [Accessed June 20, 2012].

4. Stafford, N. (2006) Scientists counter Wilmut criticisms. *The Scientist*, 15 March 2006. Available at: http://classic.the-scientist.com/news/display/23229/ [Accessed June 20, 2012].

5. Klein, A. & Moser-Veillon, P.B. (1999). Authorship: can you claim a byline? *Journal of American Dietetic Association* **99**(1): 77–79.

6. Stern, E.B. (2000). Authorship criteria: opening a dialogue. *American Journal of Occupational Therapy* **54**(2): 214–217.

7. Fleischmann, M. & Pons, S. (1989a) Electrochemically induced nuclear fusion of deuterium. *Journal of Electroanalytical Chemistry* **261**: 301–308.

8. Huizenga, J.R. (1993) *Cold Fusion: The Scientific Fiasco of the Century*. New York: Oxford University Press.

9. Fleischmann, M. & Pons, S. (1989b) Errata. *Journal of Electroanalytical Chemistry* **263**: 187–188.

10. Taylor, C. (1999) The cold fusion debacle, presented at Research Ethics Institute, 13–16 June, at North Carolina State University, Raleigh, North Carolina.

11. Brumfiel, G. (2002) Misconduct finding at Bell Labs shakes physics community. *Nature* **419**: 419–421.

12. Friedman, P.J. (1996) Advice to individuals involved in misconduct accusations. *Academic Medicine* **71**(7): 716–723.

13. Houk, V.N. & Thacker, S.B. (1990) The responsibilities of authorship, in: CBE Editorial Policy Committee, eds. *Ethics and Policy in Scientific Publication*. Bethesda, MD: Council of Biology Editors, pp. 181–184.

14. Macrina, F.L. (2000) *Scientific Integrity: An Introductory Text with Cases*, 2d edn. Washington DC: ASM Press.

15. Hackam, D.G. & Redelmeier, D.A. (2006) Translation of research evidence from animals to humans. *Journal of the American Medical Association* **296**(14): 1731–1732.

Chapter

7

Protect manuscripts

A peer reviewer is an implicit contractor

Peer reviewers are professionals who share their expertise with others by scrutinizing drafts of articles submitted to journals for publication. As members of the peer review community, we encounter peer review from two perspectives.

On the one hand, we may be asked to serve as a peer reviewer. In this role, we are given the goal of helping an editor to assess the quality of a piece. Our advice may also be solicited to help the author improve the form and substance of the draft. In either case, we must be mindful of our duty to protect the author's intellectual property.

On the other hand, we may receive comments and suggestions from colleagues who serve as peer reviewers. From either perspective, the peer review process is a sterling example of contractualism at work. When we review manuscripts we do not simply offer criticism. Rather, we offer evaluative judgments that editors may use to make decisions about the value of the piece and that the authors might use to revise it. When we read another's comments we commit ourselves to respecting their privacy and property. Peer review is a complex social activity in which both authors and reviewers have responsibilities. Reviewers must do their jobs conscientiously, and authors should at least seriously read the comments of reviewers even if their manuscript was rejected.

James R. Wilson has had two decades of experience as a journal editor. In the following essay he describes the norms of peer review.

Background essay: "Peer review," by James R. Wilson[1]

Over the past 20 years, I have accumulated considerable experience in mediating extremely acrimonious disputes between researchers acting as "severe Popperian critics" of each other's work. Much of this hard-won experience was gained during the 9 years that I served as a departmental editor and former departmental editor of the journal *Management Science*. To avoid reopening wounds which have not had much time to heal, I will not go into the particulars of any of these cases; but I feel compelled to draw some general conclusions based on these cases.

In every one of the disputes that I mediated, the trouble started with extensive claims about the general applicability of some simulation-based methodology; and then failing to validate these

---

[1] This article constitutes the last half of Wilson, J., 2002. Responsible Authorship and Peer Review. *Science and Engineering Ethics*, 8, pp. 155–174. James R. Wilson, professor of industrial engineering, North Carolina State University, jwilson@eos.ncsu.edu.

---

claims independently, reviewers and other researchers proceeded to write up and disseminate their conclusions. This in turn generated a heated counterreaction, usually involving claims of technical incompetence or theft of ideas or both. Early in my career I served as the "special prosecutor" in several of these cases. Later on I moved up to become the "judge," and in the end I was often forced to play the role of the "jury" as well. In every one of these cases, ultimately the truth emerged (as it must, of course) – but the process of sorting things out involved the expenditure of massive amounts of time and energy on the part of many dedicated individuals in the simulation community, not to mention the numerous professional and personal relationships that were severely damaged along the way [6, p. 1410].

[W]hen authors violate [Richard] Feynman's precepts of "utter honesty" and "leaning over backwards" by overselling their work, the cost to the scientific enterprise of policing these individuals rapidly becomes exorbitant.

1. Role of the peer review system

The main purpose of the peer review system is to serve the community of researchers – and ultimately to benefit society – by providing expert advice to:

- editors of archival journals who must make decisions on acceptance, rejection, or revision of papers submitted to their journals; and
- program managers of funding agencies who must make funding decisions on the research proposals submitted to their programs.

At the most basic level, the peer review system performs a quality-control function that is essential to maintaining the self-correcting character of the scientific research enterprise. The Royal Society of London is frequently given credit for introducing the concept of refereeing or reviewing scientific manuscripts when that organization took over official responsibility for publication of the *Philosophical Transactions* in 1752 [7] However, it was not until the first decade of the twentieth century that increasing specialization forced editors in virtually all scientific disciplines to seek systematically the advice of subject-area experts on the publishability of highly technical articles [8] In recent years a parallel to this development can be found in the rise of open software standards – and the principal advantage claimed for this approach to software development is that superior software products result from "peer review" by the users and developers of such software [9].

Beyond the "sifting and sorting" function described above, the peer review process can also substantially improve the quality of papers that are ultimately published. In particular, conscientious referees can provide invaluable feedback to the author on revisions that will substantially improve the clarity and readability of a paper.

However, there are some things peer review cannot do.

- Peer review cannot detect fraud.

As mentioned above, proper functioning of the peer review system depends critically on the honesty of authors. Relman elaborated on this point:

> When authors say what they did and what they observed, there must be a presumption of honesty, because reviewers and editors cannot know what occurred in the laboratory. Occasionally, internal inconsistencies or implausible results might raise suspicions of malfeasance, but it is usually difficult, if not impossible, to recognize fraud solely from perusal of a manuscript. Detection of fraud or other malfeasance is the responsibility of the author's co-workers or supervisors at the institution where the work is done, not of reviewers or editors. [10, p. 273]

The Darsee case [28] is perhaps the most well-known example of scientific fraud to occur in recent years. Dr. John R. Darsee was a young clinical investigator in the Cardiac Research Laboratory of the Brigham and Women's Hospital (a teaching affiliate of Harvard University) who was caught fabricating data by his associates and supervisors at Harvard in May 1981. A series of investigations ensued – first at Harvard (1981–1982); then at the National Heart, Blood, and Lung Institute (1981–1982); and finally at the National Institutes of Health (1983). Ultimately Darsee was found to have fabricated research publications starting when he was a biology student at Notre Dame, continuing through his medical residency and cardiology fellowship at Emory University, and ending at Harvard. Altogether 17 primary journal articles and 53 abstracts had to be retracted as a result of these investigations. Although Darsee's coauthors on the faculties of Emory and Harvard were found to have had no part in the fraud, these coauthors were unaware of Darsee's fabrications because they had little or no contact with the work that was reported in the retracted publications.

Relman [12] elaborates the lessons learned from this case concerning the imperatives of responsible authorship and the limitations of the peer review system.

- Peer review cannot certify the validity of a manuscript.

There is the widespread misconception, particularly among those outside the scientific community, that passing peer review guarantees the truth of the paper's results; and then highly publicized failures like the cold fusion episode lead to questions about the value of the peer review system. Relman put this issue in the proper perspective.

> Even at its best the system can guarantee the truth of a manuscript no more than it can the honesty of an author. Rather, its function is to hold a scientific report to the best current standards, to ensure that the design and method are acceptable by those standards, and to ensure that the data are properly analyzed and interpreted. As knowledge in the field develops, new developments will improve methods and modify older concepts. Even the best current research will probably be superseded by more sophisticated and insightful work, which might reveal unsuspected limitations or flaws in previous reports. [10, p. 276]

Clearly conscientious peer review is essential to the continued advance of science. Without it, the literature would be flooded with papers of wildly varying quality; and readers would face the overwhelming task of sifting through all this material to identify research contributions of value.

2. Problems with the peer review system

In recent years the peer review system has begun to show increasing signs of distress.

2.1. Nonperformance of editors and reviewers

By far the most serious problem with the peer review system for archival journal articles is simple dereliction of duty:

- by editors who refuse to take responsibility for "hard" editorial decisions, preferring to operate by majority vote of the referees; and
- by referees who cannot be bothered to read and evaluate carefully the work of other researchers, leaving editors as referees of last resort.

There is substantial anecdotal evidence that in some areas of science and engineering, this problem is growing worse over time; and this trend may be related to the increasingly intense competition for publications and funding [13]. Perhaps the most egregious failure of the peer review system in recent years was the publication of the initial paper on cold fusion by Fleischmann and Pons [2] in the *Journal of Electroanalytical Chemistry* just four weeks after submission; and there is some evidence that this paper was reviewed only by the editor of the journal and not by independent referees [1, pp. 219–220; 17]

Of even greater consequence is the problem of nonperformance by editors. For her pioneering work on radioimmunoassay, R.S. Yalow [14] received the 1977 Nobel Prize in Physiology or Medicine – and yet the key paper that led to this recognition was rejected by *Science* and by the

Journal of Clinical Investigation. The editor of the latter journal finally agreed to publish the paper in question only after extensive negotiations. Yalow made the following incisive remarks about the problem of nonperformance by editors.

> It is the editor's responsibility to determine whether the reviewer's reports or the rebuttals by the authors have more merit. In the cases cited the problem was not in the review process per se, but in the lack of editorial competence. On occasion I have written to remind editors that their office is not simply a letter drop, that theirs is the responsibility to act as judges between the reviewer's report and the author's response. In fact in my Nobel lecture (Yalow 1978), I published the initial letter of rejection from the *Journal of Clinical Investigation* of work that was to prove to be of fundamental importance to the development of radioimmunoassay. Eventually we reached a compromise with the editor, and the paper was published. I have since had the opportunity of writing to other editors who rejected our papers saying, "You may not become as famous as [the editor] in being identified in a Nobel lecture, but you are on the right track." [15, p. 244]

2.2. Conflicts of interest of reviewers

With increasing specialization and fragmentation of disciplines, competitors within narrow subdisciplines are more frequently called upon to evaluate each other's papers and grant proposals, creating the potential for serious conflicts of interest. In particular, such conflicts of interest may tempt referees to engage in the following types of misconduct:

- misappropriation of ideas – that is, stealing ideas from the papers and grant proposals that a referee is asked to evaluate; and
- misappropriation of priority – that is, delaying or obstructing the publication or funding of a referee's rivals so that the referee can be the first to publish a result or to receive funding for work in a particular area.

Misappropriation of ideas is particularly hard to guard against since it may occur unintentionally or subconsciously. In situations where the solution to one of the referee's own research problems is found in a paper or grant proposal sent to the referee for confidential review, permission to use the ideas in question must ultimately be sought from the author and acknowledged in papers that exploit those ideas.

Goodstein gave the following analysis of the problem of conflicts of interest of reviewers:

> Peer review is not at all suited, however, to adjudicate an intense competition for scarce resources such as research funds or pages in prestigious journals. The reason is obvious enough. The referee, who is always among the few genuine experts in the field, has an obvious conflict of interest. It would take impossibly high ethical standards for referees to fail to use their privileged anonymity to their own advantage. Most scientists do hold themselves to high standards of integrity, but as time goes on, more and more referees have their ethical standards eroded by the unfair reviews they receive when they are authors. Thus the whole system is in peril.
>
> ... Recently, as part of a talk to a large audience of mostly young researchers at an extremely prestigious university, I outlined this analysis of the crisis of peer review. The moderator, a famous senior scientist, was incredulous. He asked the audience how many disagreed with my heresy. No one responded. Then he asked how many agreed. Every hand in the house went up. [13, p. 402]

2.3. Inadequate recognition and encouragement of innovation

Examples abound of groundbreaking ideas that were rejected for publication or not funded because of the inherent conservatism (or lack of imagination?) of reviewers; in particular see McCutchen [16] and Horrobin [17]. Yalow summarized the gist of the problem with the following memorable remark.

> There are many problems with the peer review system. Perhaps the most significant is that the truly imaginative are not being judged by their peers. They have none! [15, p. 244]

Editors must be constantly on the lookout for highly innovative submissions, ensuring that referees of the highest quality are engaged in evaluating such work; and ultimately editors must make an informed judgment on the publishability of the work based on a careful reading of the work itself as well as the referees' reports on the work.

2.4. Publication bias

In the fields of education, medicine, and psychology, there is clear evidence of publication bias reflecting the direction and strength of study results [18] Such bias is the main cause of underreporting research discussed above. Other causes of bias in referees' reports include: jealousy; revenge; and prejudice against certain topics, individuals, or institutions [16] It is the job of the editor to detect such referee bias and compensate for it in making editorial decisions.

2.5. Variability of reviewers: assassins, demoters, pushovers, and zealots

Siegelman [19] coined the term demoter to describe a referee who recommends rejection of submitted papers much more frequently than the norm for "mainstream" referees, whereas a pushover recommends acceptance much more frequently than the norm for "mainstream" referees. Similarly, he coined the term assassin to denote an extreme demoter; and a zealot is an extreme pushover. Demoters and assassins contend that the standards for publication should be elevated since too many papers of marginal quality are currently being published; and thus demoters and assassins often provide lengthy reviews of a submitted paper that detail irreparable inadequacies in the paper's theoretical and experimental results or in the documentation of those results. By contrast, pushovers and zealots often seek to increase the visibility of their academic subdisciplines by making a concerted effort to increase the number of high-quality publications in those subdisciplines; and thus pushovers and zealots often provide lengthy reviews of a submitted paper that include helpful suggestions for revision. To avoid the potential for unfair treatment of authors, editors should carefully monitor the performance of reviewers, ensuring some balance in the types of referees assigned to each submitted paper.

3. Guidelines for peer review

3.1. Archival journal articles

Two of the main reasons for breakdowns in the operation of the refereeing system are
- misconceptions by referees about the job they are supposed to do; and
- misperceptions by referees about the incentives for doing a good job of refereeing, and the consequences of doing a poor job.

As Gleser [20] points out, many referees think that a manuscript must be checked line by line for errors; and seeing that this will be extremely time-consuming, they continually put off the task. On the contrary, the referee's main responsibility is to serve the editor as an "expert witness" in answering certain key questions about the manuscript – and most of these questions can be answered under the assumption that the manuscript is error-free. The eminent mathematician G.H. Hardy got to the nub of the matter by saying that a referee must answer three questions about a piece of research offered for publication [21, p. 119]:
3. Is it true?
2. Is it new?
1. Is it interesting?

Although Hardy prescribed the order of these questions, they are numbered in reverse to suggest that in many cases the work required to produce a competent review is not nearly so great as it initially appears to be, since a negative answer to Question 1 (Is it interesting?) eliminates the need for investing the time and energy necessary to give correct answers to the

Table 2. Key questions to be answered in a referee's report

1. Are the problems discussed in the paper of substantial interest? Would solutions of these problems materially advance knowledge of theory, methods, or applications?

2. Does the author either solve these problems or else make a contribution toward a solution that improves substantially upon previous work?

3. Are the methods of solution new? Can the proposed solution methods be used to solve other problems of interest?

4. Does the exposition of the paper help to clarify our understanding of this area of research or application? Does the paper hold our interest and make us want to give the paper the careful reading that we give to important papers in our area of specialization?

5. Are the topic and nature of this paper appropriate for this journal? Are the abstract and introduction accessible to a general reader of this journal? Is the rest of the paper accessible to a readily identified group of readers of this journal?

6. Are the clarity and readability of the manuscript acceptable? Is the writing grammatically correct?

7. Does the manuscript contain an adequate set of references? Is adequate credit given to prior work in the field upon which the present paper is built?

8. Is the material appropriately organized into an effective mix of text, figures and tables? Are data given in tables better presented in figures or in the text?

9. Is the work technically correct? Are the main conclusions justified by the experimental data and by logically valid arguments? Are the theorems stated and proved correctly given the assumptions? In practical applications of the theoretical results, do the authors check the validity of the underlying assumptions?

10. Are there gaps in the discussion of the experimental methods or results? If there are such gaps, can the closing of these gaps be considered (i) essential, (ii) desirable, or (iii) interesting? Are the experimental methods described in sufficient detail so that other investigators can reproduce the experiments?

11. Have the authors explicitly addressed the limitations of their study?

other two questions. Truesdell provides a cogent example of a review that concisely answers all three of Hardy's questions:

> This paper, whose intent is stated in its title, gives wrong solutions to trivial problems. The basic error, however, is not new. ... [22, p. 561]

Forscher [23], Gleser [20] and Macrina [5, pp. 62–66] provide comprehensive guidelines for refereeing; see also Table 2 below. Although some research suggests that little improvement in referees' reports results from providing referees with a checklist, training, or editorial feedback [24, 25] the generalizability of these conclusions is unclear [26, 27] On the other hand, there is some evidence that improvement in referees' reports may result from eliciting specific evaluations of separate, concrete aspects of the paper under review rather than a general global evaluation of the entire paper [28].

The questions in Table 2 are designed to elicit the desired specificity in referees' reports. If a paper passes the initial screening that consists of answering Questions 1–8 in Table 2, then it is necessary to undertake the verification of technical correctness required to answer Questions 9 and 10. If competent referees had scrutinized the initial paper on cold fusion by Fleischmann and Pons [2] with the objective of answering Questions 9 and 10 in Table 2, then the serious flaws in this work would have been uncovered immediately [1, pp. 219–220]. Finally we note that Question 11 of Table 2 requires the referee to verify that the paper includes an explicit discussion of the limitations of the study. Essentially Question 11 of Table 2 asks if the authors have adhered to Feynman's ideal of "utter honesty" and "leaning over backwards" in reporting their results. In an analysis of changes made by authors to papers that were ultimately published in the *Annals of Internal Medicine*, Purcell *et al* [29] found that the most common required revision was the inclusion of information on study limitations.

Additional tips on effective refereeing are given by Waser, Price, and Grosberg [30]. A set of questions similar to those given in Table 2 can be found on the home page of the *ACM Transactions on Modeling and Computer Simulation* by visiting <http://www.acm.org/pubs/tomacs/review/review.html>.

4.2. Grant proposals

Rosenzweig, Davis, and Brown [31] argue that it is much more damaging to a discipline to suppress important contributions than to fund or publish questionable research since new ideas cannot have any effect unless they are developed and publicized, while serious errors are usually detected and corrected. Thus they argue that reviewers of grant proposals should adopt the attitude that a proposal does not deserve funding unless it is daring, novel, or interesting; and in such cases, it is not sufficient simply to make brief, mildly positive statements of approval of the proposed research. Instead it is necessary to include in the review detailed answers to the following questions.

1. Why is the proposed research important?
2. What contribution will the proposed research make?
3. Why are the investigators qualified to do the work?

Of course similar specificity is required in discussing the weaknesses of a proposal; but it is highly desirable to guard against the well-known tendency for reviewers to provide much more detailed comments on the negative aspects of a proposal than on the positive aspects since such an imbalance tends to introduce an excessively conservative bias into the deliberations of review panels. Rosenzweig, Davis, and Brown summarize their recommendations thus:

> In order to convey a more accurate impression of our collective labors, we all need to make a conscious effort to tolerate diverse ideas and unconventional approaches, and to promote independence and originality. Robert Reich [former U.S. Secretary of Labor in the Clinton Administration] has written that "Technological innovation is largely a process of imagining radical alternatives to what is currently accepted." Thus it can thrive only if dissent is tolerated. In our reviews, we must encourage that dissent and emphasize the advances it will make possible. . . . The scientific enterprise . . . is in its very nature mutualistic and collaborative. . . . It is up to us . . . to use the peer review system carefully and wisely. Only then can it serve the goal that we all share: the rapid advancement of our discipline. 31, pp. 154–155]

Spier [32] contends that when peer review of grant applications results in sponsorship of truly innovative research, this fortunate outcome probably occurs in spite of the review process rather than because of it. He suggests that some proportion of research funding (say, 10%–20%) should be devoted to long-term support for key researchers who are identified by a radically new selection process, possibly involving randomized project selection or a lay panel that will reflect pressing social priorities. On the other hand, Chubin asserts that

> Wise stewards and editors make defensible decisions based on peer advice most of the time. If they did not, we would not still pay homage – in word and deed – to peer review. [33, pp. 111]

To address the problems of the peer review system, Chubin calls for a more "scientific" approach to public accountability of the operation of this system. As in the case of peer review of archival journal articles, significant improvements in peer review of grant proposals will require formulation of effective guidelines for reviewers – especially in written evaluations of potentially innovative proposals.

5. Carrots and sticks in the peer review system

At all levels of the scientific enterprise, it is recognized that reviewing manuscripts and grant proposals is one of the most important ways in which individual researchers can contribute to the development of their discipline. McCutchen observed that reviewing of journal articles and grant applications gives reviewers the intellectual pleasure of interacting with authors and proposers, as well as education that, I suspect, has led to more advances than generally realized. These rewards are legitimate [16, p. 158].

Since the best referees generally receive the best papers and proposals to review, those individuals enjoy the benefits of continual professional enrichment and renewal. Moreover, high-visibility editorial positions are usually filled from the ranks of prompt and insightful reviewers; and most universities and many other research organizations regard appointment to such positions as grounds for promotion and other forms of professional advancement.

The most serious consequence of bad refereeing is the long-lasting damage to an individual's reputation in the eyes of editors and program managers, who increasingly maintain computerized records on the performance of reviewers [34]. Some editors even go so far as to maintain two lists of referees, say the "A" list of good referees and the "B" list of bad referees; and when authors from either list submit a paper for review, the editor selects referees for that paper from the list to which the author belongs.

To further enhance the incentives for good reviewing, editors should provide timely feedback to referees on (a) the strengths and weaknesses of their reviews, and (b) the issues identified in other referees' reports on the same paper. As a professional courtesy, editors should include such feedback with their letters of appreciation to referees. For major journals with high rates of submission, some selectivity may be required to make this suggestion practical; in particular, editors might provide detailed editorial feedback to referees only in cases for which (i) the paper is judged to be a major contribution to the literature, or (ii) the editorial decision-making process is particularly difficult. Moreover, editors should strive to ensure that individuals who provide prompt and thorough refereeing will receive comparable service when those individuals submit their own papers for review.

6. Conclusions

In essence this article's central thesis is simply this: the proper functioning and continued advancement of the scientific enterprise depends critically on individual scientists living up to the standards of ethical conduct so memorably articulated by Feynman – not only in the design, execution, and documentation of their research projects, but also in their response to the challenges of responsible, professional peer review.[2]

[2] Acknowledgments: This work was supported by NSF Grant SES-9818359. Special thanks go to Tom Regan, Rebeca Rufty, Margaret King, and Nell Kriesberg (North Carolina State University) for many enlightening conversations on research ethics. Thanks also go to Stephanie Bird (MIT), Frank Davidoff (Executive Editor, Institute for Healthcare Improvement; Editor Emeritus, Annals of Internal Medicine), and the anonymous referees for numerous suggestions that substantially improved this paper.

References for Wilson

1. Huizenga, J.R. (1993) *Cold Fusion: The Scientific Fiasco of the Century*. Oxford University Press, New York.

2. Fleischmann, M., and Pons, S. (1989a) Electrochemically induced nuclear fusion of deuterium. *Journal of Electroanalytical Chemistry* **261**: 301–308.

3. Fleischmann, M., and Pons, S. (1989b) Errata. *Journal of Electroanalytical Chemistry* **263**: 187–188.

4. Taylor, C. (1999) *The cold fusion debacle, presented at Research Ethics Institute*, 13–16 June, at North Carolina State University, Raleigh, North Carolina.

5. Macrina, Francis L. (2000) *Scientific Integrity: An Introductory Text with Cases*, 2nd edn. ASM Press, Washington DC.

6. Wilson, J.R. (1997) Doctoral colloquium keynote address: Conduct, misconduct, and cargo cult science, in: Andradóttir, S., Healy, K.J., Withers, D. H., and Nelson, B. L., eds. Proceedings of the 1997 Winter Simulation Conference, Institute of Electrical and Electronics Engineers, Piscataway, New Jersey, pp. 1405–1413. Available via <www.informs-cs.org/wsc97papers/1405.PDF> [accessed February 26, 2002].

7. Kronick, D.A. (1991) Peer review in 18th century scientific journalism, in: Peer Review in Scientific Publishing: Papers from the First International Congress on Peer Review in Biomedical Publication, Council of Biology Editors, Chicago, pp. 5–8, also available as: Kronick, D.A. (1990) Peer review in 18th century scientific journalism. *Journal of the American Medical Association* **263**: 1321–1322.

8. Burnham, J.C. (1991) The evolution of editorial peer review, in: Peer Review in Scientific Publishing: Papers from the First International Congress on Peer Review in Biomedical Publication, Council of Biology Editors, Chicago, pp. 9–26, also available as: Burnham, J.C. (1990) The evolution of editorial peer review. *Journal of the American Medical Association* **263**: 1323–1329.

9. Raymond, E.S. (2000) The cathedral and the bazaar [online], available on the web via <www.tuxedo.org/~esr/writings/cathedral-bazaar/cathedral-bazaar> [accessed February 26, 2002].

10. Relman, A.S. (1990) The value of peer review, in: CBE Editorial Policy Committee, eds., *Ethics and Policy in Scientific Publication*. Council of Biology Editors, Bethesda, MD, pp. 272–277.

11. Culliton, B.J. (1983) Coping with fraud: The Darsee case. *Science* **220**: 31–35.

12. Relman, A.S. (1983) Lessons from the Darsee affair. *The New England Journal of Medicine* **308**: 1415–1417.

13. Goodstein, D. (1995) Peer review after the big crunch. *American Scientist* **83**: 401–402.

14. Yalow, R.S. (1978) Radioimmunoassay: a probe for the fine structure of biologic systems. *Science* **200**: 1236–1245.

15. Yalow, R.S. (1982) Competency testing for reviewers and editors. *The Behavioral and Brain Sciences* **5**: 244–245. J.R. Wilson 174 *Science and Engineering Ethics*, Volume **8**, Issue 2, 2002.

16. McCutchen, C.W. (1997) Peer review: Treacherous servant, disastrous master, in: Elliott, D.E., and Stern, J.E., eds. Research Ethics: A Reader, University Press of New England for the Institute for the Study of Applied and Professional Ethics at Dartmouth College, Hanover N.H., pp. 151–164, also available as: McCutchen, C.W. (1991) Peer review: Treacherous servant, disastrous master. *Technology Review* **94**: 27–40.

17. Horrobin, D.F. (1991) The philosophical basis of peer review and the suppression of innovation, in: Peer Review in Scientific Publishing: Papers from the First International Congress on Peer Review in Biomedical Publication, Council of Biology Editors, Chicago, pp. 250–259, also available as: Horrobin, D.F. (1990) The philosophical basis of peer review and the suppression of innovation. *Journal of the American Medical Association* **263**: 1438–1441.

18. Dickersin, K. (1991) The existence of publication bias and risk factors for its occurrence, in: Peer Review in Scientific Publishing: Papers from the First International Congress on Peer Review in Biomedical Publication, Council of Biology Editors, Chicago, pp. 92–104, also available as: Dickersin, K. (1990) The existence of publication bias and risk factors for its occurrence. *Journal of the American Medical Association* **263**: 1385–1389.

19. Siegelman, S.S. (1991) Assassins and zealots: Variations in peer review. *Radiology* **178**: 637–642.

20. Gleser, L.J. (1986) Some notes on refereeing. *The American Statistician* **40**: 310–312.

21. Halmos, P.R. (1985) *I Want to Be a Mathematician*. Springer-Verlag, New York.

22. Truesdell, C. (1951) Review of "Equations of finite vibratory motions in isotropic elastic media. Surface force sufficient to maintain equilibrium," by García, G. (1950) *Actas Acad. Ci. Lima* **13**: 29–38, *Mathematical Reviews* **12**: 561.

23. Forscher, B.K. (1965) Rules for referees. *Science* **150**: 319–321.

24. Callaham, M.L., Wears, R.L., and Waeckerle, J.F. (1998) Effect of attendance at a training session on peer reviewer quality and performance. *Annals of Emergency Medicine* **32**: 318–322.

25. Callaham, M.L., Knopp, R.K., and Gallagher, E.J. (2002) Effect of written feedback by editors on quality of reviews: Two randomized trials. *Journal of the American Medical Association to appear*.

26. Jefferson, T., Alderson, P., Wager, E., and Davidoff, F. (2002) The effects of editorial peer review: A systematic review. *Journal of the American Medical Association to appear*.

27. Jefferson, T., Wager, E., and Davidoff, F. (2002) Measuring the quality of editorial peer review. *Journal of the American Medical Association to appear*.

28. Strayhorn, J., McDermott, J.F., and Tanguay, P. (1993) An intervention to improve the reliability of manuscript reviews for the Journal of the American Academy of Child and Adolescent Psychiatry. *American Journal of Psychiatry* **150**: 947–952.

29. Purcell, G.P., Donovan, S.L., and Davidoff, F. (1998) Changes to manuscripts during the editorial process. *Journal of the American Medical Association* **280**: 227–228.

30. Waser, N.M., Price, M.V., and Grosberg, R.K. (1992) Writing an effective manuscript review. *BioScience* **42**: 621–623.

31. Rosenzweig, M.L., Davis, J.I., and Brown, J.H. (1988) How to write an influential review. *Bulletin of the Ecological Society of America* **69**: 152–155.

32. Spier, R.E. (2002) Peer review and innovation. *Science and Engineering Ethics* **8**: 99–108.

33. Chubin, D.E. (2002) Much ado about peer review, Part 2. *Science and Engineering Ethics* **8**: 109–112.

34. Abelson, P.H. (1992) Integrity of the research process. *Science* **256**: 1257.

How to proceed as a peer reviewer

Actively pursue opportunities to serve as a peer reviewer. The experience will help you to become more informed about the state of art in your field. Clarify with your editor or mentor whether the review is anonymous or open and scrupulously protect the confidentiality of the manuscript. Do not take ideas from it and include them in your own work.

Take home lessons

- Read carefully any specific instructions you are given.
- Remember that your primary task is to make judgments about the quality of the manuscript or grant proposal and to evaluate its scientific or scholarly significance.
- Ask for further informal advice about any unclear matters, such as whether the review should be exceptionally stringent or lenient, or whether your review should focus on this or that particular problem or section of the manuscript.
- Decline to review papers that have data or results that directly overlap with your work on the basis that you have a conflict of interest.
- If you believe you have been treated unfairly by a reviewer, write to the journal editor to express your concern.

Clarify statistics

8

The image of the solitary biologist standing in a field counting butterflies and recording the numbers in a notebook still conjures up a picture of "real science" for some of us old timers. Research procedures are vastly different now. Typically, single individuals don't produce data on their own – or record them only by hand; rather, interdisciplinary groups use computers and other electrical devices, amassing and recording their findings on software spreadsheets and in databases. Consequently the production, management, mining, and stewardship of data are processes rife with social, ethical, political, and legal implications. The moral issues associated with the interpretation of statistics are complex.

To get the ball rolling, consider just one introductory example. Journals generally seem unwilling to publish negative findings. If your study does not produce positive results, should you explore hypotheses about relationships in the data that were not part of your original design? If you switch mid-stream to a new statistical method in order to try to find some positive results, you may be mining, milking, or dredging data. In this way you may be able to suggest some interesting relationships and spur additional research, but your work may not be useful in proving any hypothesis. There are limits to the number of statistical methods and tests that may legitimately be used to explore a data set. In general, you should stick to the methods identified in your original plan for data analysis. If after the data are collected you adopt novel methods you may be guilty of making post hoc inferences. Such inferences themselves are not illegitimate but you must adopt appropriate methods to explore them. And the dangers are significant because it's so easy to find misleading patterns. Caution is essential when looking for correlations the set was not constructed to reveal.

Let's look now in more detail at the ethical issues associated with statistical analysis.

Collect data responsibly

There's no way around it. You need to spend time attending to your records. Your own publications depend on it, the ability of others to reproduce your results requires it, and the possibility that you might reap financial benefits from it makes it indispensable. Your data are intellectual property, and you have a claim to the data, albeit a limited claim. Having a complete research record will also be critical if you ever encounter a situation in which a person or group accuses you of misconduct. In any case, a careful record is required by federal regulations, including, in the US, the policies of the Health Insurance Portability and Accountability Act (HIPAA) Privacy and Security Rules.

Research Ethics: A Philosophical Guide to the Responsible Conduct of Research. Gary Comstock.
Published by Cambridge University Press. © Cambridge University Press 2013.

When you gather data, you almost certainly will store them in an electronic form. The best way to ensure the safety and confidentiality of the information set is to limit access to it. Use strong passwords and change them often. Regularly review who is permitted to access it. Responsibility for stewardship of the data does not end with collection and analysis; our duties extend to our interpretation and public representation of what we have found.

One must design research protocols carefully if one expects to produce valid results. A key decision is arriving at the sample size, known as n. In any particular research project or study, it's desirable that n be chosen to maximize the probability of achieving significant results given the willingness of the study's researchers to tolerate error and its estimations of effect sizes. When researchers calculate n thoughtlessly, or when a study does not carefully formulate n, the research results are likely to be inconclusive. This risk is especially large when researchers don't collect sufficient data or they change midstream the parameters and hypotheses established at the beginning of the study.

Let's see how this discussion relates to a real-life example. Suppose you and a few others are hired to interview grocery store shoppers about their preferences. You are good at the work and quickly complete more protocols than any of the other half-dozen assistants. The manager of the research project complements you and asks if you would be willing to train a new interviewer. You are pleased and quite willing to take on the new job. Meanwhile, you overhear another interviewer interpreting a question differently than you have been interpreting it. You ask around, and discover that your interpretation is idiosyncratic; other interviewers are not only providing explanations that are at odds with yours, but they are also eliciting responses that differ significantly from the results you've been getting. What should you do? Try to convert the other interviewers to your interpretation without consulting the manager? Change your interpretation to match theirs? Send an email to the Institutional Review Board, inform it of the problem, and ask that the study be suspended until an investigation can begin? Well, you should probably do none of the above. Begin with the research manager. Explain the problem. Ask for clarification of the interview item. Suggest the manager meet with all of the interviewers to discuss the dilemma. Collaboratively reach a consensus reading of all of the survey items.

. . . and guard its confidentiality

Audit your data often. Check to make sure you have recorded them properly, compare them to the original sources, and be on the lookout for errors. Errors can result, for example, from using two or more notation systems for recording the data, miscalibrating a machine, improperly reading a gel, or misunderstanding a figure. Backup the data in a secure room separate from the room in which the main computer is located and free of environmental hazards. Avail yourself of public data repositories if appropriate. Retain the record for as long as necessary, at least 3 to 7 years, so that others can reproduce the results and check it for veracity.

It is common practice to keep one's data on a personal computer. To ensure that the data stay confidential, keep the computer in a locked room and, we repeat for emphasis, use a strong password. To ensure that the integrity of the data is preserved, have one individual enter the data and another individual clean and validate them. To protect against theft and fire, back up your files onto secondary servers in a building other than the one housing your computer(s), and stay current with software updates to your operating system.

Be attentive, as well, to the unique parameters of certain kinds of research. Research with human subjects, for example, often produces data that can be traced to specific persons. To protect the confidentiality and preserve the anonymity of those involved in the research, researchers must do more than save their files in locations they think will be hard to find. They may assign numbers to the data while stripping out all names, keep a list that matches names to numbers on a secure server, and encode the data, providing the data-key only to those who need it. They may also limit access to the data, changing passwords and access codes whenever there is a change in who is permitted to view the data.

The NIH advocated data sharing in a policy it published in 2003 (National Institutes of Health 2003). The policy, designed to promote scientific inquiry as well as build capacity to replicate findings, specifies that Principal Investigators submitting proposals larger than a half million dollars in direct costs in a single year must describe how they plan to share their results. This policy is important, because it requires timely release of findings and assists graduate students in publishing their work. Do not release data before they are published; doing so may facilitate other researchers reaching premature conclusions if they read unfinalized drafts.

Case study: "What educated citizens should know about statistics and probability," by Jessica Utts[1]

... I have selected seven topics that I have found to be commonly misunderstood by citizens, including the journalists who present statistical studies to the public. In fact the researchers themselves, who present their results at the scientific meetings from which the journalists cull their stories, misunderstand many of these topics. If all students understood them, there would be far less misunderstanding and confusion in the public eye. In fact the public is often cynical about statistical studies, because these misunderstandings lead to the appearance of a stream of studies with conflicting results. This is particularly true of medical studies, where the misunderstandings can have serious consequences when neither physicians nor patients can properly interpret the statistical results.

A summary of the seven topics covered in this article is presented first, followed by a more in-depth explanation with examples for each topic:

1. When it can be concluded that a relationship is one of cause and effect, and when it cannot, including the difference between randomized experiments and observational studies.
2. The difference between statistical significance and practical importance, especially when using large sample sizes.
3. The difference between finding "no effect" or "no difference" and finding no statistically significant effect or difference, especially when using small sample sizes.
4. Common sources of bias in surveys and experiments, such as poor wording of questions, volunteer response and socially desirable answers.
5. The idea that coincidences and seemingly very improbable events are not uncommon because there are so many possibilities.
6. Understanding that what may appear to be a trend is just a part of a cycle in a time series.
7. Understanding that variability is natural, and that "normal" is not the same as "average."

---

[1] Reprinted from *The American Statistician* May 2003, vol. 57, no. 2, pp. 74–79. Copyrighted 2003 by the American Statistical Association. All rights reserved. Jessica Utts is professor and chair of statistics, University of California, Irvine, jutts@uci.edu.

1. Cause and effect

Probably the most common misinterpretation of statistical studies in the news is to conclude that when a relationship is statistically significant, a change in an explanatory variable is the cause of a change in the response variable. This conclusion is only appropriate under very restricted conditions, such as for large randomized experiments. For single observational studies, it is rarely appropriate to conclude that one variable caused a change in another. Therefore, it is important for students of statistics to understand the distinction between randomized experiments and observational studies, and to understand how the potential for confounding variables limits the conclusions that can be made from observational studies.

As an example of this problem, an article appeared in *USA Today* titled "Prayer can lower blood pressure" (Davis, 1998). The article reported on an observational study funded by the United States National Institutes of Health, which followed 2,391 people aged 65 or over for 6 years. One of the conclusions reported in the article read:

> Attending religious services lowers blood pressure more than tuning into religious TV or radio, a new study says. People who attended a religious service once a week and prayed or studied the Bible once a day were 40% less likely to have high blood pressure than those who don't go to church every week and prayed and studied the Bible less.

> (Davis, 1998)

The headline and the displayed quote both indicate that praying and attending religious services actually causes blood pressure to be lower. But there is no way to determine a causal relationship based on this study. It could be that people who are healthier are more able to attend religious services, so the causal relationship is the reverse of what is attributed. Or, it could be that people who are more socially inclined are less stressed and thus have lower blood pressure, and are more likely to attend church. There are many other possible confounding variables in this study that could account for the observed relationship. The problem is that readers may mistakenly think that if they alter their behavior with more prayer and church attendance, it will cause their blood pressure to lower.

. . .

2. Statistical significance and practical importance

Students need to understand that a statistically significant finding may not have much practical importance. This is especially likely to be a problem when the sample size is large, so it's easy to reject H0 even if there is a very small effect. It is also a common problem when multiple comparisons are done, but only those that achieve statistical significance are reported. As an example, the *New York Times* ran an article with the title "Sad, Lonely World Discovered in Cyberspace" (Harmon, 1998). It said, in part:

> People who spend even a few hours a week online have higher levels of depression and loneliness than they would if they used the computer network less frequently . . . it raises troubling questions about the nature of "virtual" communication and the disembodied relationships that are often formed in cyberspace.
> (Harmon, 1998)

It sounds like the research uncovered a major problem for people who use the Internet frequently. But on closer inspection, the magnitude of the difference was very small. On a scale from 1 (more lonely) to 5, self-reported loneliness decreased from an average of 1.99 to 1.89, and on a scale from 0 (more) to 3 (less), self-reported depression decreased from an average of .73 to .62.

. . .

3.   Low power versus no effect

It is also important for students to understand that sample size plays a large role in whether or not a relationship or difference is statistically significant, and that a finding of "no difference" may simply mean that the study had low power. For instance, suppose a study is done to determine whether more than a majority of a population has a certain opinion, so the test considers H0:p=0.5 versus Ha:p>0.5. If in fact as much as 60% of the population has that opinion, a sample size of 100 will only have power of 0.64. In other words, there is still a 36% chance that the null hypothesis will not be rejected. Yet, reporters often make a big deal of the fact that a study has "failed to replicate" an earlier finding, when in reality the magnitude of the effect mimics that of the original study, but the power of the study was too low to detect it as statistically significant.

As an example with important consequences, a February 1993 conference sponsored by the United States National Cancer Institute (NCI) conducted a meta-analysis of eight studies of the effectiveness of mammography as a screening device. The conclusion about women aged 40–49 years was "For this age group it is clear that in the first 5–7 years after study entry, there is no reduction in mortality from breast cancer that can be attributed to screening" (Fletcher *et al.*, 1993*)*. The problematic words are that there "is no reduction". A debate ensued between the NCI and American Cancer Society. Here are two additional quotes that illustrate the problem:

> A spokeswoman for the American Cancer Society's national office said Tuesday that the . . . study would not change the group's recommendation because it was not big enough to draw definite conclusions. The study would have to screen 1 million women to get a certain answer because breast cancer is so uncommon in young women.
>
> (*San Jose Mercury News*, Nov 24, 1993)

> Even pooling the data from all eight randomized controlled trials produces insufficient statistical power to indicate presence or absence of benefit from screening. In the eight trials, there were only 167,000 women (30% of the participants) aged 40–49, a number too small to provide a statistically significant result.
>
> (Sickles and Kopans, 1993)

The confidence interval for the relative risk after 7 years of follow-up was 0.85 to 1.39, with a point estimate of 1.08, indicating that there may be a small reduction in mortality for women in this age group, or there may be a slight increase. (See Utts, 1999, p. 433.) The original statement that there was "no reduction in mortality" is dangerously misleading.

The lesson to convey in this context is that students should be wary when they read that a study found no effect or relationship when the researchers expected there to be one. Generally, this conclusion is newsworthy only when it contradicts earlier findings or common wisdom. It is important in such cases to find out the size of the sample and, if possible, to find a confidence interval for the results. If the confidence interval is wide or if it tends to be more to one side of chance than the other, there is reason to suspect that the study may not have had sufficient power to detect a real difference or relationship.

. . .

4.   Biases in surveys

There are many different sources through which bias can be introduced into surveys.
Some of the more egregious are difficult to detect unless all of the details are understood. For example, a Gallup Poll released on July 9, 1999, based on a random sample of 1016 US adults, asked two different questions in random order, each of which could be used to report the percentage of people who think creationism should be taught

in public schools in the United States. The two questions and the proportion that answered "Favor" were:

Question 1: Do you favor or oppose teaching creationism ALONG WITH evolution in public schools? (68% Favor)

Question 2: Do you favor or oppose teaching creationism INSTEAD OF evolution in public schools? (40% Favor)

Notice that depending on one's own opinion, these results could be misused to advantage.

Someone in favor of creationism could report that 68% think it should be taught, while someone opposed to creationism could report that only 40% think it should be taught. There are many examples of how question wording, question order, method of sample selection and many other issues can bias survey results. See Utts (1999) or Utts and Heckard (2002) for lengthy discussion and examples.

5. Probable coincidences

Most people have experienced one or more events in their lives that seem to be improbable coincidences. Some such events are so surprising that they attract media attention, often with estimates of how improbable they are. For instance, Plous (1993) reported a story in which a Mr. and Mrs. Richard Baker left a shopping mall, found what they thought was their car in the parking lot, and drove away. A few minutes later they realized that they had the wrong car. They returned to the parking lot to find the police waiting for them. It turned out that the car they were driving belonged to another Mr. Baker, who had the same car, with an identical key! Plous reported that the police estimated the odds at a million to one.

The problem with such stories and computations is that are based on asking the wrong question. The computation most likely applies to that exact event happening. A more logical question is, what is the probability of that or a similar event happening sometime, somewhere, to someone. In most cases, that probability would be very large. For instance, I was once on a television talk show about luck, with a man who had won the million dollar New York State lottery twice, and the host of the show thought this demonstrated extraordinary luck. While it may have been wonderful for that individual, Diaconis and Mosteller (1989) report that there is about an even chance of the same person winning a state lottery in the United States in a 7-year period. That was precisely the interval between the two wins for this person.

. . .

Remember that there are over six billion people in the world, with many circumstances occurring to each one daily. Therefore, there are surely going to be some that seem incredible. In fact if something has only a one in a million probability of happening in a given day, it will happen, on average, to over 6000 people in the world, each day. When the media reports an incredible coincidence, psychic prediction, and so on, it should be viewed from this perspective.

6. Confusion of the inverse

Most teachers of statistics know that probability can be very confusing to students, and that intuition about probability is not very good. Psychologists have identified a version of this problem that leads to important misunderstandings, called "confusion of the inverse." The basic problem is that people confuse the conditional probability $P(A/B)$ with the conditional probability $P(B/A)$.

As an example, Eddy (1982) presented this scenario to 100 physicians:

One of your patients has a lump in her breast. You are almost certain that it is benign, in fact you would say there is only a 1% chance that it is malignant. But just to be sure, you have the patient undergo a mammogram, a breast X-ray designed to detect cancer.

Table 8.1. Breakdown of actual status versus test status for a rare disease

	Test is malignant	Test is benign	Total
Actually malignant	800	200	1,000
Actually benign	9,900	89,100	99,000
Total	10,700	89,300	100,000

You know from the medical literature that mammograms are 80% accurate for malignant lumps and 90% accurate for benign lumps. In other words, if the lump is truly malignant, the test results will say that it is malignant 80% of the time and will falsely say it is benign 20% of the time. If the lump is truly benign, the test results will say so 90% of the time and will falsely declare that it is malignant only 10% of the time.

Sadly, the mammogram for your patient is returned with the news that the lump is malignant. What are the chances that it is truly malignant?

Most of the physicians responded with an answer close to 75%. But in fact, given the probabilities presented, the correct answer is only about 7.5%! Eddy reported: "When asked about this, the erring physicians usually report that they assumed that the probability of cancer given that the patient has a positive X-ray was approximately equal to the probability of a positive X-ray in a patient with cancer (1982, p. 254)." In other words, the physicians confused the probability of a positive test given that the woman has cancer with the probability that the woman has cancer given that the test was positive.

Most medical tests have low false positive and false negative rates, yet the probability of having the disease, given that a test result is positive, can still be quite low if the initial probability of having the disease is low. In that case, most positive test results will be false positives.

I find that the easiest way to illustrate this concept for students is through what I call a "hypothetical hundred thousand" (Utts and Heckard 2002, p. 228), which is a table showing the theoretical breakdown of results for 100,000 people. Table 8.1 illustrates the breakdown using the numbers for the example Eddy presented to the physicians. Notice that of the 10,700 patients whose test is malignant, only 800, or about 7.5% actually had a malignancy. Because there were so many more women with benign lumps than malignant lumps, the 10% of them with a false positive test made up the large majority of positive test results.

. . .

7. Average versus normal

The seventh concept students need to understand is that of natural variability and its role in interpreting what is "normal." Here is a humorous example, described by Utts and Heckard (2002). A company near Davis, California, was having an odor problem in its wastewater facility, which they tried to blame on "abnormal" rainfall:

> Last year's severe odor problems were due in part to the extreme weather conditions created in the Woodland area by El Nino [according to a company official]. She said Woodland saw 170 to 180 percent of its normal rainfall. "Excessive rain means the water in the holding ponds takes longer to exit for irrigation, giving it more time to develop an odor."
>
> (Goldwitz, 1998)

The problem with this reasoning is that yearly rainfall is extremely variable. In the Davis, California, area, a five-number summary for rainfall in inches, from 1951 to 1997, is 6.1, 12.1, 16.7, 25.4, 37.4. The rainfall for the year in question was 29.7 inches, well within the "normal" range. The company official, and the reporter, confused "average" with "normal." This mistake is very common in reports of temperature and rainfall data, as well as in other contexts. The concept of natural variability is so crucial to the understanding of statistical results that it should be reinforced throughout the introductory course.

. . .

The issues discussed in this article constitute one list of common and important misunderstandings in statistics and probability. There are obviously others, but I have found these to be so prevalent that it is likely that millions of people are being misled by them.

. . . I serve on many PhD exam committees for students who are doing research across a wide range of disciplines. There are two questions I ask every student. One is to explain the meaning of a *p* value. The other has to do with replicating a study with an important finding, but using a smaller sample size – the researcher is surprised to find that the replication study was not statistically significant. I ask students to give possible explanations. I am sorry to report that many students have difficulty answering these questions, even when they are told in advance that I'm going to ask them. I will know we have fulfilled our mission of educating the citizenry when any student who has taken a statistics class can answer these questions and similar ones on the topics in this article and related conceptual topics.

References for Utts

Clark, H. H., & Schober, M. F. (1992). Asking Questions and Influencing Answers. In *Questions About Questions*, ed. J. M. Tanur. New York: Russell Sage Foundation, pp. 15–48.

Davis, R. (1998). Prayer can lower blood pressure. *USA Today*, August 11, 1998, 1D.

Diaconis, P., & Mosteller, F. (1989). Methods for studying coincidences. *Journal of the American Statistical Association*, **84**, 853–861.

Eddy, D. M. (1982), "Probabilistic Reasoning in Clinical Medicine: Problems and Opportunities," in *Judgment under Uncertainty: Heuristics and Biases*, eds. D. Kahneman, P. Slovic, and A. Tversky. Cambridge, UK: Cambridge University Press, chap. 18.

Fletcher, S. W., Black, B., Harris, R., Rimer, B. K., & Shapiro, S. (1993). Report on the international workshop on screening for breast cancer. *Journal of the National Cancer Institute*, **85**(20), 1644–1656.

Goldwitz, A. (1998). *The Davis Enterprise*, March 4, 1998, A1.

Harmon, A. (1998). Sad, lonely world discovered in cyberspace. *New York Times*, August 30, 1998, A3.

Magliozzi, T., & Magliozzi, R. (2001). How AAA's Foundation for Traffic Safety Misused

Otherwise Good Data, online at http://www.cartalk.cars.com/About/Drive-Now/aaa.html.

Perkins, K. D. (1999). Study: age doesn't sap memory. *Sacramento Bee*, July 7, 1999, **A1**, A10.

Plous, S. (1993). *The Psychology of Judgment and Decision Making*. New York: McGraw Hill.

Stickles, E. A., and D. B. Kopans (1993). Deficiencies in the analysis of breast cancer screening data. *Journal of the National Cancer Institute*, **85**(20), 1621–1624.

Stutts, J. C., Reinfurt, D. W., Staplin, L., & Rodgman, E. A. (2001). The role of driver distraction in traffic crashes. Technical Report; available online at www.aaafoundation.org, May 2001.

Tanur, J. (ed.) (1992), *Questions About Questions: Inquiries into the Cognitive Bases of Surveys*. New York: Russell Sage Foundation.

Utts, J. M. (1999). *Seeing Through Statistics*, 2nd edn. Pacific Grove, CA: Duxbury Press.

Utts, J. M., & Heckard, R. F. (2002). *Mind on Statistics*. Pacific Grove, CA: Duxbury Press.

Weber, G. W., Prossinger, H., & Seidler, H. (1998). Height depends on month of birth. *Nature*, **391** (6669), Feb 19, 754–755.

Conclusion: some reservations about contractualism

We now switch gears, turning attention away from the particular topics of the last few chapters and returning to the ethical theory introduced in Part B. We'll end this part in the same way that we ended Part A, with some brief thoughts about the adequacy of the ethical theory that has been guiding us.

As we have seen, contractualism has several strengths. Like egoism, it insists on what Rawls calls "the separateness of persons" (Rawls 1971). This is a virtue in an ethical theory, because it makes us pause whenever we try to justify harming an individual on the grounds that others will benefit. Contractualism does not allow us to consider persons as receptacles of utility, nor does it allow us to maximize utility without regard for how individuals will fare under the proposed policy. Rather, it insists that we respect individuals by listening to all reasonable objections one might make on their behalf and by following through with the arrangements we have made with them.

That said, however, contractualism is not without fault. In fact, it has one major shortcoming; it seems to underestimate the scope of morality, because it may include only a portion of human beings in its circle. Contractualists believe we have direct obligations only to those humans capable of using language and reason and who can participate in debates about the justifiability of their actions. But why should the group of humans included in the moral community be restricted in this way? Why aren't the interests of infants, children younger than the so-called "age of accountability," the severely cognitively impaired, and the elderly senile morally considerable? Because of their cognitive limitations, these people cannot be contractors. Consequently, contractualism has no way to condemn mistreatment of these people if the mistreatment does not break any agreements between contractors and misfortunate humans, who, after all, do not know how to contract.

This facet of the theory is very difficult to accept. For consider just one of its implications, that we would be free to harm feral children in scientific experiments. Feral children are children raised without human contact, such as Victor of Aveyron, found in 1899 in the woods of France. Allegedly raised by wolves until he was 11 years old, Victor lacked language entirely and was seemingly incapable of acquiring it. Clearly, feral children cannot understand contractual agreements and some of them may not even have the potential to acquire the capacity in question. Were we, without telling anyone, to decide that Victor would be better off dead than exposed to the vicissitudes of culture, and if we then painlessly and humanely euthanized him in order to study his brain post-mortem, would we have done anything wrong from a contractualist point of view?

The answer is no. Victor, we are assuming, is not a contractor and is unable to become a contractor. The problem is not just that Victor is not yet party to any agreements. Rather, it's that he lacks any potential to become a party to any agreements. If we do not make any promises to him after finding him, then he is not a contractor. If he could not understand such promises if we did make them, then he can never become a contractor, either. If we have not entered into any implicit agreements about how we would treat feral children we might happen to find then those children are not even potentially parties to any contracts. Therefore, being neither free nor rational in the relevant senses, Victor could not object to being euthanized nor, arguably, could anyone else so argue on his behalf. But this result is deeply troubling. The fact that contractualism leaves the way open to euthanization of noncontracting humans is a good reason to be suspicious of the theory.

The same point can be put in a slightly different way. Contractualism works well when moral questions involve our interests – the interests, that is, of the community of researchers and our loved ones. All of us have language, rationality, and morality. But when we ask about the interests of those outside the research community, those like Victor, contractualism seems to come up with the wrong answers. For contractualism tells us we have no direct duties to noncontractors (although, in fairness, it can easily argue that we have indirect obligations to them). But why don't we have such duties? Don't our duties extend to individuals beyond our tribe of rational contractors?

Fairness alone seems to dictate that we owe strangers something, even those strangers we may not care about, even those who are not even potential members of our linguistic community. A third moral theory does not have this problem. The family of theories we'll call moral rights theories all require that justice be done to those who are not fully rational. The fact that Victor is sentient, makes choices, and has a dignity of his own gives him moral rights and his possession of those rights makes it wrong for us to humanely euthanize him even if no one else ever knows that we have done so. The rights perspective insists on including all mentally challenged humans in the moral circle.

The two moral frameworks discussed to this point have their strengths and weaknesses. A weakness of egoism, you'll recall, is that it does not recognize the interests of anyone other than the self. A weakness of contractualism is that it does not recognize the interests of humans incapable of making and keeping promises. The framework to which we turn in Part C addresses these deficiencies by emphasizing the rights of all, including the rights of children, the senile elderly, strangers, and the mentally incapacitated.

Take home lessons

- Ensure the safety and confidentiality of data by limiting access, using strong passwords, and changing passwords regularly.
- To ensure the integrity of the data, have different individuals enter and clean the data, and keep secure backup copies in separate physical locations.
- Unless your grant requires immediate release of data, don't release data before they are published because others may draw premature conclusions from it.
- Don't equate correlation with causation.
- Carefully choose your study's sample size to avoid inconclusive research results due to lack of sufficient data collection.
- Keep in mind the differences between typical or normal and average – and between statistical significance and practical importance – especially when your sample size is large.
- Absence of evidence, goes the saying, is not evidence of absence. Observe Utts' distinction between no difference and no statistically significant difference, especially when your sample size is small.
- Avoid bias in surveys by wording questions carefully.
- Define all methods of analysis before you begin to collect data, avoid making post hoc inferences, and guard against using one method after another until you happen upon a significant result.

Bibliography

National Institutes of Health, 2003. *Final NIH Statement on Sharing Research Data*. Available at: http://grants.nih.gov/grants/guide/notice-files/NOT-OD-03–032.html.

Rawls, J. 1971. *A Theory of Justice*, original edn. Cambridge, MA: Belknap Press.

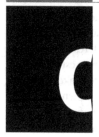

Respect strangers' rights

Whereas egoism guided our explorations in Part A and contractualism served to structure Part B, a third theory will guide us in Part C. Moral rights theorists focus on the protections deserved by all beings who have autonomy and, therefore, are entitled to have their choices protected – or who have interests and, therefore, are entitled to have their welfares protected. Like contractualists, moral rights theorists emphasize the fact that individuals have their own distinct conceptions of the good life, that people make and ought to keep promises, and that moral decisions should be made on the basis of reasons that are acceptable to free and equal persons. Unlike contractualists, moral rights theorists do not limit their concerns to those individuals capable of making contracts. Rights theorists who highlight interests recognize that some individuals are not capable of understanding reciprocal agreements, and yet those individuals have the right to be protected. The point of this chapter is to introduce the broad outlines of moral rights.

We hear people claiming their rights every day, whether it's a right to privacy or free expression or private property. Imagine a new graduate student in good standing, Jermaine. Jermaine, we say, has a right – a moral right – to enter graduate school. His right consists of at least two components. First, he has the privilege to go to school because he is free of any duties not to do so. Now, we can imagine situations in which he would not have this privilege, for example, if he had failed to submit proof of his undergraduate degree or if he had not paid his tuition. But Jermaine, as we say, is in good standing, and all such conditions have been removed. He is at liberty to go to class. Second, he has a valid claim against those who would deprive him of this liberty because he has submitted all of the required forms and completed all of the steps necessary to be admitted. Should anyone try to prevent him from walking into his classes, Jermaine has good grounds to object to their actions and he is entitled to seek the assistance of authorities as he goes about the lawful pursuit of his interests.

Moral rights theories recognize privileges and valid claims that arise from contracts. In this way moral rights theories are consistent with contractualism; both theories recognize contractors, potential contractors, and individuals with whom contractors could hypothetically make agreements. But rights theorists go further. They typically recognize the rights of all human beings whether or not they are contractors, potential contractors, or included in the contracts of others. Here, then, is the first difference between the two views; rights theories protect a larger number of beings than do contractualist theories.

A second difference has to do with the way in which each theory justifies its claims. Contractualism explains why the agreements we make with each other are binding. Rights

Research Ethics: A Philosophical Guide to the Responsible Conduct of Research. Gary Comstock.
Published by Cambridge University Press. © Cambridge University Press 2013.

theorists, noting that not every human being can make agreements, rest their theory on the nature of persons as free agents (the so-called "will theory" that emphasizes autonomy) or they rest their theory on the nature of persons as subjects of a life (the so-called "interest theory" that emphasizes welfare). Whereas contractualism is grounded in the covenants people establish with each other, rights theories are grounded in the capacity of sentient individuals to make their own free choices or to have a welfare (that is, the capacity to have the kind of life in which things can go well or badly for the individual). Whether the rights theory emphasizes autonomy or interests, it insists that we respect the dignity of individuals even if those individuals lack the intelligence or cognitive resources to enter into contracts.

If these claims seem puzzling, an example might help. Some human beings are not capable of understanding contracts: children, the senile elderly, the cognitively handicapped, the irreversibly demented. None of these individuals is cognitively equipped to make sense of agreements. Philosophers call individuals in this group moral patients to distinguish them from contracting agents. No patients, according to contractualism, have moral standing. A contractor may elect to take responsibility for a given patient and may then make claims on the patient's behalf. But if the patient is not a party to any contract and not of interest to any person who is a party to the contract, then we have no duties – direct or indirect – to the patient.

This situation strikes rights theorists as odd and regrettable. For them, patients have moral standing and others have direct obligations to patients even if the patients are not included in any contracts. According to the rights theorist – but not the egoist or contractualist – we must attend to moral patients simply because of their nature as beings with memories, aspirations, feelings and goals. In sum, the justification of rights theories rests on the nature of individual agents and patients rather than agreements we have reached among ourselves.

Here's another way to think about it. For rights theorists, a child's moral standing is built into the fabric of the ethical universe, so to speak, in much the same way that gravity and entropy are built into the fabric of the physical universe. The mentally enfeebled have rights that are intrinsic to them as humans; their rights to have their interests respected do not depend on some authority giving them rights or on their first contracting with others in the hope that others will give them rights.

According to rights theory, basic moral rights are natural because all humans have the same basic rights and all humans have those rights equally. No matter how young or old you are, how intelligent or ignorant, and no matter your race, religion, or political views, you are a member of the human family. The human family consists of a group, and the members of this group at least think that they have free will and are autonomous. What free will means is debatable, but a common interpretation is this: free to "do otherwise," able to act on your immediate wants and desires if you wish but also able to make a difference in the causal chain, choosing not to act on your immediate desires should you so decide. Choice, on the will theory, is central; we can decide to defer acting on our first impulse and free ourselves of our instinctual urges to pursue more remote, categorical, interests.

This, or something very close to it, is what rights theorists mean when they claim to ground their theory in human nature. Contractors and non-contractors alike have the capacity to act on the basis of deliberation. We can look ahead, envision different possible outcomes of each action open to us, survey the various principles that would give us good reasons to undertake this or that action, and then act on the basis of the principle we find most persuasive. We need not act egoistically for we can act altruistically, benevolently. Our rational capacity gives us dignity, a quality others must respect when they are deciding how to act toward us.

Moral rights differ from legal rights. All humans have moral rights, even if certain municipalities' legal codes do not recognize them. The laws of some societies do not allow women to own property or run for political office. In other cultures, the law disenfranchises certain ethnic minorities. But from the fact that someone lacks a legal right in a given culture it does not follow that they have lost their moral rights in that culture, too. To the contrary, a person's moral rights cannot be taken away from him or her. And this is true even if a despotic religious authority or deluded democratic majority declare that members of a certain group lack rights.

The philosopher Tom Regan describes rights using a vivid metaphor. Think of rights, he says, as a big fence around your body. There's a "no trespassing" sign hanging on it. Anyone who tries to go through that fence is violating you. On this view, if someone has a right not to be violated in scientific experiments then others are being told, Stay out! This is my body; you have no permission or valid claim to enter it. Rights are generally understood to be very strong claims. Rights can be surrendered, as when a landowner gives someone permission to come onto their property. Rights can also be overridden, even in the absence of the owner's permission, but to over-ride a moral right requires a very good reason. You may now be wondering about the status of nonhuman animals. If cognitively impaired humans have moral rights because, despite their impairments, they are nonetheless sentient and have memories and desires, then do animals have moral rights if they similarly are sentient and have lives of their own? Regan, the founder of animal rights philosophy, is very clear about his answer to this question. Yes, animals have rights even though they cannot contract with others. For animals are no different in this respect from human patients who cannot contract with others. Misfortunate humans have basic moral rights even if they lack mental sophistication. So, insists Regan, do animals; animals have moral rights insofar as they have cognitive states that are at least as sophisticated as misfortunate humans.

We will return to the animal issue – a complicated and contentious issue – in Chapter 13. For the present, let us set it to one side and restrict our focus to *Homo sapiens*. For many human beings are not capable of entering into contracts. According to contractualism, moral patients fall outside the sphere of direct moral consideration, and that fact alone makes moral rights theories unhappy with contractualism. Rights theorists insist, as we have said, that children and the demented are all part of the moral community. As Regan puts it, they are "subjects-of-a-life" (Regan 1983). They feel pleasure and pain, are conscious, and have lives of their own. Even if they are not rational or autonomous, events can go well or badly for them. How we act toward them can help them or harm them. According to rights theories, patients have moral rights equal in strength to the rights agents have, even if patients do not have all of the same rights that agents have.

Now, what moral rights, we might ask, do agents have that children or the handicapped lack? There are many such rights. For example, there is the right to vote, the right to go to college, to drive a car, to drink beer, and to serve in the military. Normal adult humans are capable of doing these things and to the extent that they take an interest in doing them they have a right to do them. But patients may not be capable of doing them and, consequently, may not have the right to do them. Still, and here's the heart of the matter, patients have other moral rights, such as the right not to be used as a tool to achieve the greater good of others.

Graduate students have various legal rights

Here is a definition of legal rights.

Legal rights are powers bestowed by juridical bodies to permit or prohibit specific actions.

Social institutions create legal rights, judicial systems interpret legal rights, and police enforce them. Legal rights can be unfairly distributed, as when one gender but not the other has the right to vote. Legal rights vary from one locality to the next. As such, they are defeasible; they can be taken away from you by an authority and against your will, as when felons forfeit their right to vote. In democratic societies, legal rights often include the right to own property and move freely about in public places. Graduate students have whatever legal rights have been given them by their local and federal governments and the universities they attend must acknowledge and honor these rights. Should an institution prohibit a graduate student from publishing a politically unpopular opinion in the student newspaper, for example, the student may be able to sue the institution on the grounds that the institution has violated the student's First Amendment rights.

Universities may also give students additional powers and entitlements beyond the students' legal rights. Graduate students, for example, are almost always entitled to meet with their professors, to participate in lab meetings, to receive mentoring, to form clubs, engage in extracurricular activities, and to be granted their degree after completing their requirements. And yet, depending on the institution, a student may not have one or more of these rights. For example, if you are a graduate student with instructional duties at Duke University or the University of North Carolina at Chapel Hill and you have a grievance against a faculty member, you have a right to speak with that university's ombudsperson, a person designated to act as a neutral mediator in disputes. On the other hand, if you are a student at North Carolina State University, you have no such right. (North Carolina State University does not have an ombudsperson.)

Since universities differ in their policies and regulations, a student at one institution may lack a legal right possessed by a student at another institution. Returning to the First Amendment example, notice that a graduate student writing for a newspaper at a public institution may have a right not to have their writing censored. Yet a student writing for a paper at a private university may not have the same entitlement. The latter student may be subject to censorship if they write material that administrators find objectionable. They may even have their funding withdrawn if administrators do not approve of the content of their articles. Another example: graduate students confined to wheelchairs may find they have a right to accommodations at universities in some countries and not in other countries. Legal rights vary between institutions and between jurisdictions.

Yet all have the same moral rights

Moral rights theories vary in how they construe rights. In some accounts, rights are discovered rather than created, equal rather than unequal, and universal rather than local. In these accounts, rights are in some important sense "natural," as if God or Nature endowed our species with powers and entitlements that cannot be taken away from us arbitrarily. Natural rights do not depend on authorities or institutions granting the right to us; such groups can only recognize rights in us. Furthermore, the distribution of moral rights is not variable among a population because all individuals have the same moral rights and they have them in equal degrees. You may surrender a moral right if you wish, you can forfeit a right, and it can be overridden by competing moral considerations. But you cannot have a right taken away from you against your will by an intervening authority unless you have done something to justify such an act. You might, for example, abuse someone in a particularly egregious fashion. In cases such as armed robbery and rape, for example, the offender presumably has surrendered his moral right to move about freely, for instance, and the authorities can justifiably lock him up.

Unlike legal rights, moral rights do not vary from institution to institution. While students at North Carolina State University, for example, have no legal rights to speak with an ombudsperson, they nonetheless have a moral right not to be exploited, they retain their right to have their grievances heard by someone in power. NC State, of course, recognizes these rights; even though it lacks an ombudsperson, it provides other procedures, formal and informal, for aggrieved students. Why? Because when NC State grad students are wronged by a faculty member or administrator, their basic humanity is challenged and their dignity compromised. Such violations must be addressed.

So far, we have explained the wrongness of research misconduct using egoistic (Part A) and contractualist (Part B) schemes. Egoism and contractualism account in many ways for our sense that the consequences of cheating are unacceptable. If we're egoists, we hold that misconduct is wrong insofar as it interferes with our achievement of our goals. If we're contractualists, we believe that misconduct is wrong insofar as it violates the terms of hypothetical agreements.

But is there a dimension of the wrongness of cheating that these views don't capture? Suppose Elizabeth Goodwin had succeeded in falsifying the photos on her grant application. Suppose that her students had not turned her in and, furthermore, that none of them were ever caught. Suppose, too, that the lab's project was funded, that all of its members proceeded to publish important papers, and that each student secured a competitive teaching position. In sum, let's imagine that Goodwin's misconduct resulted in no harm at all and very good consequences indeed for everyone involved. Goodwin's actions, we are supposing, maximized aggregate happiness. Still, isn't there something wrong in what she did? If you think so, one reason might be that you feel that her action failed to show respect for humanity, for humans in general, even if no one human being was harmed by it.

People who lie and cheat make honest people, even those not directly affected by the lying and cheating, feel as if their own value is degraded. Dishonest people also may indirectly put honest people at a disadvantage, because everyone needs access to reliable information if they are to make good decisions. If lying and cheating are widely tolerated it will eventually become impossible to make good decisions. The reason is that no one will be able to trust any information that is relayed to them. Perhaps this is the cause of our conviction that others owe us the truth. Goodwin ought not to lie in her grant proposal whether or not she has previously contracted with others to tell the truth – and whether or not she can maximize aggregate happiness by lying.

Douglas MacLean makes the point clearly. He writes:

> Respect for persons and their status as free agents with wills of their own and the capacity to understand and guide their actions by reasons implies that we need and have a right to know the truth, insofar as we can, in order to guide our reasons and actions. When someone lies to us, even if the overall consequences are good, they deprive us of the basis we need to apply our reasons and values to figure out what to do. Lies deflect our beliefs from what is true; they prevent us from living and acting "in the real world." It is for reasons like this that most of us believe we have a right to know the facts, even if they are painful to us or to others.
>
> (MacLean 2010)

Moral rights theorists point to a dimension of the ethics of lying not covered by egoism or contractualism. Something about the act of perpetuating falsehoods seems wrong in itself, even if the consequences of lying are on balance good for everyone involved. We might call this thing that we detect about lying its "intrinsic" wrongness.

When Mary Allen came to believe that Goodwin had altered a photo on a grant application, she may have felt that Goodwin's misconduct was intrinsically wrong. Allen seems to have felt that the act would be wrong even if it had never been discovered, even if Goodwin had never previously committed and would never subsequently commit another such act.

What might be the source of Mary Allen's feeling? For her, the question seems to have a theological answer: God sees such "hidden" acts and disapproves of them. For others, hidden acts are wrong because they are direct affronts to the kind of being that humans are, namely beings who need to understand the world clearly, and yet who are easily misled by appearances. It is hard enough to make one's way in the world when others deal honestly with us. When they purposely distort our view of the world, however, they can make it nearly impossible for us to achieve any of our purposes. That is why our sense of justice is offended by lies, and even by lies that seem to harm no one in particular.

One way to describe the situation is to say that people naturally seek – and hence value – the truth. When others try to trick us into adopting false or distorted views, they fail to respect that natural inclination. To put it another way, we seem to have a right against others that they tell us the truth, whether or not the law requires it of them, and whether or not truth-telling will lead to the best consequences overall. For this reason, we might need something like a notion of moral rights to explain why lying is intrinsically wrong.

In Part B, we noted that, according to contractualism, all contractors are equals. For moral rights theorists like Regan, all subjects of a life are equals. Being another's equal does not mean that one has the same entitlements. We are each the moral equal of Mark Zuckerberg, founder of Facebook, but we are not each entitled to his stock shares. Rather, to say that you and I are the moral equals of Mark Zuckerberg means to say that we have the same amount of dignity and worth that he has.

Those who defend moral rights theories go farther on this point than do contractualists. The equality of each human being is based not on one particular feature of us, such as our rationality. It is based instead on the fact that each of us is a psychological unity with goals and memories, hopes and desires of our own, and a life that can go well or badly for us. There are, as we have said, several kinds of moral rights theories, but a prominent way to define the general approach emphasizes the dignity of all subjects of a life (Regan, 1983). Regan builds his theory on the fundamental insight of the German philosopher Immanuel Kant, that we should always treat persons as ends-in-themselves, and never instrumentally, never using others as means to one's own ends only. In Kant's definition, only persons – fully autonomous agents – have moral rights. For Regan, non-autonomous humans and nonhuman animals capable of being harmed also have moral rights. Both Regan and Kant view people generally as independently valuable and as bearers of inherent rights, and not simply as subjects we can use to advance our own projects. A corollary belief is in something that philosophers call "the good will" – the proper attitude of respect for the integrity and intrinsic value of each person. We should always act in a way that expresses the right intentions, the right "will," a good will. We demonstrate this good will when we recognize – in thought and action – that people have the ability to make their own choices.

Egoism and contractualism begin with our natural inclinations and preferences. Moral rights theories, on the other hand, deny that our preferences make a good starting point for ethics. Acts have moral value only if they are done in the right spirit, for the right reason. Suppose Goodwin had meant to keep her misconduct secret all along. However, talking to Padilla on the phone one day she has a slip of the tongue and accidentally discloses that she falsified a photo in the proposal. This inadvertent disclosure might be judged good by a contractualist looking at the consequences of the slip-up and deciding that the slip-up led to circumstances in which people actually fulfilled their agreements. But moral rights theories would not judge the disclosure of the truth as good in itself because it was not performed with the right motives. According to Kant, it is not possible to justify acts of wrongdoing – or right doing, for that matter – if those acts are performed from suspect motives.

What rights do we have? Moral rights are often called human rights and the United Nations Universal Declaration of Human Rights (1948) lists the following (among others):

- the right to life, liberty, security of person and freedom of movement
- the right to an education
- the right to equality before the law
- the right to presumption of innocence until proven guilty
- the right to legal recourse when one's rights have been violated, even if the violator was acting in an official capacity
- the right to appeal a conviction
- the right to be recognized as a person before the law
- the right to privacy and protection of that privacy by law
- the right to freedom of thought, conscience, opinion, expression, and religion
- the right to freedom of assembly and association.

The Declaration contains both positive and negative rights. Positive rights are valid claims about what we are permitted or required to do and indicate ways in which rights holders should be helped. Negative rights are valid claims about what we are permitted or required not to do and are cashed out in terms of prohibitions against harming the holder of the right. The list above proclaims positive rights to security and education, and negative rights against states not to interfere with citizens. States may not harm citizens by, for example, seizing their property, presuming that detainees are guilty, outlawing peaceful assemblies, or inhibiting freedom of thought or religion.

We can define negative rights as follows:

If it is true that a person P has a right to X, then it would be wrong to deprive P of X or to prevent P from Xing on purely consequentialist grounds.

For example, if George has a right to express his opinion that a scientific experiment his lab is considering conducting in a developing country is too risky for its subjects, then it would be wrong to prevent George from expressing his opinion on the grounds that his expressing himself may have the consequence of making a lot of people worse-off than they'd be if George were kept from expressing himself. No one may legitimately invalidate George's claim to free speech, according to the moral rights principle, by arguing on consequentialist grounds that allowing George to speak freely will lead to great unhappiness.

Countries that sign the UN Declaration are committed to the recognition of these rights for all of their citizens. But how exactly are these rights justified? This is a difficult question and, as we shall see at the end of Chapter 12, not a question that has been decisively answered by defenders of moral rights. But let us set forth the case here.

Moral rights theories are views that hold that one should always respect the dignity of others

Historically, rights were seen as coming from God. When God created the world, goes the account, God created a hierarchy of beings, with God at the top, the king in the middle, and the king's subjects at the bottom. (Animals were below the king's subjects.) Insofar as the reigning monarch conferred rights on subjects, the derivation of their rights was clear: people had rights because the king had given those rights to them, and the king had the power to confer those rights because the king had received the power to do so from God. If some people had rights that others lacked, it was because the king had not given everyone the rights in question.

This line of reasoning is hardly convincing today. Even contemporary theorists who tie morality to God tend to think that moral rights are dependent not on a sovereign – earthly or heavenly – but on the nature of each individual person, a nature we all share. That is to say, moral rights are intrinsic to us and we possess them whether or not a superior power has seen fit to grant them to us.

For those living in democratic and pluralistic cultures, a more plausible response is that moral rights are grounded in human nature, that is, in the metaphysical characteristics of what it is to be a person. Who – or what – are persons? As we have suggested, we are autonomous agents, animals capable of making free choices, selecting our own values, and exercising control over our actions. To be this kind of animal is to be the kind of animal that has intrinsic worth and deserves respect. It is to be the kind of animal that has moral rights.

Control is central to this understanding of what it means to be a person. When we are free to make our own decisions we are, all other things equal, better off than when others are in control of us. Compare how you feel when others tell you what to do and how you feel when you make your own decisions. When someone else, a king or tyrant or even an overbearing parent, makes choices for us, we are not well positioned to achieve our categorical interests, make something of ourselves, or lead a rewarding life. Kant argued that when others make decisions for us, they violate our dignity. He famously argued that each human being must be treated as an end, as an independent maker of decisions and generator of value. To treat someone as a means to your own ends is to disrespect them by restricting their freedom to pursue their own independently determined goals.

We can see how this view of human nature leads to strong negative rights, starting with the right against others that they not take away your capacity to make your own decisions. If someone interferes with your movement around town, for example, or steals your credit cards, they have made intrusions on your privacy and autonomy. If you have a negative liberty right that others not impede you in moving freely about, then others have the corresponding duty to respect this right of yours. In short, rights entail duties.

According to the interpretation of rights that we are using, rights must be relatively easy to understand, simple in form, not difficult to apply, and straightforward in their policy implications – features that make rights useful and teachable to children. On this view, rights are like trump cards. In card games, when clubs are the trump suit, even the lowly two of clubs will beat the ace of hearts. Similarly, according to this conception of moral rights, arguments based on absolute rights always defeat arguments based on consequences.

Even if great consequences will come to 100 people by trampling on one person's right, the hundred are not justified in exploiting the one for their own ends (Regan, 2000).

When individual rights claims conflict with claims about maximizing the well-being of many others, the rights claims take precedence, according to most rights theories. Many examples from the history of research make this point. For example, in Part B we discussed the controversial US Public Health Service syphilis trials at Tuskegee. You'll recall that we did not have an easy time explaining why the study was objectionable if we confined ourselves to the traditional concerns of a narrow contractualism. The theory seemed destined to give us the wrong results by claiming that the study may have been permissible if no explicit or implicit agreements were broken. By contrast, if we apply moral rights theories to this case we immediately get the right answer. Withholding life-saving penicillin from syphilitic patients in a researcher's care violates the men's basic rights even if the men have signed contracts saying that they agree to be used in this way. The fact that the research will provide important knowledge about the course of the disease (assuming that the research does provide such knowledge) is not a consideration that overrides their right not to be used as means to others' ends. Moral rights theories make this point dramatically and emphatically because they take us so quickly, efficiently, and convincingly to the correct conclusion in such cases. Clearly, moral rights theories have a central role to play in research ethics, and especially in deliberations about the experimental use of humans.

So far so good. But what do we do when moral rights conflict? How should we decide which right takes precedence in cases where two rights are present? The answer is often not clear.

Consider the following example. As the details of the case are somewhat complicated, we will have to take some time explaining the facts.

Case study: human pesticide toxicity testing

In the late 1990s, US consumers became concerned with the levels of pesticides on fruits and vegetables. As a consequence, Congress directed the Environmental Protection Agency (EPA) to add a safety factor to its risk assessments of pesticide residues on food. EPA was told to reduce by ten-fold the amount of pesticide residue allowable on fruits and vegetables. The motivation behind the policy was a desire to protect children, pregnant women, and other members of the population who might be more susceptible than healthy adults to small amounts of pesticide residues. The pesticide industry reacted by saying that current limits already sufficed to protect all consumers, and a ten-fold reduction was unnecessary. A further massive reduction in tolerable limits, complained the industry, would constrain the efforts of farmers to control crop pests, increase consumer food prices, and – although the industry did not say so – reduce agricultural chemical manufacturers' profits.

Industry offered a counter-proposal. Rather than continue to test pesticides on animals, as in current practice, and then reduce the amount by an additional ten-fold safety factor, industry representatives proposed to test pesticides directly on humans. It argued that science has no way to determine the differences of tolerable pesticide levels in mice and rats compared to tolerable levels in infants and children. To adequately protect infants and children, we ought to test the pesticides on them.

Critics of industry were upset. They believed not only that all of us have a moral right not to be put at risk of harm for the good of others but, in addition, that this right prohibited the use of humans as guinea pigs in pesticide testing. But industry could have argued in response that citizens – especially children living in poor households with limited food budgets – have a competing right to benefit from government-sponsored research, research that might reduce the price of food. According to this analysis, one person's right not to be put at risk of harm in a scientific experiment conflicts with another person's right to benefit from lower food prices resulting from government research. Which right takes precedence?

To answer such questions, we must look closely at the respective weight of the rights involved. For example, is the negative right of an experimental subject not to be put in harm's way more essential to maintaining one's dignity than the positive right of a poor child to social benefits? Is it more important to reduce the price of fresh vegetables by a few cents or to refrain from testing pesticides on people? It is an important question, but to answer it we must have information about the facts of the children's current well-being, the magnitude of the decrease in the price of vegetables, the doses of pesticides to be received by the subjects, the facts provided to those subjects about the risks to which they will be exposed, the history of pesticide testing on humans, and alternative possibilities for improving the lot of poor children apart from testing chemicals on healthy people.

Before we introduce further facts of the case we must state an important presupposition of the following discussion. We will henceforth suppose that the industry critics are right, that all humans have a negative moral right not to be put at risk of harm without their consent in order to achieve greater goods for others. This right, a kind of right to inviolability, we will call the *Do no harm* right. *Do no harm* meets the conditions we mentioned earlier. It provides an easily-understood rule the application of which to actual cases is straightforward enough to guide behavior. As a right, it trumps all non-rights based ethical considerations. *Do no harm* does not allow scientists to test pesticides on children even if, as is the case in this instance, their parents or proxies have given informed consent.

Do no harm is not a new invention. It, or something like it, has been used by the medical community for thousands of years (cf. the Hippocratic Oath). Now, suppose a scientist submits a research proposal to test pesticides experimentally on people. On the basis of *Do no harm*, reviewers of the proposal would seem to be justified in rejecting the proposal out of hand. After all, pesticides are poisons; they are meant to kill their targets; and we traditionally test pesticides on animals rather than people for something like the reason articulated in *Do no harm*. An experiment to test poisons on people seems as obvious a violation of *Do no harm* as we can imagine.

But is it? Congress directed the EPA to add the ten-fold safety factor to its risk assessments of pesticide residues to protect children and other vulnerable members of the population. It was, in effect, trying to protect these citizens' rights not to be harmed. So, we may legitimately suppose that we have here a case of conflicting rights. Now, for the facts.

Prior to the passage in 2002 of the Food Quality Protection Act (FQPA), risk assessments for pesticides depended on animal studies usually involving rodents, rabbits, or dogs. To acknowledge the differences between humans and the experimental species in use, policy-makers required that the algorithm include an additional ten-fold uncertainty factor. The assumption was that humans might be ten times as sensitive to pesticide residues on food as any mouse or rat. The uncertainty factor therefore reduced the amount of synthetic chemical residues permitted for humans to a tenth of what had been found to be safe for rodents. For example, methyl bromide gas is an effective fumigant for protecting apples against post-harvest insect damage. To determine how much gas we can safely use on the apples, we conduct experiments to determine the no observable effect level (NOEL) for laboratory animals. In an experimental setting, scientists feed the animals increasingly large amounts of the chemical and note the largest dose at which no effects are observed. Suppose these tests establish NOEL at 500 parts per million (ppm) for the animal species (US Government 2006). Now we apply the uncertainty factor to account for the variability between humans and the animals. After this simple calculation, NOEL is 50 ppm for humans (500/10). Until 2002, this figure was the accepted figure.

In 2002, however, the FQPA added a second ten-fold uncertainty factor to account for the variability among humans because of discrepancies in ages, immunity levels, body shapes, and physiological vulnerabilities to toxins. So the NOEL was again divided by ten. Overnight, the NOEL was reduced from, say, 50 ppm to 5.0 ppm (50/10). Such a policy clearly represented a burden to farmers and grocers, who had to reduce dramatically the amount of pesticides in use. The burden resulted from the possibility of greater crop losses, more complicated agricultural practices to control pests, lower profits, and so on.

The pesticide industry responded to the EPA's new directive by arguing that the second uncertainty factor would be unnecessary if toxicity tests were conducted directly on humans. Industry experts, after all, agreed that physiological reactions to toxins in one species (experimental mice) are not a valid inferential basis for extrapolations to the physiological reactions of another species (humans). The most accurate way to determine the highest actual level of safe exposure to pesticides residues on food, said industry representatives, is not to test the chemicals on animals and then add an arbitrary factor of ten as a cushion. It is, rather, to use humans in the tests.

Within 2 years of the congressional directive to the EPA, a series of experiments were conducted in which informed adult experimental subjects were intentionally exposed to pesticides. It is not obviously wrong to conduct such tests; in fact, Phase 1 clinical trials routinely deliberately expose subjects to potentially harmful chemotherapeutic agents. Before the end of 2004, at least 15 new human toxicity studies were submitted to EPA's Office of Pesticide Programs.[1] Soon thereafter, the Environmental Working Group began a campaign opposing the research on ethical grounds. One might easily imagine that they objected to human pesticide toxicity testing on the grounds that it violates *Do no harm*.

We return now to our original question about conflicting rights. How would such a disagreement be decided? We would have to examine the arguments on both sides. There are several reasons one might offer to support the position that pesticide testing offends *Do no harm*. In fact, one might argue that the burden of proof is on the person who thinks the testing does not violate *Do no harm* because pesticides are toxic; they are designed to kill the animals at which they are targeted; and they can cause cancer in consumers who eat the foods on which they have been sprayed. Why would anyone think that testing such substances on children does not violate children's rights?

One might buttress this argument by pointing out that no one asserts that the testing benefits the research subjects enrolled in the tests, subjects who are, after all, not suffering from any disease that giving them a pesticide might help to ameliorate. Nor does anyone

---

[1] Personal correspondence with John M. Carley, Program Analyst, US Environmental Protection Agency, Office of Pesticide Programs, 11/2007. Carley notes that since EPA's promulgation of the rule in February 2006 "the controversy has largely died down ... and no proposals for new research involving intentional exposure of human subjects to pesticides to identify or quantify toxic endpoints have been submitted to the agency for several years."

know what harm may come from cumulative exposures. What are the chances that the subjects would escape being harmed by long-term unpredictable effects of exposure? Finally, even though the subjects will be asked for their informed consent, those subjects will be under various kinds of pressures. Even if a parent willingly signs an informed consent release on behalf of their child, should society allow children to be placed in this position? The opponents of pesticide testing apparently thought not.

On the other hand, once we have detailed scientific information about testing we may have good reason to think the testing either is a justified violation of *Do no harm* or does not violate any moral rights. With a full understanding of the procedures in hand, we may come to agree with industry that the amount of pesticide used in the trials will be so small that the experimental subjects are at no serious risk of harm at all. For these subjects ingest pesticides during the course of their everyday diet and experience no adverse effects. If the amount of pesticide they are given during pesticide testing in the lab is less than they receive every day outside the lab, then it may well be that the testing does not violate *Do no harm*.

Here are some facts that lend some support to the suppositions of the previous paragraph. About half of the 15–20 studies submitted to EPA between 2000 and 2003 using humans followed a single-rising-dose model and studied acute effects. In these studies the initial dose was set so low that adverse effects were unexpected – and none were found. In most of these studies no observable effects were reported even at the highest dose tested. For these reasons, the National Research Council of the National Academy of Sciences concluded that the US Environmental Protection Agency was justified in testing pesticides on humans under certain conditions (Committee on the Use of Third Party Toxicity Research with Human Research Participants Science, Technology, and Law Program, National Research Council, 2004).[2]

Commenting on the apparent safety of most of the trials, John Carley, an analyst in the EPA's office of pesticide programs, notes that "in only a couple of the studies was any adverse effect reported," and those effects – the effects noted in the report of the anti-pesticide-testing advocacy group, "The English Patients" (Environmental Working Group, 1998) – were sweating, light-headedness, and headache lasting no longer than 4 hours. No nausea, no trembling. The symptoms observed are classified in the risk assessment literature as "minor and reversible," moving Carley to observe that, "It has been argued that this study design is a model of risk minimization, since the subjects experience no adverse effects."

It appears, therefore, that one could design the trials so as not to violate *Do no harm* and, in fact, this may already have been done. What conclusion can we draw from this case? Here's one. Whereas we ought to encourage people across cultures to act instinctively on the basis of *Do no harm* because it is a moral right, we must nevertheless also insist that we look at all the facts. For it may be that great good can be achieved by an action that seems to violate *Do no harm* and yet, on further analysis, the action does not violate the right at all. Furthermore, if we are certain about all of these claims – about the claim that the testing poses no risks to human subjects and the claim that the magnitude of benefits from the testing is potentially huge – then we ought not to act instinctively on the basis of the moral right. The reason is that the apparent violation of the right is not a violation. And the poor child's right to benefit from cheaper food prices

---

[2] The conditions do not seem unusual or particularly difficult to satisfy; the experiments must "meet the most stringent scientific and ethical standards, ensuring that research participants are protected and that the studies are scientifically necessary and valid."

produced by publicly financed scientific research may be a right we can respect, if it is a right, without running afoul of the experimental subject's right not to be harmed.

Of course, the argument in these pages has established no such conclusion. There are many factors we have stipulated and many assumptions that need defending. We haven't, for example, shown that pesticide tests will have any effect whatsoever on the price of food, nor have we explored the question of whether our imagined pesticide study might nonetheless run afoul of other human rights. If it involved children under age six or mentally incapacitated patients, for example, one might object to it on moral rights grounds. Children and the cognitively impaired are vulnerable populations subject to special protections because they are not yet autonomous and cannot understand scientific explanations of clinical trials. Moral rights theorists, in sum, may object to any version of pesticide testing that involves disrespecting human rights and this is true no matter how great the social goods of the trial might be. For the consequences of disrespecting a right, in a view like Regan's, are irrelevant, even if the benefits outweigh the costs one hundred to one. The ends, and this is the point, do not justify the means.

Despite the complexities involved in applying moral rights theories, the theories have many obvious strengths. They emphasize the separateness of persons, they guard our dignity, and they provide reliable guidance in practical matters more often than not. For these reasons we will employ the theories throughout Part C as we explore the use of humans in research, the rights of mentors and mentees, intellectual property, and conflicts of interests.

Take home lessons

1. Right actions are actions that respect persons and their autonomy or interests.
2. Identify all parties whose rights might be violated by an action you are considering.
3. Distinguish legal rights from moral rights.
4. If rights conflict, ask which rights are the most important and act so as to minimize violations of them.
5. In conducting research, protect the rights of experimental human subjects.

Bibliography

Committee on the Use of Third Party Toxicity Research with Human Research Participants Science, Technology, and Law Program, National Research Council. 2004. *Intentional Human Dosing Studies for EPA Regulatory Purposes: Scientific and Ethical Issues.* Washington DC: The National Academies Press.

Environmental Working Group. 1998. *The English Patients: Human Experiments and Pesticide Policy.* Washington DC: Environmental Working Group. Available at: www.epa.gov/scipoly/sap/meetings/1998/december/english.pdf.

MacLean, D. 2010. Lying: An Ethical Introduction. Unpublished manuscript, quoted with permission.

Regan, T. 2000. Research Ethics: An Introduction. Unpublished manuscript, quoted with permission.

Regan, T. 1983. *The Case for Animal Rights.* Berkeley: University of California Press.

US Government, 2006. Electronic Code of Federal Regulations § 180.123. Available at: http://ecfr.gpoaccess.gov/cgi/t/text/text-idx?type=simple;c=ecfr;cc=ecfr;sid=90d2cc399ba54a4e1b47dd49fc1b055a;region=DIV1;q1=apple;rgn=div7;view=text;idno=20061213;node=20061213%3A1.0.6.

Chapter 9

Inform subjects

Suppose your research group has been collecting data for 2 years when an associate convinces the team to investigate an additional hypothesis. The hypothesis strikes everyone as intriguing, and you collectively decide to add ten new questions to a survey instrument you have people filling out online. A few months later you, a first-year graduate student, wake up in the middle of the night and realize that the group never asked the Institutional Review Board (IRB) to approve the new questions. You even have reason to believe that the Principal Investigator (PI) is aware of the situation and has decided to do nothing. What should you do? We will return to this question at the end of the chapter. First we must lay out the reasons that the informed consent of research subjects is so important.

Introduction

Researchers enroll tens of thousands of people in experiments each year. In many cases, the participants benefit profoundly from the experience. In some cases, though, some participants are harmed. How do we minimize the risks to each individual, ensure that moral rights are protected, and maximize overall well-being?

The question directs attention to one of the most important issues in research ethics because unspeakable crimes have been committed in the name of science. The Nazi doctor Josef Mengele, for example, conducted experiments on twins in which he injected dye into the eyes of brown-eyed patients to determine whether he could transform them into blue eyes (Robert Jay Lifton, *The Nazi Doctors: Medical Killing And The Psychology Of Genocide*. Basic Books, 1986). He forcibly distended the rectums of adolescents, without anesthesia, and excised tissue samples from their kidneys and prostates. When experiments were concluded, the subjects were killed by injections to the heart. The justification Mengele gave for his research was that he was trying to discover basic scientific knowledge about physiological processes in order to assist in the medical treatment of wounded German soldiers. But could such awful experiments ever be justified by appeals to their potential consequences? No reasonable observer would answer such a question affirmatively.

The Nuremberg War Criminal Trials held Mengele accountable for his deeds. In the spirit of that legal judgment and as an extension of the principle on which it is based, the Nuremberg Code of 1947 insists that all humans used in research have the right to refuse any procedure. Experimenters must obtain the voluntary informed consent of all subjects they enroll in research. The Code also stipulates that research subjects must have the legal capacity to give consent, and should be so situated as to be capable of exercising power of

Research Ethics: A Philosophical Guide to the Responsible Conduct of Research. Gary Comstock.
Published by Cambridge University Press. © Cambridge University Press 2013.

choice without the intervention of any element of force, fraud, deceit, duress, over-reaching, or other ulterior form of constraint or coercion. The Code further requires that everyone used in research must have sufficient knowledge and comprehension of the elements of the protocol that they can make an enlightened decision about their participation. Furthermore, the duty and responsibility for ascertaining the quality of consent rests not only upon the individual directing the project but on everyone who engages in it (*Trials of War Criminals before the Nuremberg Military Tribunals under Control Council Law No. 10*, Vol. 2, pp. 181–182. Washington DC: U.S. Government Printing Office, 1949).

As we will see shortly, human rights theories provide one of the strongest justifications of informed consent. Before turning to that matter, however, we must first see in more detail just what informed consent is.

What informed consent is

The principle of informed consent was developed to protect human subjects, "living individuals" in the language of the Code. Researchers must obtain informed consent from their subjects whenever the researcher intends to perform medical protocols, or to obtain "data through intervention or interaction," or to gather private information that may be tied to the person enrolled in the trial (Dept. of Health and Human Services Protection of human subjects : Title 45, Code of federal regulations, part 46, 102(f), revised June 18, 1991).

What is an "intervention" or "interaction?" The definitions are broad. "Interaction" includes any occasion when researcher and subject communicate, whether the contact is face-to-face or online. "Intervention" encompasses physical examinations in which data are gathered as well as experiments in which the subject's environment is controlled and manipulated. Regulations define identifiable private information as including:

1. Information about behavior that occurs in a context in which an individual can reasonably expect that no observation or recording is taking place
2. Information which has been provided for specific purposes by an individual and which the individual would not expect to be made public (45 CFR 46.102(f)).

Institutional review boards (IRBs) were created after the 1979 Belmont Report from the US Department of Health, Education, and Welfare to review research proposals and ensure that all research under the IRB's jurisdiction protects human subjects from unwarranted risk. IRBs are charged with protecting experimental subjects' rights and guarding against the possibility that investigators will use subjects primarily for the researcher's financial gain. The Boards facilitate the review of scientific proposals by colleagues, providing a venue for a more-or-less impartial analysis of the proposed protocol. Experimental subjects can be put at risk if the risks are freely assumed, are outweighed by benefits, and subjects are selected according to criteria that are fair, just, and inclusive (see Title 45 of the Code of Federal Regulations, part 6 (Dept. of Health and Human Services 1992)).

Why it's complicated

Informed consent is complicated for four reasons.

First, whereas different issues arise in each discipline, the members of the IRB cannot be specialists in all disciplines and yet they must apply the same ethical principles to each proposal. The criteria upon which the IRB guidelines are built reflect three principles articulated in the Belmont Report:

respect for persons, or recognition of the personal dignity and autonomy of individuals; beneficence, or the obligation to protect persons from harm by maximizing anticipated benefits and minimizing possible risks of harm; justice, or the obligation to ensure that the benefits and burdens of research are distributed equitably and that subjects are not chosen simply because they are available, cost effective, or easy to enroll (National Commission for the Protection of Human Subjects of Biomedical and Behavioral Research 1978).

The IRBs have the difficult task of applying these principles to all proposals that come before them, and often their members lack expertise in the methods and objectives of the discipline from which the proposal originates. For example, the questions an IRB member must consider when dealing with questions from a medical researcher testing a new cancer drug differ significantly from the questions that arise when a psychology researcher is proposing to conduct online surveys with undergraduate students.

The diversity of issues is reflected in the diversity of training programs offered by the Collaborative Institutional Training Initiative (CITI), an online training website for those using human subjects. CITI has at least two dozen separate educational tracks for different purposes. Those conducting social and behavioral sciences research have a different track from those doing biomedical and stem cell research or internet surveys. Those dealing with international audiences have a different track from those who intend to enroll prisoners, children, minors, public elementary school students, or pregnant women, in their studies.

Second, informed consent is complicated because researchers debate the meaning of the term. Some hold that informed consent refers specifically to the mental state of an autonomous agent. On this reading, informed consent is only present when subjects have been fully informed about the purpose of the study and its potential risks and benefits, and are aware that they may withdraw at any time. Subjects, that is, must be entirely free in their decisions to participate. If subjects have for any reason not made careful and deliberative choices, then their informed consent is lacking even if all policies and procedures have been fulfilled. Others hold that informed consent refers more narrowly to a social practice in which policies have been followed correctly. Here, informed consent is possible whenever the relevant rules of the institution conducting the experiment have been followed. Do we have informed consent of a subject whenever researchers have satisfied all of the relevant rules? Or can we follow all the rules – and obtain the subject's signature on the form – and still not have the subject's informed consent?

Third, informed consent is costly. Researchers and IRB members complain that scientific progress is impeded by the amount of paperwork required and the unreasonable attention paid to what is claimed are trivial details (Gunsalus *et al.* 2006). As Grady (2010) writes,

> Excessive or "hyper" regulation is seen as seriously affecting or stifling research productivity without adding mean meaningful protections for participants (Gunsalus *et al.* 2006). According to Bledsoe *et al.*, "IRBs have disrupted student careers, set back tenure clocks, and blunted the essence of many intellectual traditions. Facing demands that spiral to the level of sheer impracticality, faculty and students . . . face a stark choice: to conduct innovative research in their fields or to meet the requirements of their IRB" (Bledsoe *et al.* 2007).

Fourth, informed consent may stand in the way of research to benefit populations whose members cannot give their consent. Children, the cognitively limited, elderly patients with dementia – these people lack the ability to understand researcher's methods and procedures.

For that reason they are unable to give informed consent, and yet they need our help nonetheless. The Helsinki Declaration addressed this issue by reasoning that vulnerable populations could be enrolled in research protocols as long as they were represented by legally authorized proxies who would protect the subject's best interests (World Medical Association 1964). The Helsinki document opened an important door to studies on disorders unique to those, for example, with dementia or Alzheimer's disease.

As if these difficulties weren't enough, a new complication has arisen in the past few years. There are few, if any, studies of the extent to which IRBs actually succeed in protecting the rights of experimental human subjects (Grady 2010).

Why it's hard to get

It is difficult to obtain informed consent because the subject's context so heavily influences their decisions. If subjects "agree" to participate in an experiment simply because they think an authoritative figure wants them to do it, have they really consented?

Stanley Milgram's work at Yale University beginning in 1961 kicked off a long string of experiments that show how much influence authorities have on our allegedly free choices. The Milgram experiments also raised ethical questions of their own because the protocol required that Milgram deceive his subjects about the purpose of the study. How can one obtain a subject's informed consent if one does not fully disclose all of the risks and benefits of the experiment to the subject? To explore these questions, let's look at what Milgram did.

In the 1950s and early 1960s, social psychologists puzzled over the behavior of Nazi medical researchers who had exploited Jewish, homosexual, and Roma patients throughout the 1940s. Common wisdom considered it abnormal that German doctors would obey immoral commands (such as those Mengele no doubt issued) and thought the doctors' actions needed an explanation. Some people explained the individual researchers' behavior as a response to the charisma of individual psychopaths, such as Hitler, and a fascist "personality cult." Others explained it as a collective phenomenon and appealed to allegedly aggressive traits of the so-called "Germanic personality."

In a contrarian thesis, however, Hannah Arendt proposed that nothing needed to be explained, that the Nazi's abominable disregard for human rights was to be expected. Arendt argued that evil was "banal," that is, it was boring, obvious and commonplace (Arendt 1963). Milgram set out to test Arendt's thesis. He designed controlled experimental conditions in which subjects would be pressured by an authority figure to do something immoral. If Arendt was wrong, reasoned Milgram, subjects would refuse to obey orders that offended the subject's conscience even if the orders were delivered by authority figures in white coats.

Milgram's experiments always involved three people. Two were actors and Milgram's confederates. The first played an authority figure, a university research scientist. He (it was always a male) would try to manipulate the subject into performing actions that the subject would normally find morally objectionable. The second confederate was the "learner" to the experimental subject's "teacher." In each experiment, the scientist (usually Milgram himself) would tell the learner and the teacher that they were going to participate in an investigation of the role of punishment in learning (Milgram 1974). The teacher first helped the learner memorize words and then would punish the learner with a series of electrical shocks, from 15 to 450 volts, whenever the learner got a word wrong.

The experiment was effectively designed to ensure that the teacher believed that the learner was receiving electrical shocks. It is important to understand, however, that the learner never received any shocks. He only acted as if were being shocked. At each wrong answer, the "voltage" was set higher. As the teacher heard the learner's cries of pain, the teacher often hesitated to administer the next shock. Here was the crux of the experiment, for at each sign of resistance by the teacher, the scientist would authoritatively instruct that the experiment "must go on," and demand that the teacher continue with the punishment.

Milgram hypothesized that most teachers would cease to follow orders once they had progressed about a third of the way up the range. He thought no one would administer a shock above level 20 (350 volts). He based his prediction on the comments made by psychiatrists, college students, and middle-class adults when the experiment was explained to them and they were asked to predict their own break-off points. Typical remarks included "... I myself am scared stiff of shocks and I couldn't give shocks to people that were protesting ...", "I can't stand to see people suffer," and this:

> ... since the subject volunteered, and I volunteered, and since the experimenter has no physical authority over me, the subject should be released when he is at such a point that he asks to be released, and I would release him.
>
> (Milgram 1974)

These three respondents predicted that if they were called upon to be the teacher, they would disobey orders, respectively, at 90 volts, 150 volts, and 150 volts. Table 9.1 gives the predictions of 39 psychiatrists, 31 college students, and 40 middle-class adults who were not in the study but were asked to say how they would behave if called upon to be teachers.

Notice that no more than eight of the 110 total subjects expected to administer shocks beyond level 13 (195 volts). No one predicted that they would continue beyond level 20 (350 volts).

Milgram was allowed to proceed with his experiment and his actual results are found in Table 9.2.[1] The first three columns are reprinted from Table 9.1 for comparison purposes. The three columns on the right show results from three separate trials.

In Test 1, the teacher was physically separated from the learner, who was located in another room. In this "remote" condition, no teachers defected until level 20, or 300 volts, at which point five people refused to go on. The two important numbers here are 26, the number out of 40 who administered a level 30 shock (450 volts), and 65.0%, the percentage of teachers who were completely obedient. Nearly two-thirds of all teachers continued to shock the learner all the way to the end of the scale. In Tests 2 and 5 the teacher was allowed to hear the learner yelling ("Please stop! I told you I had a heart condition!") and banging on the wall, but the results were similar to Test 1. Under orders from the authority, teachers administered electrical shocks that they had every reason to believe were harmful if not fatal.

Given the prevailing view of human nature in the 1950s, the importance of Milgram's discoveries can hardly be overestimated. Arendt was right. Obedience to immoral commands of authorities is normal, to be expected, and not an aberrant behavior that needs an explanation. The default condition of at least two-thirds of us is that we are highly susceptible to environmental conditions (the other third is more capable of resisting immoral commands). Under certain conditions, that is, most of us lack the capacity to act on principles we would

---

[1] Used with permission of my colleague, James Svara, who created Tables 9.1 and 9.2 as summaries of information in two tables published in Milgram 1974, pp. 29 and 35. Working with Van Kloempken, then a graduate student at North Carolina State University, Svara created a classroom exercise that employs these tables. In the exercise, students imaginatively play the role of an IRB member reviewing a proposal from a Dr. Milgram at Yale who is seeking IRB approval for his obedience studies.

Table 9.1. Individuals predict their own breakoff points (Milgram, p. 29): predicted results

Shock level		Psychiatrists	College students	Middle-class adults
No shock		2		3
Slight	1	1	1	
	2			
	3			1
	4	1		1
Moderate	5	6	4	7
	6	1	3	1
	7	4		1
	8	4	1	3
Strong	9	1	3	2
	10	14	12	9
	11		1	2
	12	2	6	3
	13	2		1
	14		1	
	15			1
	16			1
Intense	17			1
	18			
	19			
	20	1		3
Extreme intensity	21			
	22			
	23			
	24			
Danger: severe	25			
	26			
	27			
	28			
XXX	29			
	30			
Number of subjects		n = 39	n = 31	n = 40
Avg. max. shock level		8.20	9.35	9.15
% "obedient"		0.0%	0.0%	0.0%

defend under normal circumstances. And yet the two-thirds of teachers who shocked their learners did not do so happily. They squirmed and grimaced and laughed nervously, showing extreme discomfort about what they were doing. So their actions were not the results of twisted maniacal minds. They were the results of minds that wanted to go along and get along. If we are such conformists, so easily swept up into others' projects, however corrupt, what confidence can we place in our ability to think for ourselves and to act independently?

Table 9.2. Maximum shocks administered (Milgram, p. 29): predicted vs. actual results

Shock level		Predicted results			Actual results		
		Psychiatrists	College students	Middle-class adults	Test 1	Test 2	Test 5
No shock		2		3			
Slight	1	1					
	2						
	3			1			
	4	1		1			
Moderate	5	6	4	7			
	6	1	3	1			1
	7	4		1			
	8	4		3			
Strong	9	1	3	2	1		
	10	14	12	9		5	6
	11		1	2	1		
	12	2	6	3	1		1
Very strong	13	2		1			
	14		1				
	15			1			
	16			1			
Intense	17			1			
	18						2
	19				1		
	20	1		3	5	1	1
Extreme intensity	21				4	3	1
	22				2		1
	23				1	1	
	24				1	1	
Danger: severe	25				1		1
	26						
	27						
	28						
XXX	29						
	30				26	25	26
Number of subjects		$n=39$	$n=31$	$n=40$	$n=40$	$n=40$	$n=40$
Avg. max. shock level		8.20	9.35	9.15	27.00	24.53	24.55
% "obedient"		0.0%	0.0%	0.0%	65.0%	62.5%	65.0%

Test 1: the subject could not see or hear the "victim."
Test 2: the "victim" yelled at higher levels to be released.
Test 5: the "victim" yelled at higher levels that he had a heart condition and demand to be released. (At a certain high level the "victim" went completely silent.)

Milgram's experiments inspired a flurry of psychological studies over the next several decades. One of these studies was Jerry Burger's "Replicating Milgram: Would People Still Obey Today?" (Burger 2009). Unlike Milgram, who completed his work before IRBs were instituted, Burger had to obtain permission from his IRB to do the study, and had to obtain informed consent from all of his experimental subjects. And what did Burger find? His results were virtually the same as Milgram's. Milgram drew this lesson from his work:

> Often, it is not so much the kind of person a man is as the kind of situation in which he finds himself that determines how he will act. (Milgram 1974)

The Milgram experiment raised profound questions about human psychology and dramatically re-shaped how psychologists thought about free will. But the experiment itself had raised ethical questions.

Consider the consequences of a research program in which subjects are intentionally deceived into thinking they are killing someone. Milgram's "teachers" were not informed about the true reason for the experiment into which they were being enrolled because Milgram could not have successfully tested his hypothesis about the role of authority in obedience without keeping his teachers in the dark about the fact that the learner was not actually being shocked. Milgram's work raises many ethical questions. The question most relevant to this chapter, however, is this: how much weight should we put in a subject's decision to engage in research? Milgram shows that about two-thirds of us can easily be manipulated into doing whatever a man in a white coat tells us we ought to do. That's a sobering result and it suggests that people may not ethically approve of doing what they are apparently freely agreeing to do. How much faith, then, can an honest researcher put in a subject's assertion that the subject wants to be in an experiment – even if the subject has "freely" signed a consent form?

Why it matters

Informed consent matters for two reasons.

First, our social role as a researcher requires that we recognize the autonomy of our experimental subjects. Not to inform people of the fact that participating in research exposes them to potential risks is not only to fail to protect their well-being. It also fails to show them the respect they deserve as free agents. To honor your experimental subjects' rights, identify and minimize risks to them; protect their privacy; and ensure that any risks of psychological, professional, or physical harm that remain are proportionate and reasonable to the potential benefits of the research, especially for vulnerable populations. Provide sufficient information so that each subject can make an informed decision about whether to participate. Obtain their voluntary informed consent, typically in writing, prior to beginning the project. Use scientifically valid designs and methods that will collect the data necessary to test the hypothesis. Justify any use of deception, and allow subjects to withdraw at any time.

Second, being associated with a research project puts us in the role of educators. If we do not explain to our subjects the procedures to which they will be exposed we do not put them into a position where they can exercise and develop their freedom. Almost inevitably, experimental subjects in research have certain choices open to them. We can assist and empower subjects by helping them to understand where and when they can exercise their capacities as free beings. In so doing, we play a role in their exercising their autonomy. Rational agency is not a capacity with which we are born; it must be developed. Not to seek our subjects' informed consent in research matters denies them an opportunity to grow into the sort of beings they are.

The background reading by Douglas MacLean highlights and explains this under-appreciated dimension of informed consent, and suggests that a more extensive informed consent process could help subjects strengthen and refine their autonomy.

Background essay: "Informed consent and the construction of values," by Douglas MacLean [2]

Informed consent is a fundamental component of moral justification. It distinguishes love-making from rape, employment from servitude, and life-saving surgery from felonious assault with a deadly weapon, to mention just a few examples. At a more general level, consent distinguishes democratic from authoritarian governments, and it justifies a capitalist economic system. Efficiency is important but freedom is what makes capitalism most appealing, as producers choose what to produce, and consumers choose what to buy. Consent is required to justify activities that impose a risk of harm or death on others.

. . .

When disparities of power or the effects of new technologies threaten the effectiveness of consent democratic governments intervene with regulations aimed at reinforcing the conditions of consent or establishing procedures for obtaining it. Laws that give citizens and consumers access to information or that protect a variety of freedoms of expression are examples of government activities aimed at making consent more effective.

. . .

What gives consent its transforming and justifying power? Perhaps this question has not received much attention because the answer seems obvious though difficult to articulate clearly. I will argue that the value of consent is less obvious than it is often taken to be. This fact has some important implications for determining policies and regulations that make the consent of those on whom risks are imposed more effective.

The value of consent in promoting well-being and in promoting freedom

Consent requirements have obvious instrumental value (Scheffler 1985). If we assume that people generally know their own interests better than others know them, then consent requirements can be effective means for ensuring that the interests of those affected by decisions are given due weight in making those decisions. If we also assume that people are generally less willing to be treated in morally unacceptable ways themselves than they are to treat others unacceptably, then consent requirements also have value as an effective tool for deterring morally unacceptable behavior. You will be less likely to trample my interests in pursuit of your own if you need my consent before you act.

Consent requirements may also have a more direct and noninstrumental value in promoting well-being. In some settings, consent procedures may reduce alienation, hostility, and other destructive attitudes stemming from lack of inherent trust. The result may be to make cooperation more likely or, for example in clinical medical settings, to improve the prospects of a good outcome. Giving consent may promote a person's self-esteem, his sense of personal responsibility for his own recovery, and his feelings of identification and solidarity with those trying to help him. Being given a voice in the choice of actions that will affect one may also contribute directly to a

---

[2] Reprinted from S. Lichtenstein & P. Slovic, eds. *The Construction of Preference.* New York: Cambridge University Press, 2006. Douglas MacLean is Professor of Philosophy, University of North Carolina, Chapel Hill, maclean@email.unc.edu.

person's well-being in a more general way, for a life deprived of such a voice would be deficient or servile in important ways that would affect a person's happiness.

But neither the instrumental value of consent in promoting well-being nor the direct value it may have as a constituent of a person's well-being can be the whole story of its justification. At least part of that story must appeal to a different kind of consideration altogether. The act of giving consent is a way of incorporating a person's will into decisions that affect her personally and into collective actions of which she is a part. Consider the fact that sometimes people really don't know what is good for them, and others may be able to intervene or act more effectively to protect them or make them better off. In many such situations, however, we tend nevertheless to insist that a free and rational person be given the right to consent to actions that will affect her. It is often important to let people choose, even if we have good reason to expect that they will make bad, harmful, or simply nonoptimal choices. Consent matters in these contexts not only as an effective means for getting our interests promoted and desires satisfied, but also to give us a voice in decisions that affect us or are made in our name. We cannot fully comprehend this aspect of the value of consent by appealing to the various ways that consent promotes happiness or well-being. Rather, part of the value of consent has to do with autonomy. Both at an individual level and in collective decision-making, it is through consent that we realize our nature as free agents. If this is correct then consent procedures must be designed not only to promote well-being but also to protect and enable us to realize our freedom. In what follows, I try to explain these remarks and explore their implications.

Informed consent in the physician–patient relationship

To help fix intuitions, I will focus on medical or healthcare decisions, although the claims I will be defending are meant to be general and not tied in any essential way to this domain. This is an area, however, in which the value of informed consent has received much thought and discussion. One standard view sees consent as having two components: informing and consenting. The healthcare professional is responsible for the former and the patient for the latter. This view of the value of consent has been clearly stated by Gorovitz (1982):

> The doctrine of informed consent is simple and clear on the surface. Physicians do the sorts of things to their patients that people in general cannot justifiably do to one another. If the patient understands what the physician proposes to do and, thus informed, consents to its being done, then the medical intervention is not imposed on the patient in violation of the patient's autonomy; rather, that medical intervention is properly viewed as a service provided to the patient at the patient's request. Not only does this procedure of gaining informed consent respect the patient's autonomy, but it also protects the physician against the charge of imposing treatment on a patient who did not want that treatment – it protects the physician, in other words, against the charge of assault. On the face of it, the requirement should be applauded on all sides. (p. 38)

Gorovitz (1982) is aware that informing patients about their alternatives can be difficult and costly, and he is also sensitive to the kinds of duress and pressures that can undermine the value of a patient's consent. He allows that paternalistic actions can sometimes be justified, but he argues that the threshold must be high before we allow the principle of benevolence to override the principle of autonomy. "Respect for persons –for their liberty and their right to express their individuality by pursuing a freely chosen course of action – supports the Principle of Autonomy" (p. 42).

. . .

The standard model of informed consent described by Gorovitz (1982) . . . presupposes that at least the patient is aware of her values and preferences, but we have reasons to doubt this assumption. . . . Patients may be confronting a decision under considerable stress, and they may also face a variety of complex prospects about conditions that are difficult to imagine or compare. In an excellent article that explores different models of the physician–patient relationship,

Emanuel and Emanuel (1992) consider a common clinical case. A 43-year-old premenopausal woman, recently divorced and gone back to work, discovers a breast mass, which surgery reveals to be "a 3.5-cm ductal carcinoma with no lymph node involvement that is estrogen receptor positive" (p. 2223). What are her options? Mastectomy or lumpectomy with radiation have identical 80% 10-year survival rates, and lumpectomy without radiation results in a 30% to 40% risk of tumor recurrence. Lumpectomy with chemotherapy prolongs survival for premenopausal women who have axillary nodes involved in the tumor, but the effects of chemotherapy on women with node-negative breast cancer is unclear. Individual studies suggest that there is no benefit from chemotherapy, but the National Cancer Institute believes that there may be a positive impact. A clinical trial is under way to study the issue further, which this woman is eligible to enter. Chemotherapy would prolong treatment by many months, but it would also bring the benefits of receiving the best medical care for the duration of the trial and contributing to the advance of scientific knowledge about breast cancer and its treatments. How should this woman incorporate this information into a decision about which treatment she will consent to receive?

We can assume that she values her health, but she also cares about her appearance, self-image, and life outside the hospital. The idea of separating fact from value in the presentation of the alternatives seems unhelpful if not impossible. A more reasonable consent process would involve the physician in a discussion that would help the patient articulate her values and apply them to the facts and prospects that a good decision would have to take into account.

. . .

A challenge to the assumption of existing preferences

Although the deliberative model that E.J. Emanuel and L.L. Emanuel (1992) defend is very different from the informative model described by Gorovitz (1982), both models in the end (although to varying degrees) share what I shall call the assumption of existing preferences. If patients do not have values that they can apply directly, almost mechanically, to the information they receive, they at least have deeper or more general values that can be mined, interpreted, and fitted to the alternatives they confront to generate preferences or choices that reflect those values. Surely we can safely assume that most 43-year-old women who learn that they have breast cancer want to survive and live an active life. The point I want to challenge is not whether people have any underlying values that they bring to their decisions, but the extent to which their values can be regarded as preexisting and thus independent of the descriptions of their prospects. The assumption of existing preferences presupposes a strong degree of independence. If we have reason to doubt this independence, as I believe we do, then the value of consent and the deliberative model will have to be seen in a different light.

The strongest reasons for doubting the assumption of existing preferences comes from psychological research in behavioral decision theory, which explores the empirical bases of human judgment and choice. I want to focus on a particular aspect of this research, but to do this I must first describe briefly the broader context into which it fits.

Some of the most interesting research in behavioral decision theory shows how preferences are causally influenced in predictable but nonrational ways, with the implication that most of us can be led to make choices that we would also admit are not rationally justifiable. These predictable but nonrational determinants of preference track descriptions of choice situations that do not correspond to any features of the situation that most people would regard as relevant to their goals or interests. Psychologists call these influences framing effects (see Kahneman & Tversky, 2000). Some evolutionary story can probably be told to explain this tendency and show that it helped us survive the competition of natural selection, but this fact provides limited comfort when compared with the overall consequences of our susceptibility to framing effects.

The standard (but not uncontroversial) theory of rational choice – utility theory – consists of a set of axioms that define existence and coherence conditions for preferences. The main theorem of utility theory says that rational preferences maximize expected utility. This means that if an individual has preferences that are coherent, in the sense defined by the axioms, then it is possible to assign utilities and probabilities to the alternative possible outcomes so that the most preferred alternative is the one that maximizes expected utility. Utility theory sees rationality, therefore, in terms of preferences for outcomes or states.

Now consider the following experiment (Kahneman & Tversky, 1979):

Example 1: the isolation effect

Problem 1: assume yourself richer by $300 than you are today. You have to choose between
- a sure gain of $100
- 50% chance to gain $200 and 50% chance to gain nothing.

Problem 2: assume yourself richer by $500 than you are today. You have to choose between
- a sure loss of $100
- 50% chance to lose nothing and 50% chance to lose $200.

These two problems offer equivalent prospects in terms of wealth. Each offers a choice between a sure gain of $400 and a gamble with an equal chance to gain either $300 or $500. If wealth completely defines the outcomes in these problems, then a rational person should choose the same option in both of them. But, in fact, most people choose the sure gain in Problem 1 and the gamble in Problem 2. This is a framing effect. We are led to see the prospect in Problem 1 as a choice among gains and the prospect in Problem 2 as a choice among losses, and most people tend to value perceived gains and losses differently.

. . .

Framing effects and methods for eliciting preferences

Suppose we wanted to determine which of two objects was heavier. We could place them on either side of a balance scale, which is a method of direct comparison, or we could weigh them independently on a spring scale that registers the weight of each and use that comparison to determine which is heavier. The ordering of the objects according to weight should be the same either way. It doesn't matter for this purpose what metric is used or whether the scales are accurate.

Now suppose that the weighings produced a different result, such that object A was heavier when put on the balance scale, but object B registered a greater weight on the spring scale. What would we think? We would probably think that something was wrong with one of the scales, and we'd look around for another one to determine which object was really heavier. But suppose now that further weighings produced the same result. Every balance scale we could find indicated that A was heavier than B, but B registered more kilos or pounds than A on every spring scale. We would be deeply puzzled. This result would upset a basic assumption we make about the physical world, that the relative weights of two objects do not vary with the kind of scale we use to determine those weights. With no other hypotheses available to explain these results, we would be forced to conclude that the weights of (at least these) objects were not independent of the scales used to measure or compare those weights. But, we might continue to wonder, which object is really, objectively heavier? It seems that this question has no answer. Surely it does no good to run off to a hundred scales to see what a majority of them tell us. The concept "heavier than" would seem not to be independent of the process of measurement. It is, we might say, constructed out of the measurement process and thus relative to it.

Now this fantasy about the relative weights of physical objects and the meaning of "heavier than" strains credibility from the start. Indeed, our experience convinces us that the basic properties of the physical world (or at least the common-sense physical world of medium-sized objects) are independent of our acts of perceiving and measuring them. But the psychological evidence indicates that preferences are not like this and that the assumption of existing preferences is simply not true.

Why should it be otherwise? There is little intuitive reason to think that preferences should simply be an ordering of objective states of the world. Our desires and values, after all, are to a considerable degree determined by how we describe and conceive things and by their relation to our subjective position in the world. It is not unreasonable to think that to have a preference for a prospect, we have to perceive our relationship to it in some way and that coming to see our relationship to it differently will affect our preferences.

We can now begin to appreciate the implication of these thoughts for the value of informed consent. We express our freedom when we consent to activities that affect us because we construct our values and preferences in ways that incorporate those activities into states of affairs that we endorse or reject. This is what the value of autonomy means in this context. Consent is part of a process of preference or value construction, which explains why it has the power to justify what happens to us.

A deliberative model of shared decision-making should be the goal of . . . consent-giving relationships, therefore, because this is the only model that is suitable for constructing preferences and values. . . . Physician and patient [and researcher and subject] work together to construct values in a deliberative process leading to consent. Getting information about the prospects we face is an important component of that process, but there is simply no neutral way in which to package, deliver, and integrate that information into an expression of consent. The act of informing is part of the value-construction process, not merely a pre-condition of it.

References for MacLean

Emanuel, E.J. & Emanuel, L.L. 1992. Four models of the physician-patient relationship. *JAMA: The Journal of the American Medical Association*, **267**(16), 2221–2226.

Gorovitz, S. 1982. *Doctors' Dilemmas: Moral Conflict and Medical Care*. New York: Macmillan.

Kahneman, D. & Tversky, A. 1979. Prospect theory: an analysis of decision under risk. *Econometrica*, **XLVII**, 263–291. Available at: http://www.princeton.edu/~kahneman/docs/Publications/prospect_theory.pdf [Accessed June 20, 2012].

Scheffler, S. 1985. The role of consent in the legitimation of risky activities. In M. Gibson, ed. *To Breathe Freely*. Totowa, NJ: Rowman & Littlefield, pp. 75–88.

A deliberative model of informed consent such as MacLean recommends can help subjects more fully to exercise their freedom. It can also help researchers to fulfill their social responsibilities (see Chapter 15). MacLean's model is useful not only for thinking about needed reforms in medical research protocols. It should also stimulate debate in the social sciences about the methods and goals of survey instruments. Should survey-takers regard their activities not simply as exercises for gathering opinions but also as occasions for education, too? Whether and how such goals might be incorporated into social scientific research are unclear. More thought is needed.

How to get experimental subjects' informed consent: sample form

The template below contains much of the information currently required by most institutional IRBs for enrolling subjects in surveys. It is based on a form created by the

Committee on the Protection of Human Subjects at California State University, Fresno (California State University, Fresno).

Informed consent form

You are invited to participate in a study conducted by Dr. Jane Smith of Central State University. We hope to learn [state here the purpose of the study – what is it designed to discover or establish?]. You were selected as a possible participant in this study because [state reason for selecting this subject].

If you decide to participate, Dr. Smith and her team will [describe the procedures to be followed, including their purposes, how long each one will take, how often they will be repeated]. [Describe the risks, discomforts, inconveniences, and benefits reasonably to be expected. If benefits are mentioned, add:] We cannot guarantee, however that you will receive any benefits from this study.

[Describe appropriate alternative procedures that might be advantageous to the subject, if any. Any standard treatment that is being withheld must be disclosed.]

Any information that is obtained in connection with this study and that can be identified with you will remain confidential and will be disclosed only with your permission or as required by law. If you give us your permission by signing this document, we plan to disclose [state the persons or agencies to whom the information will be furnished, the nature of the information to be furnished, and the purpose of the disclosure].

[If the subject will receive compensation, describe the amount or nature.] [If there is a possibility of additional cost to the subject because of participation, describe it.] [If there are risks to the subjects, state them explicitly.]

Your decision whether or not to participate will not prejudice your future relations with Central State University [and the named cooperating agency or institution, if any]. If you decide to participate, you are free to withdraw your consent and to discontinue participation at any time without penalty. The Committee on the Protection of Human Subjects at Central State University has reviewed and approved the present research.

If you have any questions, please ask us. If you have any additional questions later, Dr. Smith [give a phone number or address] will be happy to answer them. Questions regarding the rights of research subjects may be directed to John Jones, Chair, CSU Committee on the Protection of Human Subjects, 555 123 4567.

You will be given a copy of this form to keep.

You are making a decision whether or not to participate. Your signature indicates that you have decided to participate having read the information provided above.

_____ Signature and date

_____ Signature of witness and date

_____ Signature of investigator and date

We return now to the example with which the chapter started. As we have seen, every member of a research team has a duty to call attention to problems as soon as they occur. If a graduate student becomes aware of a breach of protocol, they must take corrective action. The next step in our case, therefore, must be to discuss the issue with the principal investigator. If the head of the project does not then communicate with the IRB, the student must pursue the matter by consulting first with other members of the group and eventually with higher administrators if necessary in order to ensure that the moral rights of the survey subjects are protected.

Take home lessons

To honor your experimental subjects' rights, follow these basic guidelines:

- Identify, minimize and communicate risks to the person on whom the research is being conducted, making sure to protect their privacy.
- Ensure that any risks of psychological, professional, or physical harm that remain are proportionate and reasonable to the potential benefits of the research, especially for vulnerable populations.
- When enrolling subjects do not discriminate on the basis of gender, race, religion, or ethnicity.
- Disclose all information specific persons need to make fully informed decisions to ensure that each one individually understands the procedure, and obtain voluntary written agreement to the terms prior to starting the project.
- Ensure that methods and design are scientifically valid and will succeed in collecting appropriate data to test the hypothesis; justify any deception involved.
- Allow subjects to withdraw from the project at any time.

Bibliography

World Medical Association. 1964. WMA Declaration of Helsinki - Ethical Principles for Medical Research Involving Human Subjects. Available at: http://www.wma.net/en/30publications/10policies/b3/ [Accessed March 9, 2012].

Arendt, H. 1963. *Eichmann in Jerusalem: A Report on the Banality of Evil.* New York: The Viking Press.

Bledsoe, C.H., *et al.* 2007. Regulating creativity: research and survival in the IRB iron cage. *Northwestern University Law Review*, **101**(2), 593–641.

Burger, J.M. 2009. Replicating Milgram: would people still obey today? *American Psychologist*, **64**(1), 1–11.

California State University, Fresno, n.d. Sample informed consent form. Available at: http://www.csufresno.edu/humansubjects/resources/informed_consent.shtml [Accessed August 21, 2011].

Dept. of Health and Human Services, U.S. 1992. Protection of human subjects: Title 45, Code of federal regulations, part 46, revised June 18, 1991., Bethesda, Md.: Dept. of Health and Human Services, National Institutes of Health, Office for Protection from Research Risks,. Available at: http://www2.lib.ncsu.edu/catalog/record/NCSU1257084.

Grady, C. 2010. Do IRBs protect human research participants? *JAMA: The Journal of the American Medical Association*, **304**(10), 1122–1123.

Gunsalus, C.K., *et al.* 2006. Mission creep in the IRB world. *Science*, **312**(5779), 1441.

Kahneman, D. & Tversky, A., eds. 2000. *Choices, Values, and Frames*, 1st edn. Cambridge University Press.

Milgram, S. 1974. *Obedience to Authority: An Experimental View.* Taylor & Francis.

National Commission for the Protection of Human Subjects of Biomedical and Behavioral Research. 1978. Belmont report: ethical principles and guidelines for the protection of human subjects of research. Bethesda, Md.: The Commission.

10

Mentor inclusively

A mentor is a counselor

A mentor is a counselor into whose hands is entrusted the teaching of the next generation. Odysseus, preparing to leave for war, entrusted the care of his son, Telemachus, to his friend, Mentor. Each junior researcher must have a mentor, an advisor or professor or principal investigator to watch out for them, to encourage and challenge them. Junior researchers need advice both on technical aspects of their research and on the broader social aspects of making a good life as a professional. Because it involves a relationship of unequal power, mentoring is difficult enough when the junior and senior persons involved share a cultural background, gender, and ethnic identity. When the relationship involves individuals of groups traditionally under-represented in research, the activity requires special care and attention. Here we first consider the marks of a healthy mentoring relationship and then explore the challenges and opportunities inherent in the gender and racial diversity of mentors and mentees.

Who is a good mentor? He or she is someone with integrity who takes as their primary responsibility the development of the mentee's academic and research skills. A good mentor fosters an atmosphere of openness and mutual respect, commits to helping the mentee through to the end of the mentee's project, has significant research experience, and is an excellent teacher. Good mentors know the literature of the field, are in touch with principal authors and opinion-makers, and are respected by their colleagues. They give constructive criticism and encouragement through difficult times; they help mentees to develop conference presentations and alert them to postdoctoral opportunities and job openings. They ensure that a mentee's advisory committee is formed expeditiously and meets at least once a year.

Mentoring generates two kinds of obligations, individual and collective. We focus first on the individual level. Here, both teachers and students have it within their power to meet their duties whether they are the younger student being helped along or the more experienced colleague who is doing the helping. Our background essay explores this matter.

Research Ethics: A Philosophical Guide to the Responsible Conduct of Research. Gary Comstock.
Published by Cambridge University Press. © Cambridge University Press 2013.

Background essay: "Mentoring," by Ellen Hyman-Browne (Deceased), Michael Kalichman and Daniel Vasgird[1]

I.   Mentoring and its importance in the education and training of science professionals

Mentoring is one of the primary means for one generation of scientists to impart their knowledge to succeeding generations. More than textbooks and formal classes, the relatively informal, though complex and multidimensional, relationships between mentors and their trainees prepare the next generation of science professionals.

In her 1977 speech at the Nobel Banquet, prizewinner Rosalyn Yalow addressed the students of Stockholm, identifying them as "the carriers of our hopes for the survival of the world and our dreams for its future." Yalow spoke of an ever-widening circle of learning. She said, "If we are to have faith that mankind will survive and thrive on the face of the earth, we must believe that each succeeding generation will be wiser than its progenitors. We transmit to you, the next generation, the total sum of our knowledge. Yours is the responsibility to use it, to add to it, and transmit it to your children" [1].

Rosalyn Yalow's own success in science, and the success of her trainees, exemplifies the long tradition in science and medicine of one's willingness to sponsor, support, and encourage another's career development.

As suggested by Yalow, both the mentor and the trainee have responsibilities for the success of the process. These will be explored here as aspects of the responsible conduct of research, and in addition we will discuss ethical issues in the conduct of mentoring, and mentoring itself as a means to transmit ethical standards of professional conduct.

Mentoring has received increasing attention in the past decade, and subsequently a body of literature has emerged describing the mentoring process and discussing its potential benefits and problems. Issues regarding fair access to mentors and the impact of a lack of mentoring on women and minorities are especially important. At some institutions, guidelines and formal programs have been put in place to deal with these concerns. This module explores these and other facets of mentoring, with the goal of increasing understanding of and attention to this important matter.

II.   Description of mentoring: the complexity of the role and the many forms it takes

A mentor is someone who has experience with the challenges that trainees face, the ability to communicate that experience, and the willingness to do so. A mentor takes a special interest in helping another person develop into a successful professional. In Greek mythology, Mentor was a trusted friend of Odysseus and helped to advise Telemachus, the son of Odysseus.

The role of a mentor is different from that of a supervisor or adviser, although these formal academic roles can lead to a mentoring relationship. The essence of mentoring has been described in a report by the National Academy of Sciences as being an adviser, teacher, role model, and friend [2]. We would add one more component to that mix: advocate.

---

[1] Reprinted from Responsible Conduct of Research, Mentoring, Columbia Center for New Media Teaching and Learning, n.d. Available at: http://ccnmtl.columbia.edu/projects/rcr/rcr_mentoring/introduction/index.html (accessed March 17, 2012). Ellen Hyman-Browne, deceased, was Research Compliance Officer, Children's Hospital, Philadelphia. Michael Kalichman is Director of the Research Ethics Program, University of California, San Diego, kalichman@ucsd.edu. Daniel Vasgird is Director of the Office of Research Integrity and Compliance, West Virginia University, daniel.vasgird@mail.wvu.edu.

A mentor might be a faculty adviser, a laboratory director, a fellow student, another faculty member, a wise friend, or simply another person with experience. For our purposes, a trainee or protégé in the research setting includes anyone in a junior or apprentice position, such as an undergraduate or graduate student, a postdoctoral fellow, or a junior faculty member.

The significance of the mentor-trainee relationship is examined in a book about Nobel laureates by Harriett Zuckerman, Scientific Elite, in a chapter entitled "Masters and Apprentices in Science" [3]. The laureates reported to Zuckerman "that for them the principal benefit of apprenticeship was a wider orientation that included standards of work and modes of thought." Zuckerman found that ". . . apprenticeship was a time of what social scientists call socialization. Socialization includes more than is ordinarily understood by education or by training: it involves acquiring the norms and standards, the values and attitudes, as well as the knowledge, skills, and behavior patterns associated with particular statuses and roles. It is, in short, the process through which people are inducted into a culture or subculture."

Zuckerman reasoned that the process of socialization experienced by the laureates occurred in mutually reinforcing ways: ". . . the masters' own performance provided a model to be emulated; the masters evoked excellence from the apprentices working with them, and they were severe critics of scientific work . . . the masters generally served as role models, teaching less by precept than by example. By themselves adhering to demanding standards of work, they sustained the moral authority to pass severe judgments on work that failed to meet comparable standards" [3, p. 126].

Like the Nobel laureates described by Zuckerman, and like Telemachus in mythology, a trainee will benefit most from close ties over an extended period of time with a mentor who is personally committed to the relationship. Some commentators on this subject emphasize the personal nature of the mentor–trainee relationship. Others caution that boundaries are important. In either case, no two mentors will behave in exactly the same way – each brings to the task his own strengths and preferences. But every good mentor will act from a sense of responsibility and a commitment to the future of the trainee.

III. Roles, activities, and functions

William Silen, MD, Dean for Faculty Development and Diversity and the Johnson & Johnson Distinguished Professor of Surgery at Harvard Medical School, describes a rare species: "the truly complete mentor." This is "a single individual who is able to serve as an advisor/guide, developer of talent/coach, opener of doors/advocate, role model, interpreter of organizational or professional rules, protector, rule setter/boss – and carries on all of these functions on a long term basis" [4].

A rare species indeed. Few of us can claim the time or the skill to perform all of these roles for one other person; and it seems virtually impossible in the context of today's large laboratories, filled to the brim with graduate students and postdocs.

But to appreciate potential contributions of mentors it is helpful to consider the wide range of needs to be met. First and foremost, mentors in the sciences should help trainees develop as capable researchers. A mentor can contribute to the technical development of the trainee in many aspects of research, including methods, directions, creative thinking, completing academic or professional requirements, and scientific communication.

A second essential need for trainees is career development and preparation for the job market. This includes an understanding of the current job market, opportunities to make contacts with leaders in the trainee's field of research, active introduction into the network of people working in his or her discipline, and an awareness of the range of career options. A mentor may also advise a new scientist on career moves in terms of applying for grants, what grants to apply for, and how to submit a strong grant proposal.

Another focus of mentoring is the socialization of trainees. Such socialization should include guiding ethical development as well as fostering an understanding of the political, economic, and social elements of interacting within the academic community and instilling a sense of collegiality. This training includes promotion of skills for teaching, communication, working in teams, leadership, management of people, interacting with others, listening, expressing ideas, administration and planning, and budget management.

A particularly important mentoring role is that of advocate. Silen used the term "protector," but, however one phrases it, there are times when the mentor has to step forward and defend or advocate for the trainee. A specific academic example might be the situation in which a mentor's doctoral student is in the midst of his or her comprehensive examinations and has been instructed to rewrite an essay many times for a particular question. A member of the review panel for the exam has a reputation for demanding perfection from students and keeps sending the essay back. After the mentor reviews it thoroughly and perhaps discusses it with others, it is clear that the student's answer is well worth a pass or better. In that situation, it would not be inappropriate for the mentor to step in to move the process along. Other advocacy initiatives could stem from complaints from one's trainee about harassment or unequal treatment by others.

Clearly, the above list is long, but all of these elements, and more, are components that are necessary in order to survive and succeed in academia. A complete list of such elements should be limited only by the needs of the individual trainee. Any situation in which one person's knowledge or skill is greater than another's is a potential starting point for a mentoring relationship.

Although every trainee may need a "truly complete mentor," this may actually be a composite of more than one individual. Not all established scientists can bring the requisite time, knowledge, and interest to the full range of issues that are likely to be important to each trainee. Each mentor and each trainee have responsibilities that, if fulfilled, will optimize the effectiveness of the relationship for both.

IV. Mentoring on ethics and responsible conduct of research

One crucial role for a mentor is to assist the trainee in understanding and adhering to the standards of conduct within his or her profession. Within a small research group, this can often happen through example, impromptu counsel, and the free-flowing exchange of thoughts and ideas. But today many research groups are too large or competitive for this to occur. Whether or not this change in scale has impeded the extent to which new scientists become aware of prevailing standards of conduct, it appears that issues of responsible conduct are not discussed frequently enough.

"...nearly 40% of postdoctoral research fellows ... reported having had no guidance in ethical research from a scientific mentor ..."

For better or worse, whether by personal habit or increased demands, the current default method of teaching the traditions and standards of science is by unwitting and serendipitous example. Unfortunately, without discussion of ethical principles and the purposeful assurance that everyone is included, this approach to training is seriously flawed. The principles of decision-making are not explicit and are therefore open to interpretation (and misinterpretation), and many important roles of scientists (e.g., peer review or negotiating collaborations) are not observed by the trainee. The available evidence strongly argues against relying on this approach to training.

The importance of mentoring for training in the responsible conduct of research has been recognized in several national reports on the integrity of research. For example, a report from the Institute of Medicine [5] noted the importance of mentors and specifically recommended that departments and research units should monitor the supervision and training of young scientists to ensure that it is adequate. In 1992, a Panel on Scientific Responsibility and the Conduct of Research concluded that "Research mentors ... are responsible for defining, explaining, exemplifying, and requiring adherence to the value systems of their institutions." Similarly, a more recent report emphasized the importance of continued mentoring for postdoctoral researchers (Committee on Science, Engineering, and Public Policy, 2000 [6]).

Responsible conduct is more than the desire to do the right thing or the reading of relevant regulations and publications. It is also important that trainees recognize the wide range of accepted practices, and that some of these practices may be preferable to others. Furthermore, trainees need to understand that acting responsibly depends on an appreciation that standards can vary between and within disciplines, can change over time, and in some cases are not yet clearly defined. For trainees to understand the varied and evolving nature of these standards, it is necessary that experienced scientists clearly convey their understanding of accepted practices in the conduct of research.

V.   The ethics of mentoring

The mentor–trainee relationship can be abused in many ways as a result of the inherent imbalance of power. Mentors have more knowledge, experience, and status, and in most cases are in a position of authority over the trainee. Even a mentor who is not very senior has a great deal of power relative to a trainee. The trainee has much to gain from the mentor's support and advocacy, and fear of jeopardizing that support makes the relationship especially imbalanced. Perhaps the greatest power disparity exists for a trainee from a foreign country.

A mentor can use this power to exploit the trainee – for example, in refusing to give proper credit for the trainee's contributions or in seeking to obtain personal or even sexual favors. A common complaint of trainees is that they are required to spend so much time working on the mentor's research that there is little time left for their own.

Perhaps the greatest complexity occurs in the mentoring of graduate students. Where does the responsibility of the supervisor end and that of the trainee begin? What about the responsibilities of the advisory committee and the entire graduate program faculty for the success of graduate research training? Is there a difference between a research supervisor and a research mentor? If there is a difference, are the duties associated with mentoring optional? How much does a faculty member "owe" to the duty of research supervision, as opposed to what they owe themselves and their other academic duties? Whose responsibility is it to protect students from poor advisers?

Boundaries between a faculty member's financial and career interests and their responsibilities to their advisees create additional problems. Jonathan Cole posed an important question in this context: in the role of research adviser in determining a research topic, if there is a choice between a topic that may lead to a patent and one that is more "intellectually interesting and challenging," is it appropriate for the adviser to push the student toward the topic with patent possibilities because of the potential financial rewards? Cole suggests that such a constraint on the student's topic would be inappropriate [9].

In the case of industry-funded research, it may be in the sponsor's interest to delay publication of results for as long as 2 years. A faculty member must consider the consequences for any graduate student or trainee involved in such research. If there are constraints on publication, the trainee should be made aware of them before choosing to participate in the research, and both the mentor and the trainee must consider the impact of such delays on the trainee's career prospects.

A mentor may, rather than exercise his or her power "over" a trainee, withhold power, disengaging and failing to serve as champion, sponsor, or protector. If a mentor is threatened by the success of a trainee, he may undermine the confidence of the trainee. Other problems can arise when a trainee is ignored or neglected, communication is inadequate, there is a lack of feedback, or the mentor gives extremely harsh criticism.

"Toxic mentoring" is a label that has been used to describe these problematic relationships. Dr. William Silen published an article in Mentations, a Harvard Medical School publication, entitled "Tormentor of the Year, A Cautionary Tale" [10]. Silen suggests that, "[a]t the same time we proffer kudos upon outstanding mentors, it behooves us to call attention to those who engage in actively negative mentoring, which for want of a better term we shall refer to as 'tormenting.' Perhaps an award should be given to 'Tormentor of the Year.'"

Whether we call them toxic mentors or tormentors, those who take advantage of or ignore trainees must be reminded that they have a special obligation to foster the intellectual development and independence of the next generation of scientists. The most effective mentor ensures that her trainee gets the maximum appropriate credit for any joint publications; encourages the trainee to attend national or international conferences, workshops, and symposia and to present research at such events; promotes the trainee's work among colleagues; and helps the trainee create important professional networks.

The guiding principle should be the interest of the trainee. Departments and schools have a role in setting out reasonable expectations for the mentor and the trainee, as well as in suggesting strategies to make the relationship as productive and mutually satisfying as possible. Virtually all studies of and guidelines for research advising and mentoring stress the importance of structuring the research process carefully – establishing deadlines for various milestones in the process, scheduling regular meetings with the adviser and the trainee, and dealing with issues of authorship and intellectual property.

VI. The responsibility to mentor minorities and women

Those who seek to broaden the representation of minorities and women in the research professions increasingly look to mentoring to help achieve that goal. Traditionally, white trainees are more likely than minority trainees to have a mentor, and men are more likely than women to have a mentor. Correcting this imbalance is a logical step, given the significance that mentoring has in career development, and the importance of maximizing the potential of all members of the scientific community.

The Outer Circle: Women in the Scientific Community (edited by Harriet Zuckerman, Jonathan R. Cole, and John T. Bruer [W.W. Norton & Company, New York, 1991]) explores the reasons that women, in general, may not have been as productive in scientific careers as men. Research tracking the accomplishments and tenure outcomes of assistant professors at two universities is described by Mary Frank Fox: "To the extent that women are excluded from collegial channels and collaborative opportunities, their productivity can suffer" [11]. In one study, it was found that only 25% of the women, compared with 52% of the men, had co-authored papers with senior professors. Furthermore, a significantly larger percentage of those who had collaborated were promoted, compared with those who had not collaborated. In a second study, it was found that collegial interactions – specifically, collaboration in co-authoring and mentoring relationships – related to both productivity and promotion rates.

Discussing another study of career processes in science, Fox concludes, ". . . collaboration with a mentor affects pre-doctoral productivity and job placement, which, in turn, influence later productivity. But the mentor also influences productivity independent of these indirect effects. For those who collaborate with a mentor, the mentor continues to affect the student's productivity." Mentoring socializes a trainee into the culture of science and initiates a young scientist into the scientific community. Historically, women and minorities have been excluded from this process, which has obviously limited their possibilities "to do research, to publish, to be cited – to show the crucial marks of productivity in science."

Many programs have been developed to correct the imbalance in mentoring opportunities. For example, Harvard Medical School created the Office for Diversity and Community Partnership, to promote increased recruitment and the retention and promotion of underrepresented minority faculty, and to oversee all diversity activities involving Harvard Medical School faculty, trainees, students, and staff. The inaugural issue of *Mentations*, the newsletter of the office, contains an announcement of the first annual Harvard Medical School Award for Excellence in Mentoring [12]. In addition to recognizing the importance of mentoring through an award, this office also conducts programs on mentoring and handles requests for assistance and information about mentoring.

The Association for Women in Science [13] began a mentoring project in 1990, with the ultimate goal of increasing the number of women who attain bachelor's degrees and advanced degrees in science and engineering and achieve successful careers as science and engineering professionals. It was designed to integrate female students into the scientific community by helping them identify and overcome the obstacles that prevent them from continuing in science. In addition, MentorNet [14], a mentoring network for women in engineering and science, states as its mission "to further women's progress in scientific and technical fields through the use of a dynamic, technology-supported mentoring program; and to advance women and society, and enhance engineering and related sciences, by promoting a diversified, expanded and talented workforce." MentorNet seeks to achieve this by providing students with mentoring to enhance their presence in fields where they remain underrepresented, and to facilitate their entry into scientific and technical careers.

VII.   Responsibilities of trainees

Most young or aspiring scientists have at least a modest conceptualization of their ultimate career aspirations and have internalized the usual worries that accompany those dreams. Few, however, will be fortunate enough to have one or more ideal mentors step in to help. The obvious solution is to seek out more senior scientists, and sometimes peers, who have the experience that is lacking. Finding someone who will be an effective mentor is primarily a responsibility of the trainee.

1.   Identify career plans

In seeking a mentor, the first step for a trainee is identifying particular needs. What are his or her career plans? Trainees should assess their skills, talents, and interests, and seek advice from someone who is knowledgeable about suitable career options. Someone who can help with this initial look at career plans may be, or may become, a mentor, but this is not essential. (The IDP referred to earlier can help in this regard: http://www.faseb.org/LinkClick.aspx?fileticket=fhdgO6SYtjM%3d&tabid=433.)

2.   Locate prospective mentors

Having identified general career interests, a trainee should seek as prospective mentors people who have succeeded in making the transition from where the trainee is now to where the trainee hopes to be. This means identifying people who know and have overcome the challenges to success. For example, for some women it would be invaluable to seek out women who have met the challenges that they are likely to face.

Characteristics to look for in potential mentors include experience in areas relevant to the trainee's personal and career development, an interest in the trainee and his or her career, a willingness to make the time to meet with the trainee, and an ability to provide the trainee with useful advice, not a rigid set of demands. In addition, an ideal mentoring relationship depends on the compatibility of the personalities of the mentor and the trainee. Assessing such qualities and the interpersonal skills of the prospective mentor is much more difficult than gauging someone's success as a researcher. However, because research is defined by personal as well as professional relationships, these qualities are as important as any other criteria in identifying a supervisor, thesis adviser, or mentor.

Finding a compatible mentor, adviser, or supervisor is more likely to be successful when trainees first do their homework and ask questions of senior students. What do previous trainees or employees report of their experience working with the prospective mentor? What is the quality of the trainee's interactions with the prospective mentor? How do other faculty and staff feel about the prospective mentor? What is the track record of the prospective mentor, e.g., rate of degree completion and time to degree?

3. Distinguish between supervisors and mentors

Not everyone embodies the characteristics needed in a good mentor. While the terms "mentor," "thesis adviser," and "research supervisor" are frequently used interchangeably, it is important to note that thesis advisers and research supervisors are not necessarily mentors. For example, thesis advisers are responsible for ensuring that students fulfill departmental and institutional requirements for the graduate degree and for providing advice about research directions, methods, and publication. Mentors, on the other hand, provide information beyond scientific concepts and laboratory techniques – information that is essential for professional success, such as how to obtain funding, manage a research lab or group, use time effectively, and understand departmental politics and institutional committees.

Although supervisors ideally are mentors, that is not always the case. In some cases, a thesis adviser or head of a research group will provide much of the mentoring that trainees need. If not, then initiating a discussion with a supervisor about authorship criteria, the funding process, or mentoring itself might stimulate the supervisor to become a better mentor. However, whether or not a supervisor is an effective mentor, it is unlikely that one person alone can provide all that is needed.

4. Be clear about needs and expectations

A mentoring relationship should not be a passive one for either the mentor or the trainee. From the trainee's perspective, it is necessary to take an active role in identifying and communicating his or her needs and expectations in the mentoring relationship. At the same time, the mentor's advice should not be accepted without question. Although a mentor can provide a unique and invaluable perspective, the trainee has the responsibility to evaluate the mentor's advice in light of his or her own values, goals, and experience.

5. Keep learning about effective mentoring

It is important for trainees to continue learning about the mentoring process to optimize their own experience and also to prepare them to be effective mentors. A good starting point would be the resources and mentoring guides listed at the end of this module.[2] However, it should be more than this, and the suggestion might be made to one's program or department head to add mentoring as a topic for seminars or colloquia.

VIII.   Responsibilities of mentors

Just as scientific trainees have a responsibility to seek mentors, scientists have a complementary responsibility to become mentors. Taking an active role in helping to train the next generation of scientists should not be optional – it should be part of the definition of a scientist. For this reason, the enterprise of science depends on effective communication not just about the science but about the practice of science, standards of conduct, and ethical and social responsibility. This obligation extends to all members of the community, not just senior researchers. For example, it is likely that a newly arrived undergraduate student could benefit from the mentoring of a graduate student, technician, or even a more senior undergraduate.

---

[2] This refers to the larger online module from which this essay is taken: "Responsible Conduct of Research, Mentoring," Columbia Center for New Media Teaching and Learning, n.d. Available at: http://ccnmtl.columbia.edu/projects/rcr/rcr_mentoring/introduction/index.html (accessed March 17, 2012).

1. Be available

At the core of mentoring responsibilities is the simple admonition to make oneself available. Woody Allen once said that 80% of success is simply showing up, and mentoring is no different. However, some researchers make the mistake of thinking that somehow mentoring will take over their professional lives and leave no time for their research responsibilities. It doesn't have to be this way, nor should it. In the span of a few minutes, a mentor can give her trainees a feeling of empathy by being attentive to a few key elements, such as careful listening and keeping in touch.

Careful listening is the art of hearing exactly what someone is trying to tell you without first evaluating. Try to focus on the nuances of word emphasis and body language. Through careful response and a few well-placed questions, the way is open for clear communication and a feeling of support and encouragement.

Keeping in touch means regularly communicating with your trainees. Try to give at least a few minutes to your trainees every other day or so. These short exchanges can help one stay aware of what is going on and anticipate problems before they grow.

Another way to ensure that trainees feel acknowledged is through multiple mentoring. Mentors differ, and not everyone will fully reciprocate a trainee's commitment. This can often be managed through multiple mentoring systems, which can allow, through a division of labor, for differences in style, skills, and availability.

2. Allow for differences in personalities

Successful mentoring, as with any close personal relationship, depends on the personalities of the parties involved. Some trainees learn readily with a minimum of nurturing or guidance, or at least prefer to believe that they require a minimum of help. In such cases, frequent and probing discussion initiated by a mentor may be perceived as invasive and micromanagerial. Other trainees may require the reassurance of being closely monitored and receiving frequent feedback, both positive and negative. Conversely, some mentors will be uncomfortable with offering advice or initiating discussions unless first asked by a trainee, and other mentors will readily volunteer information and advice without any clear indication that help would be welcomed.

The most effective mentoring is likely to occur when the personalities of the mentor and the trainee are a good match. In an effort to act as a mentor, a research supervisor or thesis adviser should attempt to fit his or her style of interaction to the needs and personality of a trainee. Similarly, in an effort to gain the most from a mentoring relationship, the trainee should make allowances for differences between his or her personality and the mentor's.

3. Let trainees make their own decisions

The role of the mentor is to provide advice, help, and encouragement. However, the trainee should not be bound to follow suggestions made by the mentor. Ultimately, it is the responsibility of the trainee to act based on his or her own values, goals, and experience.

4. Teach by words and example

Although not all role models are automatically good mentors, the demonstration of good skills and behavior is a necessary element of mentoring. If a mentor argues for rigorous authorship criteria but fails to follow his or her own advice, then lessons learned by the trainee may include that the mentor is an unreliable source of information, that the standards of conduct in research are poorly defined, and that the mentor is, unfortunately, a hypocrite. For a mentor, the lesson is that actions speak louder than words. However, it is still important that mentors make explicit the often implicit rationale for their behavior, because the policy and philosophy that underlie even the most exemplary behavior may be esoteric to the uninformed observer. This is especially true for observers who have a different cultural background.

5. Keep learning about effective mentoring

Responsible mentors should strive to continue learning about effective mentoring, through experience and through the available resources on mentoring. It is also suggested that a discussion about and comparison of mentoring techniques be added to faculty meeting agendas or other faculty events such as retreats.

IX.   Dealing with problems in the mentor–trainee relationship

Advance planning in the form of existing procedures or guidelines for addressing problems is the ideal. When asked what would improve their situations, many graduate students and postdocs respond with a request for written guidelines – they want to know what to expect and how to deal with problems [15,16]. Indeed, many academic institutions, graduate schools, and individual departments have written strategies for dealing with problems, concerns, and conflicts. These might range from "Speak first to your immediate supervisor or the faculty member involved" to "The department graduate adviser is the person with whom you should consult."

Communication between the mentor and the trainee should be considered first; if it is successful, it may prevent a problem from growing into a more serious grievance. If the trainee needs further assistance, he or she should first ascertain whether there are appropriate school procedures. Take into account all possibilities. Each situation and individual is unique – in one case it may be wise to deal with the problem within the department; in another, the best course may be to seek assistance elsewhere in the institution. The trainee will find someone to talk to by making use of the many resources of the university. One important resource to be aware of in dealing with mentoring problems is the ombudsperson's office at the university.

X.   Award/rewards

The benefits of mentoring to the trainee, the mentor, and the organization as a whole are demonstrable [17]. For example, trainees gain an understanding of the organizational culture, access networks of communication that carry significant professional information, and receive assistance in defining and achieving career goals.

The benefits to mentors are just as great. They may gain satisfaction from the sharing of their knowledge and experience, and from having a trainee succeed and eventually become a colleague. Mentoring keeps one on top of his or her field, helps to develop a professional network, and extends the scientist's contributions. Another benefit is the increased stimulation from bright and creative protégés. Mentors also derive enhanced status and self-esteem, and benefit from joint projects leading to shared grants and authorship as well as to increased revenues. The best mentors are also likely to be able to recruit students of high caliber. The value to the overall stability of the organization results from the development of future leadership, and improved performance within a work group.

This leads one to assume that mentoring activities would be assigned a high priority. In fact, mentoring is rarely rewarded. While a few universities (e.g., Harvard, mentioned above) give awards for excellence in mentoring, mentoring achievements rarely appear on one's CV, nor be considered in tenure decisions.

In 1996, President Clinton established the Presidential Award for Excellence in Science, Mathematics, and Engineering Mentoring. This award honors individuals and institutions that have outstanding records in mentoring students in underrepresented groups on their path to significant achievement in science, math, and engineering.

Institutions that set out to support and reward mentoring activities need to obtain increased support for enhancing mentoring efforts at the highest levels. One approach is to begin by holding school- and department-level discussions on how to enhance mentoring activities. Some ideas for programs include: implementing a formal approach and matching mentors and trainees;

developing group mentoring approaches; continuing with informal mentoring but heightening awareness of the benefits of mentoring and instituting more recognition or rewards; assisting senior professionals in developing their mentoring skills; implementing additional incentives for mentoring; and including documentation of mentoring in the annual evaluation process. The effort will be returned many times over in the increased satisfaction and productivity of all involved.

References for Hyman-Browne, Kalichman and Vasgird

1. From Les Prix Nobel. Rosalyn Yalow – *Banquet Speech at the Nobel Banquet*, December 10, 1977. The Official Web Site of the Nobel Foundation. © 2003 The Nobel Foundation. http://www.nobel.se/medicine/laureates/1977/yalow-speech.html (accessed on 7/10/2003).

2. National Academy of Science (NAS). 1997. *Advisor, Teacher, Role Model, Friend: On Being a Mentor to Students in Science and Engineering*. Washington DC: The National Academies Press. http://stills.nap.edu/html/mentor/

3. Zuckerman, H. 1977. *Scientific Elite: Nobel Laureates in the United States*. New York: Free Press.

4. Silen, W. 1998. In search of the complete mentor. In *Mentations*, Vol. 5. Available at: http://www.hms.harvard.edu/dcp/mentations/fall_98/searchofmentor.html.

5. Institute of Medicine. 1989. *The Responsible Conduct of Research in the Health Sciences*. Washington DC: The National Academies Press.

6. Committee on Science, Engineering, and Public Policy, National Research Council,. 2000. *Enhancing the Postdoctoral Experience for Scientists and Engineers: A Guide for Postdoctoral Scholars, Advisers, Institutions, Funding Organizations, and Disciplinary Societies*. Washington DC: The National Academies Press.

7. Csikszentmihalyi, M., Damon, W. & Gardner, H. 2003. *The GoodWork Project*. Cambridge, MA: Presidents and Fellows of Harvard College. Available at: http://www.pz.harvard.edu/Research/GoodWork.htm.

8. Rimer, S. 2003. Finding that today's students are bright, eager and willing to cheat. *The New York Times*, Wednesday, July 2: B8.

9. Cole, J.R. The Research University in a Time of Discontent.

10. Silen, W. 1996. Tor-mentor of the year: a cautionary tale. In *Mentations*, Vol. 2. Available at: http://www.hms.harvard.edu/dcp/mentations/fall_96/torment.html.

11. Fox, M.F. 1991. Gender, environmental milieu, and productivity in science. In H. Zuckerman, J. R. Cole, and J.T. Bruer, eds. *The Outer Circle: Women in the Scientific Community*. New York: W.W. Norton, pp. 188–204.

12. http://www.hms.harvard.edu/dcp/mentations/fall_95/import.htm.

13. http://awis.org/r_mentoringmain.html.

14. http://www.mentornet.net/.

15. *At Cross Purposes: What the experiences of doctoral students reveal about doctoral education*. By Chris M. Golde and Timothy M. Dore. January, 2001. A report prepared for The Pew Charitable Trusts, Philadelphia, PA. http://www.phd-survey.org/

16. http://www.nationalpostdoc.org/.

17. Anderson, M.S., Oju, E.C. & Falkner, T.M.R. 2001. Help from faculty: findings from the Acadia Institute Graduate Education Study. *Science and Engineering Ethics*, **7**(4), 487–504.

To ensure that you understand your mentor's views about issues related to research ethics, schedule an interview with them. Tell them that you would like to discuss responsible conduct of research. To structure the conversation and make the most efficient use of your mentor's time, email the following questions to them before you meet. The questions concern authorship practices; intellectual property; gathering, storage, and dissemination of data;

educational opportunities in responsible conduct of research; and progress to degree. It is critical to your success that you know your mentor's answers to these questions. And many mentors will already have shared their views with you. But faculty members are very busy people and may forget to discuss these topics. (And some faculty, unfortunately, consciously avoid them.) If you feel awkward about initiating the conversation, let us help you. Tell your mentor that you are reading this book and the authors have assigned you this task. Feel free to saddle us with the responsibility of making demands on the faculty member's time – but have the conversation.

Exercise: "Interview your mentor," by Gary Comstock and Charlotte Bronson[3]

Assignment: Interview a mentor or advisor. Preferably, this person will be your mentor or advisor, and a principal investigator (PI) and faculty member in your department. Ask questions (below) about: (a) authorship practices, (b) intellectual property, (c) research ethics education, and (d) time to degree.

A. Authorship practices

1. Who is in your group? In the sciences, the relevant group is usually the laboratory group, but your mentor may have other ideas and, in any event, it is important for you to have clarity about this point.
2. What criteria does the group use to determine who is an author on a paper? What sort of credit is deserved by those who make the following contributions: overall project design, project funding, design of individual experiments, data collection, data analysis, data interpretation, literature searches and review, writing, editing, and preparation of figures?
3. What criteria does the group use for determining who is first author?
4. What criteria does the group use for determining who is last author?
5. What criteria does the group use for determining who receives an acknowledgement?
6. What practices does the group consider "courtesy authorship" and what is the group policy on courtesy authorship?
7. Who in the group has the right to decide authorship?
8. Have relationships ever been strained due to differing views on authorship? If so, without naming the persons involved, what happened?

B. Intellectual property

1. What classes of research records are maintained by the group (research notebooks, computer files, films, culture collection lists, etc.)?
2. What are the policies (explicit or assumed) of the group on how research notebooks are to be created and maintained? Include the following information:
   - Any specific type of notebook (bound, loose-leaf, electronic)? If the notebook is bound, is there any particular style that the lab prefers?
   - Any particular type of writing instrument (ballpoint pen, India ink pen, pencil)?
   - What type of information is to be kept in the notebook (dates, experiment number, title, purpose, approach, methods, protocols, results, data sheets, graphs, computer files, conclusions, suggestions for future experiments, signatures, etc.)?

---

[3] Charlotte Bronson is Professor of Plant Pathology and Associate Vice President for Research, Iowa State University, cbronson@iastate.edu.

- Any policies on how the above information is organized in the notebooks?
- Any policies on re-writing notes before putting them into a notebook?
- Who owns the notebooks?
- Who has access to the notebooks?
- How long must the notebooks be kept? Who must keep them? Any policies on removal of notebooks from the premises? Any policies on copying the notebooks?

3. Has the group ever suffered because of improperly or inadequately kept notes?

C. Education in research ethics

Discuss the following statement and questions with your supervisor. Both the National Institutes of Health and National Science Foundation now require that education in the responsible conduct of research should include the following topics:

a. Research misconduct
b. Publication practices and responsible authorship
c. Peer review
d. Data acquisition, management, sharing, and ownership
e. Mentor/trainee responsibilities
f. Collaborative science
g. Human subjects
h. Conflict of interest and commitment
i. Research involving animals
j. Social responsibilities of researchers.

1. How is knowledge of these issues passed on in the lab? Is it mostly informal mentoring relationships? Or are there structured occasions, such as seminars or courses?
2. Is the PI satisfied that colleagues in the department are sufficiently communicating RCR to their graduate students?
3. If the answer to #2 is negative, what more does the PI think that the department should be doing?
4. Is the PI aware of research ethics courses offered on your campus? Which course, if any, does the PI recommend that you take?

D. Progress to degree

1. How soon should my doctoral committee be formed?
2. How often should my committee meet?
3. What is the typical time to degree in the department? Among your students?
4. (If the person you are interviewing is your doctoral supervisor) Would you help me make a list of the specific tasks I must accomplish under your supervision to earn my PhD.?

We began this chapter by noting that mentoring generates both individual and collective obligations. At the collective level, the experienced gatekeepers of a profession are required to ensure that the doors to the profession are not closed to certain groups. When barriers to entry are high for, say, women or people of color or talented students who lack economic resources, mentors must address these systemic issues. Students and mentees are simply not usually positioned to be able to reform powerful social structures.

As Mary Fox noted in the background essay, "Mentoring," women in science have not had the opportunities to co-author papers with senior professors at the same rate as have men in science. In the next article, the self-named blogger "Female Science Professor" reflects on her experiences and offers advice to younger women who are beginning research careers.

Case study: "Why 'female' science professor?" by Female Science Professor [4]

In the URL of my blog, I am simply "science-professor," but the pseudonymous name I use as a blogger is "Female Science Professor." Why the extra adjective? Does it matter in my work as a scientist and a professor that I am female?

Many times it does. In fact, when I first started using the moniker, my reasons were a bit cynical. I had been so often reminded by colleagues, in their words and actions, that I was different from the "regular" (read: male) science professors, that I decided to use the extra adjective to describe myself.

Even today, being different in that way – a woman in a male-dominated profession – has often meant that my female colleagues and I are seen as less qualified than our male counterparts. Often it has meant being told that my professional achievements were likely the result of my gender, not my abilities – for example, being told that a university "had to hire a woman," that the National Science Foundation "had to give a certain number of grants to women," that an organization "had to give that award to a woman" (because deserving men had gotten the award every year for the last century), or that conference organizers "had to invite at least one woman speaker." Some of those "had to" examples might even be true, but, in most cases, what happened was that qualified women were taken seriously and allowed to achieve what they deserved without being overlooked or held to a higher standard.

Being a female science professor has meant sitting in committee meetings with men who believed that they were there because of their intellectual gifts and wisdom but that I was there because, again, there "had" to be at least one woman on the committee. It has meant having my sentences interrupted and my ideas ignored unless a man expressed a similar opinion.

It has meant being paid less than my male peers.

It has meant having people assume that my series of papers with a particular male colleague must be the work of a graduate student (me) with her adviser (my co-author).

It has meant having surreal conversations like this, typically at conferences, but sometimes during conversations with a visitor to my department:

Male Science Professor (MSP), on meeting me for the first time:

Your husband is also a scientist.

ME: Yes, that's right. He works on topics X and Y.

MSP: I don't know that work, but I do know his work on A and B (insert accurate description of my research topics).

ME: Actually, I work on those topics, my husband doesn't. His name is (different last name from mine).

MSP: I have never heard of him. The person I am thinking of has the same last name as you. It must be someone else.

ME: But you just described my research. Maybe you are thinking of my work.

MSP: Oh no, I am sure that the person with the same last name as you is a man. His work is very well known and he publishes a lot. When I heard your name, I thought it must be your husband.

---

[4] Reprinted from Advice, *The Chronicle of Higher Education*, June 15, 2010. Available at: http://chronicle.com/article/Why-Female-Science/65922/?sid=ja&utm_source=ja&utm_medium=en [Accessed June 25, 2010]. Female Science Professor is the pseudonym of a professor in the physical sciences at a large research university who blogs under that moniker and writes monthly for The Chronicle of Higher Education Catalyst column. Her blog is at http://science-professor.blogspot.com.

True story. In fact, I am that person who publishes a lot on topics A and B. I just don't happen to be a man.

Being a female science professor, particularly when I was younger, meant starting each academic term having to convince students that I was a "real" professor and therefore, if they called their male professors "Professor" or "Dr.," they should not call me "Mrs." It meant encountering graduate students and postdocs who were rudely skeptical that I had anything interesting to teach them. In one memorable instance, when I was an assistant professor, a first-year graduate student who was taking one of my courses said to me: "We're the same age. Why do you act like you know more than I do?"

Being a young female scientist meant being insulted, patronized, and intensely criticized with alarming frequency. In a few cases, it also meant being physically and verbally harassed by men who were unable to treat women as professional colleagues.

As I have gotten older and more established as a scientist, those incidents have decreased, but they have persisted to some extent even as I move deeper into my 40s. As recently as a few years ago, I was told that I was "too young" for a position of responsibility that had been given to men my age or younger many times before. A colleague who is 4 months older than me, and who got his PhD the same year that I did, was deemed old enough for the post, but I was "too junior."

Has all of this made me angry? Yes, but I do not spend my days simmering with hostility and bitterness, waiting for the next insult or slight. I love my job and I am pretty good at it – both the research and teaching aspects of it – and that fills most of my days with positive experiences that overshadow the jarring encounters with sexism. The indignities have been unrelenting at times, but they have never outweighed the excellent aspects of being a science professor.

On my blog, 80% of my posts are about general academic issues and my experiences as a professor, or specifically as a science professor. In the remaining 20%, in which I write about "women in science" issues or my personal experiences as a female science professor, I have the dual aim of venting (complaining, ranting, shaking my virtual fist at the world) and informing readers about what it is like to be a female science professor – the good and the bad.

Maybe those personal stories help others who are experiencing the same thing; maybe they are depressing because they show that even a moderately successful, middle-aged female science professor still has to cope with sexism.

When I write about those issues, I get many positive comments, but the topic also invariably generates hostile comments and email messages, some of which say that "man-hating" women like me are the cause of sexism. Although some of my readers wish I would not waste space on those hostile and absurd comments, I publish all but the most obscene and threatening ones because they demonstrate more powerfully than my little anecdotes just what we women are up against. The only other topic that generates nearly as much passion and anger as "women in science" is money.

Despite more than a decade of increasing numbers of female students in the physical sciences, it is disturbing that my profession, my scientific specialty, my university, and my department are not more populated with women. I have read many of the recent reports – there seems to be a new one every year – trying to quantify and explain the lack of women in certain fields of science, engineering, and math. I know that the reasons for the continuing underrepresentation of women, and the actions that need to be taken to alleviate the problem, are many and complex.

I am not sure why I am here and so many other women who have similar or superior skills and scientific interests are not. I do not fit the stereotype of the single, childless monomaniac who succeeds in science by acting like a man. I am married, I have a child, and I am not particularly aggressive (although I can be assertive, a handy trait).

Nevertheless, here I am: a somewhat rare beast – a midcareer female professor of the physical sciences at a major research university, wishing that I were not still so "different" from most science professors. But I'm still enjoying my job and determined to advertise my differences if doing so helps increase, in some small way, awareness of the magnitude of the problem, and thereby helps solve it.

The next essay raises questions about the possibility of racial bias in the peer review process, another area in which senior scholars must bear responsibility. Whose duty is it to ensure that researchers are not being discriminated against in the review of research proposals?

Case study: "NIH uncovers racial disparity in grant awards," by Jocelyn Kaiser [5]

It takes no more than a visit to a few labs or a glance at the crowd at a scientific meeting to know that African American scientists are rare in biomedical research. But an in-depth analysis of grant data from the US National Institutes of Health (NIH) on page 1015 in this issue of *Science* finds that the problem goes much deeper than impressions. Black PhD scientists – and not other minorities – were far less likely to receive NIH funding for a research idea than a white scientist from a similar institution with the same research record. The gap was large: a black scientist's chance of winning NIH funding was 10 percentage points lower than that of a white scientist

. . .

The NIH-commissioned analysis, which lifts the lid on confidential grant data, may reflect a series of slight advantages white scientists accumulate over the course of a career, the authors suggest. But the gap could also result from "insidious" bias favoring whites in a peer-review system that supposedly ranks applications only on scientific merit, NIH officials say.

The findings have shaken NIH. "I was deeply dismayed," says Director Francis Collins: "This is simply unacceptable that there are differences in success that can't be explained." With NIH Deputy Director Lawrence Tabak, Collins has authored a response on page 940. "Now we know, and now we have a chance to do something about it. The leadership here is absolutely committed to making that happen," Collins says.

News about the gap is drawing a mix of reactions from the African American biomedical research community and others. Some are puzzled, some are shocked, and some say the results are no surprise. "We've known anecdotally for some time that African Americans are not as successful at getting R01s," the type of NIH grant typically held by independent investigators, says Wayne Riley, president of Meharry Medical College in Nashville, Tennessee, and chair of the Association of Minority Health Professions Schools. Raynard Kington, an African American former NIH deputy director, now president of Grinnell College in Iowa, and last author of the study, says: "This shouldn't be news. What it should be is a wake-up call."

NIH officials say this analysis began a few years ago after they became concerned that minority scientists appeared to be less successful in winning grants. Although peer reviewers are not informed of an applicant's ethnicity, NIH administrators have access to such information through the investigator's profile, which includes self-reported personal information. Initially, NIH looked at awards to top-tier research institutions and found little disparity; then it decided to investigate further. In 2008, the agency contracted with Discovery Logic/Thomson Reuters and research economist Donna Ginther of the University of Kansas, Lawrence, to do a modeling study. Ginther, who has previously focused on the participation of women in science, combined NIH grants data for 2000 through 2006 with Thomson Reuters' publications data and a National Science Foundation (NSF) database that tracks PhDs. The study focused on NIH's award of a new R01, which often launches a career.

[5] Reprinted from *Science*, 2011, 333(6045), pp. 925–926. Jocelyn Kaiser is a staff writer, *Science*, jkaiser@aaas.org.

The initial surprise was that R01 proposals from black PhD scientists (including 45% non-US citizens) were extremely rare. They totaled only 1.4% of all applications, compared with 3.2% for Hispanics and 16% for Asian scientists. (By contrast, African Americans make up about 13% of the U.S. population.) About 60% of all proposals were deemed good enough to be scored; the rest were turned away with no score. Among highly scored grants, minority groups were funded just as often as white scientists. But when Ginther's team included both scored and nonscored proposals, they found stark differences: while 29% of applications from whites were funded, only 25% of Asian applications were and only 16% of those from black scientists. In raw numbers, only 185 of nearly 23,400 funded R01 grants were from black PhD scientists – less than 1%.

Ginther's team sought to account for possible confounding factors, including the applicant's training, publication record, previous research awards, type of institution, and country of origin. "We did everything but read the proposals," Ginther says. The difference in grant success rate for Asians, 87% of whom were not US citizens, disappeared when only US citizens were included. This makes sense, Kington says, because difficulties with English might make it challenging for native Asians to write a strong proposal.

But for black applicants, even after accounting for the large number of non-US citizens within that group, a 10-percentage-point gap remained because their proposals were more likely to be unscored or receive a low score. "It's shockingly different," Ginther says. While agreeing that "the general conclusion is probably right," University of Chicago professor emeritus and biostatistician John Bailar cautions that the exact size of the gap is "in question" because Ginther's team used incomplete data and relied on "a lot of big assumptions," such as linear scaling of data.

Why didn't black scientists' proposals do as well? One possibility is that more of the applications were of lower quality, Ginther says. She and her co-authors suggest that white scientists may enjoy a "cumulative advantage" in grant-writing – for example, through better access to mentors and research collaborations. Still, if that were the explanation, there should have been a gap for Hispanic scientists, too, suggests biologist Richard Morimoto of North western University in Evanston, Illinois.

Another possibility is that some reviewers infer the race of an applicant from clues, such as the college attended or the name. That knowledge could influence assessments, Collins says. "I would like to believe that flagrant, intentional racism is rare," but "more subtle kinds of bias can't be ruled out," Collins says.

One expert on racial inequality, economist Samuel Myers of the University of Minnesota, Twin Cities, calls for the same type of comprehensive analysis to be done for NSF; overall funding rates for black scientists who apply for NSF grants are about 4 percentage points lower than for whites, according to the agency's own data since 2002. "It's not a high percentage, and we don't know how statistically important it is, but we do track it," says NSF spokesperson Maria Zacharias. Looking only at research grants "would reveal a much larger disparity," Myers suggests.

Publicizing that young black scientists have such a hard time winning NIH's R01s, some leading black biomedical scientists say, may unfortunately make things worse. The paper "could have a chilling impact on our ability to mobilize and inspire young people," says Reed Tuckson, executive vice president of UnitedHealth Group in Minnetonka, Minnesota. James Hildreth, dean of the college of biological sciences at the University of California, Davis, says that at historically black universities, there's already "an intimidation factor" about submitting research proposals to NIH. "Many have the presumption that it won't be evaluated objectively or fairly." Now those fears may be warranted, Hildreth says. Adds neuroscientist Erich Jarvis of Duke University in Durham, North Carolina: "Sometimes it's good to be naive."

NIH intends to figure out what's responsible for the R01 success gap with some experiments, such as conducting reviews with no identifying information about the applicant. NIH may also have reviewers and staff undergo tests to learn about implicit biases. "We can probably never remove all of these factors that might unconsciously be influencing the assessment," Kington says, but "I'll be happy if we can do better."

To help black scientists craft stronger proposals, NIH will make an effort to include minorities in a new program that allows early-career scientists to participate in study sections to learn about the process. Mentoring could make a big difference, too, says Freeman Hrabowski, president of the University of Maryland, Baltimore County: "Even for the best of the best, we need to be giving more support." NIH is setting up two committees, one internal and one external co-chaired by Tuckson, to brainstorm about solutions.

NIH also plans to take a closer look at its training programs aimed at filling the minority scientist pipeline. The agency has a variety of programs meant to expand that pipeline, but a 2005 National Research Council study co-chaired by Bailar found that NIH wasn't compiling the data it needed to show they were working (*Science*, 20 January 2006, p. 328). The fact that black scientists submitted less than 2% of all PhD applications for R01s and that investigators from outside the United States made up nearly half of that indicates that African Americans are "even more underrepresented than we had thought," Kington says.

NIH also hopes to explore another troubling finding: black scientists benefit less from training programs than white scientists do when they apply for an R01. "A lot of questions remain to be answered," says study co-author Walter Schaffer of NIH.

To make the community more inclusive – genuinely open to women and other historically under-represented groups – requires collective action. Individual mentors should be aware of their own insensitivities and weaknesses. And we should correct them. But there is more to do, much more, when the institutional deck is stacked against entire groups. Here, mentors must band together, agitate within their departments, institutions, and professional societies, and move together aggressively to correct injustices.

Conclusion

Presumably you will have productive relationships with your mentor and they will meet regularly with you, discuss your progress toward your objectives, and encourage you to present at professional conferences. They will help you to become established as an independent thinker and ensure that you fulfill all of your departmental and institutional requirements for graduation.

However, as the differential in power between the two of you is inherently imbalanced, problems may develop. If they do, meet face-to-face with your mentor at the earliest oppor- tunity. If you feel you are being abused, request that the behavior stop. If this does not work, write down the specifics of your complaint, document that you have met with the offending person and share this email confidentially with someone you trust. If you think the mentor is amenable to change and yet the abuse does not stop, schedule a second meeting with them to ensure that they fully understand the nature and depth of your distress. In the event that problems continue, meet with the department head or director of graduate programs.

Take home lessons

- Your mentor's primary responsibility is the development of your academic and research skills.
- Mentors should foster an atmosphere of openness and mutual respect.
- Mentors should know the literature of the field and be in touch with principal authors and opinion-makers.
- Mentors should encourage you through difficult times, give you constructive criticisms, and encourage you to present your work.
- Your research committee should be formed quickly and should meet yearly, at least.

Recognize property

Introduction

Graduate students may wonder who owns the data they produce and who is responsible for mistakes in articles they help to author. Intellectual property refers to a set of rights that convey exclusive ownership of intangible assets to the people who create them. The assets in question include such things as artistic designs, scientific discoveries, and research publications. Intellectual property protects the rights of creators through legal instruments such as copyrights and patents. This chapter explores these issues, addressing the possibility of one's owning data, new knowledge, coauthored papers – even our own DNA.

Who owns your data?

Start with the question of whether students and postdocs own the data they generate. For example, suppose Sami is a postdoctoral fellow in a lab involved in a clinical trial testing a new implantable device with the potential to prevent heart arrhythmia. The lab's Principal Investigator has been supported by the National Institutes of Health. If the lead investigator is interested in patenting the machine, she may assemble the group for a discussion of each one's rights in the event that the device is patented. She might explain that in the Bayh-Dole Act of 1980, the US Congress clarified the fiduciary relationship between public universities, taxpayer-supported scientific granting agencies, and individual researchers.

Bayh-Dole allows universities to have control of the intellectual property, such as patents, generated by researchers using federal dollars. Consequently, each institution has the right to patent, develop, and commercialize technologies they produce. If a patent is granted, the university may decide to license the technology to private firms. Those firms may manufacture, advertise, and sell the product and return royalties to the university. The university can and often does return some of the royalties to the department that developed the technology.

The arrangement relieves faculty and graduate students of the burden of having to negotiate contracts with the business sector. It is up to the institution to sort out who owns what data. Typically, the university owns the data, reaps the rewards, and decides whether and how much of the financial rewards to return to the discoverers.

Some critics have alleged that Bayh-Dole has led to bad results at the public policy level, with the university selling out to industry. If you're interested in pursuing this issue further, Derek Bok's book *Universities in the Marketplace* is a good place to start (Bok 2003). On a more personal level, graduate students and postdocs should know that if they leave the university, perhaps to take up a new job, they may need the data for articles they must publish. Can they take the data with them? Universities typically do not allow anyone to take the original data, although senior researchers usually are permitted to take a copy of the data to their new institution. Postdocs might be permitted to do so as well, but this is a matter to discuss with your mentor.

Intellectual property raises many questions concerning data ownership. Our background essay addresses many of the most important questions.

Background essay: "Intellectual property," by Adam Cureton, Douglas MacLean, Jami Taylor and Henry Schaffer [1]

What is intellectual property and why should faculty and graduate students care about it? What are the relevant rules and policies regarding intellectual property? Do I own what I create as a member of a university? What are trademarks, copyrights and patentable inventions? What is the fair use doctrine and how does it apply to my teaching and research? What justifies having a system of intellectual property rights in the first place?

Introduction: property rights

Property is an asset that can be owned. We will return to what "ownership" means, but for now it is important to distinguish two broad types of assets: those that are tangible and those that are intangible. Tangible assets include items that can be seen and touched, such as real estate, cars, jewelry and clothing. Intangible or intellectual assets include books, journals, music, computer code, and other similar creative works. When we say that we own a book we could mean that we own the particular, tangible object consisting of pages, a cover, and so on. Alternatively, we could mean that we own the intangible, intellectual assets of the book, including the particular arrangements of its words, the ideas it expresses, etc.

What does it mean to own property? Ownership is merely a bundle of rights that one has with respect to an asset. Rights are a complicated philosophical concept, and we speak of rights in many different senses. For example, we speak and make sense of claims of legal rights, procedural rights, rights that contracts be fulfilled, rights to freedom of speech and expression, and so forth. We understand roughly what talk about such rights means, even if we do not endorse or agree with claims to all such rights. Without entering into a thorough philosophical discussion about the precise nature of rights, we can say generally that to have a right to something is to have a claim to it. In particular, non-intellectual property rights are claims to tangible assets, such as an automobile. What this means is that if one owns an automobile, then one has authority, within certain limits, over whether and how it is used by others.

Of course, to have a right does not mean that one has unlimited authority or a completely open-ended claim. For example, free speech rights do not include a right to yell "Fire!" in a crowded

---

[1] This essay began its life as an article written by Taylor and Schaffer for the OpenSeminar in Research Ethics online course. Available at http://openseminar.org/ethics/. It emphasizes the legal framework in the United States. It also addresses the ethical dimensions of intellectual property, and in particular the notion of intellectual property rights.

Adam Cureton is Assistant Professor of Philosophy, University of Tennessee, Knoxville, adamcureton@gmail.com. Douglas MacLean, Professor of Philosophy, University of North Carolina, Chapel Hill, maclean@email.unc.edu. Jami Taylor is Assistant Professor, Political Science and Public Administration, University of Toledo, jami.taylor@utoledo.edu. Henry Schaffer, Professor Emeritus of Genetics and Biomathematics, North Carolina State University, hes@ncsu.edu.

theater or to produce and distribute child pornography. To have a right to physical movement does not mean that you are free to punch others in the nose for no reason or to trespass on restricted private property. Similarly, to own a car or to have a right or authority over its use does not mean that you can do whatever you please with your car. You cannot drive anywhere you like, you cannot drive at any speed you choose or drive without a license, and you cannot dispose of your car in any way you want. However, within the limits established by law and other social norms, if you own a car then you have rights to its use or authority over who may use it and how and when it may be used. This is what the rights of ownership imply. When you sell your car, you are transferring those rights to the new owner.

Types of intellectual property

While the example of tangible property like cars is fairly straightforward, intellectual property is somewhat less clear. In order for intellectual property to exist, an idea must first be had or created. Of course, you cannot have a right to an idea per se. Nobody violates a right by coming up with the same idea as someone else. In order to have intellectual property, your idea must be expressed in some way, it must be instantiated. An example of instantiation occurs when an author envisions a story and then puts her idea on paper; an artist imagines a sculpture and then creates it; a musician has an idea for a song and then produces or records it. Without this concrete expression, an idea does not qualify as intellectual property.

Like real property, intellectual property comes with a bundle of rights. Ownership allows one to prohibit or restrict access to intellectual property. Ownership also allows property to be bought and sold, or rented out. For example, some computer software program licenses require the user to pay a periodic fee to maintain software usage rights.

Intellectual property is established and protected by laws. In this legal framework, there are four types of intellectual property law: copyright, patent, trademark, and trade secrets. The various types of intellectual property law receive different legal treatment. They also face oversight from different government agencies.

The laws that establish and enforce intellectual property rights are in effect ways of treating intellectual property in many of the same ways we treat tangible property. As a philosophical matter, we can ask how this kind of similar treatment is justified. Before discussing this and some other philosophical issues, we will describe several aspects of our legal framework that establish and protect intellectual property.

Types of intellectual property law

As previously noted, there are four general types of intellectual property: copyright, patent, trademark, and trade secrets.[2] The following sections briefly address the various types of intellectual property law.

1. Copyright

Copyright refers to the legal protection of original works of authorship. This covers items such as literary works, research articles, music, computer software, plays, and movies. Copyright does not cover the ideas that are conveyed in such works but instead covers the way that ideas are expressed. Copyright protections are automatically provided to the author of published and unpublished works at the moment they are affixed in a tangible medium. Examples of putting the work in a tangible medium include recording them on tape or putting them to paper.

---

[2] US Department of State, Bureau of International Information Programs. 2006. *Focus on Intellectual Property*. Retrieved May 22, 2006 from http://usinfo.state.gov/products/pubs/intelprp/.

Copyright protections are statutorily grounded in Article 17 of the United States Code. The copyright holder has the exclusive right, with respect to his or her work, to:[3]
1. Reproduce the work
2. Prepare derivative works
3. Sell, lend, distribute copies or transfer ownership
4. Perform the work publicly
5. Display the copyrighted work publicly.

For works created after January 1, 1978, the duration of the copyright is the author's life plus 70 years.[4]

Authorship determination is a seemingly simple task. Either a person authored a piece or she did not. However, an important authorship exception exists for "works made for hire." As a general rule, if an employee creates a work under the scope of her employment, then the employer is the author and copyright holder.[5] For example, if someone creates a television advertisement while working for an advertising agency, then the agency or its officers have the copyright.

This authorship exception is important in academic research because research within the context of some complicated institutional arrangements is a central fact of most academic professions. University policies on copyright ownership may vary depending on whether the work is created by faculty, staff or students. For instance, at many universities, faculty members (a class of "employees") own the copyright of their work provided that the university did not provide exceptional support in its creation.[6] However, the university typically owns the copyright of work authored or created by staff as part of their employment. Students own the copyright to their work, but if a work was created during the instructional process then the student may not be granted full copyright protection. For example, a student may not be allowed to use class or lab notes for commercial purposes. Additionally, students do not receive copyright if the work was created as a function of employment or the product of externally funded research.

There are other limitations to copyright protections. An important exception in academia is the fair use doctrine. This is a limitation on exclusive copyright ownership. The fair use doctrine allows for use of a copyrighted work for the purposes of criticism, teaching, news reporting, scholarship, and research. There are several factors in Section 107 of the US copyright law that determine whether fair use is applicable:[7]
1. The purpose of using the work, such as whether it will be used for commercial or educational reasons
2. The nature of the copyrighted work
3. The portion of the work used in relation to the work as a whole
4. The effect (if any) the usage would have on the value of the copyrighted work.

Copyright protections are also the subject of various international treaties. The Berne Convention for the Protection of Artistic Property and the Universal Copyright Convention (both signed by the

---

[3] US Copyright Office. 2004. *Copyright basics*. Retrieved January 14, 2006 from http://www.copyright.gov/circs/circ1.html#wci.

[4] Ibid.

[5] US Copyright Office. 2004. Works made for hire under the 1976 Copyright Act. Retrieved May 20, 2006 from http://www.copyright.gov/circs/circ09.pdf.

[6] For example see North Carolina State University. 2006. Copyright regulation – Copyright implementation pursuant to copyright use and ownership policy of the University of North Carolina. Retrieved May 22, 2006 from http://www.ncsu.edu/policies/governance_admin/gov_gen/REG01.25.3.php.

[7] US Copyright Office. 2006. Fair use. Retrieved May 22, 2006 from http://www.copyright.gov/fls/fl102.html.

United States) provide a loose framework that gives a small degree of international standardization in this area. However, not all countries are signatories to these treaties. There is no international copyright that protects authors regardless of geographic location. Copyright protections are dependent on the laws of each country.

2. Patents

A patent is a property right that is given to the developer of an invention. For example, Steve Jobs was co-creator of a process that allows for live content resizing on a computer display. He and co-inventors applied for and received a patent on this invention (US Patent Number 7,797,643). Patents in the USA are issued by the United States Patent and Trademark Office (USPTO). There are three types of patents:[8]
1.   Utility patents: for the discovery of new machines or processes or the improvement of existing machines
2.   Design patents: for original ornamental designs made for manufacture
3.   Plant patents: for the invention or discovery of distinct and new varieties of plants. The inventor must also be able to asexually reproduce this plant.

Unlike copyright, an inventor must apply for patent protection. If the application is granted, the inventor's patent lasts for 20 years. A patent allows the inventor the right to exclude others from making, using, offering for sale, or selling the invention in the United States.[9] It also grants the inventor power to prohibit others from importing the invention into the United States.[10]
The owner of the patent can also assign it to another entity. In the example above, Mr. Jobs and his co-creators assigned their patent to Apple. The holder of a patent is responsible for its enforcement. Patent infringements may be pursued in the Federal court system.

3. Trademarks

The United States Patent and Trademark Office is involved in another area of intellectual property, trademarks. Trademarks are words or symbols that indicate the provider of a good or service. A trademark is used to distinguish between providers.[11] For example, the golden arches logo is identified with the fast food chain, McDonalds. McDonalds holds a trademark on this logo along with phrases such as "Chicken McNuggets" and "You deserve a break today." Trademarks allow the owner to prevent others from using the same symbol or phrase. However, it does not allow the holder to prohibit another provider from selling the same good or service. For instance, McDonalds can keep other fast food restaurants from using the phrase "Chicken McNuggets." It cannot keep other fast food restaurants from selling fried chicken nuggets. Trademarks can be registered with the USPTO when service providers are engaged in interstate or international commerce.

4. Trade secrets

A trade secret is information that gives its holder a competitive advantage in the marketplace.[12] Trade secrets include such things as formulas, techniques, or other proprietary business procedures.[13]

---

[8]   US Patent and Trademark Office. 2005. *General information concerning patents*. Retrieved January 14, 2006 from http://www.uspto.gov/web/offices/pac/doc/general/index.html#ptsc.
[9]   Ibid.   [10] Ibid.   [11] Ibid.
[12] US Department of State, Bureau of International Information Programs. 2006. *Focus on Intellectual Property*. Retrieved May 22, 2006 from http://usinfo.state.gov/products/pubs/intelprp/.
[13] Hefter, Laurence, and Litwitz, Robert. 1995. Protecting intellectual property. *Prosperity Paper Series*. US Department of State, Bureau of International Information Programs. Retrieved June 7, 2011 from http://usinfo.org/trade/bg9515e.htm.

Perhaps the most famous trade secret is the formula for Coca-Cola. Another famous trade secret is the blend of herbs and spices that is used in Kentucky Fried Chicken. Unlike patents and copyrights, trade secrets are not creatures of statute. There is no governmental agency that addresses them. However, the owner of a trade secret may be entitled to damages if another person or entity improperly discloses a trade secret.[14] Trade secrets are valuable only as long as the information remains confidential.

Violations of intellectual property law

If your intellectual property rights are violated, it is generally your responsibility to assert your rights. Depending on the type of intellectual property involved, you may have a variety of ways to respond to violations. Copyright and trademark infringement carry civil penalties such as injunctions prohibiting continued violations and monetary damages. Serious cases of copyright infringement may also result in criminal prosecution by the federal government. Patent infringements are subject only to civil penalties. Therefore, a patent holder is solely responsible for enforcing her legal rights. Until recently, only civil remedies were available for the punishment of trade secret violations. However, under the Espionage Act of 1996, the federal government may undertake criminal prosecutions for trade secret theft.

In all cases of intellectual property violation, negotiation is the simplest and cheapest possible remedy. Sometimes, intellectual property violations occur as the result of innocent mistakes. A simple phone call or friendly letter notifying the perpetrator might be enough to resolve the problem. Litigation might also be an option. As previously mentioned, copyright, patent, and trademark violations are actionable in the federal court system. Alternative dispute resolution (ADR) is another means of resolving these issues.

The justification of intellectual property rights

We have defined intellectual property rights, and we have described the main ways that intellectual property rights are created and enforced in law. However, we have not said anything yet about the justification for creating and enforcing intellectual property rights. Indeed, the very idea of intellectual property rights raises some interesting philosophical questions, and there are many spirited controversies over the justification for intellectual property rights and over the extent of the protections which are afforded in law.

You may recall that some enterprising computer programmers created a web-based music-sharing network called Napster[15] in 1999. This was a platform that allowed users logged onto the web site to gain access to and download onto their computers free any piece of music that was on the computer of any other user logged onto Napster. Because of the popularity of the site, almost any recording was available to be downloaded. Some musicians and most music producers argued that Napster users were violating the ownership rights of musicians. CD sales plummeted in part because people had no reason to pay $19.95 for a recording when they could download the songs free. Lawyers were hired, suits were filed, and courts began to puzzle over the nature of intellectual property rights and what it meant to say that musicians' and producers' rights were being violated.

The truth of these claims, as we have suggested, is not altogether obvious. This is in part due to the difference between intellectual property and tangible property. Tangible property is a physical object, and if I take your property, you no longer have it. However, if I download your recording of a song, you still own that recording. You can still play and sing your song, charge people to listen to you sing, or charge a radio station to play your recording. You can still make and sell CDs of your

---

[14] Ibid.
[15] http://www.napster.com/ http://en.wikipedia.org/wiki/Napster, retrieved June 8, 2011.

music. You may lose some of the income you otherwise might have expected to receive, and this is the core argument in the efforts to close sites such as Napster. Is the exclusive right to reproduce the work given by copyright law violated by the operation of Napster and similar websites? Considering the legal aspects, this copying violates the copyright holder's exclusive right to reproduce the work. The ethical approach considers the arguments for and against different proposals of IP rights. The impact of ignoring this exclusive right is that some musicians lost income because of Napster, but other musicians profited. The latter found an outlet for their music that they did not have before. This is in part due to the profit-maximizing motives of record producers who wanted to limit the number of musicians whose work could be easily available. These mostly "indie" musicians benefited handsomely from free sharing that became a vehicle for publicizing their music. The main losses were to the profits of the large recording studios and the musicians who had already "made it." But what were their rights? Napster did not prevent them from making and selling CDs. For the most part, it prevented them from charging extremely high prices for something that is very inexpensive to produce and distribute. Legally, record producers have a right to sell recordings for whatever price the market will bear, but the philosophical question is whether the rights of musicians or record producers include a right to prohibit individuals who own a record to share it with other individuals or allow them to make copies of it. Should the benefits to the public as a whole be considered in this dispute?

Of course there are reasons in favor of establishing a system of intellectual property that will exclude other people from acting in ways that are likely to reduce the profits one can gain from one's creative endeavors, but the loss that a musician suffers when someone acts to deprive her of profits that she might receive for her recording is nevertheless different in important respects from the loss she suffers when someone steals her guitar. Intellectual property rights that exclude others from using computers or recording devices to copy music owned by others require some philosophical justification.

Here is another example of an intellectual property right. Suppose a drug company develops an effective vaccine against some widespread disease. It seeks and receives patent protection, which prohibits other companies from producing and selling the same vaccine. As a result, the developer can charge a very high price for this drug. The price supports the research that was necessary to develop the vaccine and the company's other products, and it rewards workers and shareholders handsomely. However, the price of the drug may effectively make it prohibitive for use in poor or developing countries, where the disease may be taking its greatest toll. Should these other countries respect US patent laws, or should they be encouraging domestic manufacturers to figure out how to produce a similar vaccine? And if another country develops a similar (or identical) vaccine, and sells it domestically at a price its citizens can afford, should Americans be prohibited from buying it overseas? Why should patentable products receive a kind of protection that is not available in the global competition for other products, i.e., all the products which are not protected by patents? (Corn was first domesticated and grown in Mexico during prehistoric times, but nobody thinks that Mexicans nowadays have a right to prohibit farmers in the United States from growing corn.)

These examples show the similarities between copyright and patents with respect to the protection provided to the owner, and show the questions which arise when considering the justifications for the protection.

Defining, protecting and supporting schemes of intellectual property rights enjoy widespread support. Alexander Rosenberg describes a powerful utilitarian case for assigning strictly enforced intellectual property rights because doing so, he argues, provides enormous utilitarian benefits and may even be necessary for us to continue living even minimally tolerable lives.[16] Economists

[16] Alex Rosenberg. 2004. On the priority of intellectual property rights, especially in biotechnology. *Politics, Philosophy and Economics* 3 (1):77–95.

have long known that once land, labor and capital are fixed, technology and "good ideas" will be needed to meet the needs and wants of an ever-growing population. The trouble is that it is impossible to predict where the next good ideas will come from or what they will be. According to Rosenberg, we therefore cannot depend on central planning from government agencies to identify, still less to solve, the problems we face now and in the future; we must instead institute a market and price-system to give people the most efficient information and incentives to go out and find and develop the next big thing. The most effective way to create the right kind of incentives is to assure entrepreneurs, inventors, research firms, and artists that they will be able to profit from their efforts and their ideas. This means protecting their interests by granting them exclusive rights to the benefits of their efforts, at least for a certain period of time. Thus, Rosenberg argues, we have good reason to "privatize" ideas so that those who spend the time, energy and money needed to come up with them are able to reap the rewards of their blood, sweat and tears. They are afforded an intellectual property right in their invention, song or drug that prevents others from using it without paying up. Without the assurance created by intellectual property rights, Rosenberg claims, few of us would put out the effort to come up with a good idea for fear that it would just be copied by people who did not invest the same time and energy as we did. Indeed, without intellectual property rights, those who did come up with new ideas would probably choose to keep them secret as long as possible, for fear that the ideas would be "stolen," in which case there is likely to be duplication of research efforts, increased industrial espionage, and other ways of wasting economic resources. Without intellectual property rights, Rosenberg argues that there would be serious under-investment in good ideas, including ones that have great potential to make almost everyone significantly better off. Rosenberg goes even further and claims that if we were to abrogate the intellectual property rights of, say, a drug company that has discovered a cure for malaria in order to provide the medication to the millions of people today who have that disease but cannot afford to pay the price charged by the firm that owns the patent, we would end up scaring drug companies away from investing in "third-world" diseases, where they may not get as great a return on their investment as they would focusing on "first-world" problems such as male-pattern baldness or erectile dysfunction.

As strong as this argument is, it is not entirely uncontroversial to assign intellectual property rights such a central role in our social and legal systems. Doubts about the value of treating intellectual property like tangible property are long-standing and have been propounded recently by Lewis Hyde, who takes a historical look at the idea of intellectual property and argues that current laws and policies regulating intellectual property are on the whole unjustified.[17] These policies have the effect of establishing a new "enclosure movement" that diminishes what has historically been part of the public domain in order to exploit and profit from monopolies. The idea behind this criticism of privatizing intellectual developments appeals to ancient ideas of citizenship and republicanism, in which all citizens benefit from the interconnections that exist in a culture of shared knowledge and understanding. Thus, Thomas Jefferson insisted that "The field of knowledge is the common property of mankind." Another critic of intellectual property rights was Benjamin Franklin. Hyde's book describes Franklin's invention of the lightning rod, which involved Franklin's collaborating with three colleagues in a common laboratory set up in the Pennsylvania State House. Although the experiment did establish something original – that electricity behaved like a fluid with positive and negative charges – Franklin reported his result in *The Pennsylvania Gazette* without taking any credit for the discovery or mentioning that he had invented the lightning rod. He also did not seek a patent for it. Franklin claimed that he had drawn on a common stock of knowledge and was committed to "produce something for the common benefit."

---

[17] Lewis Hyde. 2010. *Common as Air: Revolution, Art, and Ownership* (Farrar, Straus & Giroux, 2010).

In a famous letter to Isaac McPherson, Jefferson questioned whether copyright laws ought to exist at all. "He who receives an idea from me, receives instruction himself without lessening mine; as he who lights his taper at mine, receives light without darkening mine." Nevertheless, in debates leading up to the drafting of the Constitution, according to the historian Thomas Darnton, "Jefferson was persuaded by Madison that a strictly limited copyright would indeed 'promote the progress of science and the useful arts,' as the Constitution was to proclaim. By enjoying a short-term monopoly on the publication of their writings, authors would be encouraged to share their ideas in print." The original copyright act of 1790 set the term at 14 years, renewable once. Today, copyright lasts for the life of the author plus 70 years or, as a result of The Copyright Term Extension Act of 1998, even longer. This does not appear to be consistent with the "limited time" stated in the Constitution, and is the source of controversy about the balance between the protection of authors and the benefits to the public. The law greatly extending the term was prompted by the fact that the monopoly on Mickey Mouse was about to expire. As Darnton remarks, "When asked how long he thought copyrights should last, Jack Valenti, the lobbyist for Hollywood, quipped, 'Forever, minus a day.' Valenti has won; Jefferson has lost."[18] Because of the rise of the internet and the popularity of entities like *Wikipedia*, however, not to mention the revenues collected on pharmaceuticals which are protected from competition by patents, these issues are as lively today as they ever were.

Another recent example further demonstrates some of the potential bad effects of strong intellectual property rights and some of the beneficial effects of forgoing the protections that rights create. In 2003, a group of scientists and executives from government agencies, industry, universities, and non-profit groups agreed to collaborate on research aimed at understanding and eventually treating Alzheimer's disease.[19] The challenge that each research team faced was to find biological markers that show the progression of Alzheimer's in the human brain. Although it wasn't known exactly what these markers would show, many researchers suspected that they would unlock some of the mysteries about the cause, progression, and possible treatment of the disease. While working independently, the researchers were not making much progress because of the large amount of data that was needed. Given the hurdles they faced, the group decided to pool all of their information and to make it publicly available. This kind of collaboration was unprecedented in medical research in the age of intellectual property rights. As one scientist involved in this work remarked, "It's not science the way most of us have practiced it in our careers. But we all realized that we would never get biomarkers unless all of us parked our egos and intellectual-property noses outside the door and agreed that all of our data would be public immediately." The National Institute on Aging, along with some other foundations, companies, and universities, put up the money needed to create the database, and, as reported in *The New York Times*, "The effort is bearing fruit with a wealth of recent scientific papers on the early diagnosis of Alzheimer's using methods like PET scans and tests of spinal fluid. More than 100 studies are under way to test drugs that might slow or stop the disease." This kind of open collaborative effort is now serving as a model for understanding and eventually treating Parkinson's disease.

The "Open Source"[20] movement in computer software and related areas is a longer-standing example of a community trading the revenue possibilities of intellectual property protection for increased progress. A newer similar movement with respect to books and other digitally authored

[18] Thomas Darnton, "A Republic of Letters," a review of Lewis Hyde, *Common as Air*, *The New York Times*, August 20, 2010.

[19] The information about this effort, and the quotations in this paragraph, are from Gina Kolata, "Sharing of Data Leads to Progress on Alzheimer's," *The New York Times*, August 12, 2010.

[20] http://www.fsf.org/ http://en.wikipedia.org/wiki/Open_source; http://www.ncsu.edu/it/open_source/, retrieved June 9, 2011.

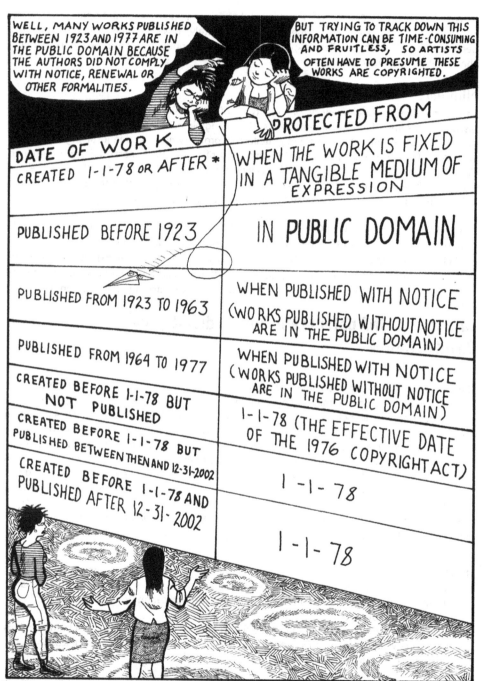

Figure 11.1. Copyright law (Reprinted with permission from *Bound By Law* © 2006, 2008 Keith Aoki, James Boyle, Jennifer Jenkins (Aoki *et al.* 2008) at http://www.law.duke.edu/cspd/comics/. Accessed March 24, 2012).

material is the Creative Commons[21] effort. All of these are consistent with intellectual property law, as are the medical research efforts mentioned immediately above, and the change has primarily been with respect to the intellectual property owners' willingness to license their work without charges in an open manner.

Summary

This article offered a brief overview of some types of intellectual property along with a brief discussion of some of its ethical dimensions. The intangible nature of intellectual property contributes to the difficulties in defining intellectual property rights and in justifying them. The variations of intellectual property and their ethical justifications have moral, legal and economic dimensions that are important to consider as well. It is hoped that by shining a light on these topics, it will help students and practitioners to become more cognizant of these vital issues and better able to manage their own encounters with intellectual property.

The last part of this chapter takes up a critical question in the development of new biotechnology: whether we ought to allow private ownership of the human genome.

Who owns your DNA? Who should own it, if anyone? David Resnik explores the question in "DNA Patents and Human Dignity," asking whether we run the risk of commodifying and degrading humanity if we allow ownership of human body parts such as our genes.

Case study: "DNA patents and human dignity," by David B. Resnik[22]

. . .

The purpose of this paper is to clarify and analyze the claim that DNA patents violate or threaten human dignity.[23] I will argue that patents on human DNA do not violate human dignity because they do not treat human beings as complete commodities. However, since human DNA patenting uses market rhetoric to describe human body parts, it does treat human beings as incomplete commodities and, therefore, may threaten human dignity by taking us further down the path of human commodification. By applying market language to human DNA, we may come to hold less respect for the value of human life. On the other hand, since market rhetoric already pervades many aspects of science, medicine, and society, the threat posed by DNA patenting is neither new nor unique. DNA patenting is but one aspect of a larger, more profound conflict between the free market and respect for human dignity. It is not clear that banning human DNA patenting would address this larger issue.

. . .

The claim against patents on human DNA can actually be divided into two distinct claims:
- The very practice of patenting human DNA treats human beings as having only a market value; human DNA patenting represents the complete commodification of human beings and violates human dignity.
- The practice of human DNA patenting could lead to further commodification of human beings (the "slippery slope"); human DNA patenting is a form of incomplete commodification that threatens human dignity.

---

[21] http://creativecommons.org/, retrieved June 9, 2011.

[22] Reprinted from *The Journal of Law, Medicine & Ethics*, 2001, 29(2), pp. 152–165. David B. Resnik is Bioethicist and Institutional Review Board Chair, National Institutes of Health Sciences, resnikd@niehs.nih.gov.

[23] The passages are excerpts, with deleted material indicated by ellipses.

It is important for our purposes to distinguish between violations of human dignity and threats to human dignity. Violations of human dignity are actions that treat people as having only extrinsic worth or only a market value; threats to human dignity are actions that may lead to violations of human dignity. For example, raping a person violates that person's dignity [44]. A motion picture that glorifies rape threatens human dignity because it could cause people to rape. Selling a person as a slave violates that person's dignity; exploitative labor practices, such as indentured servitude or paid child labor, threaten human dignity because they could lead to practices that are the equivalent of slavery.

Most of the kinds of actions that violate human dignity are clearly immoral and many are also illegal, such as murder, rape, assault, theft, and slavery. It would appear that we have a much higher tolerance for actions that merely threaten human dignity, since we do allow many practices, institutions, and objects that threaten human dignity to continue, such as pornography, television violence, advertising, unpaid labor, surrogate pregnancy, and professional athletics. However, we often regulate these practices in order to prevent them from leading to violations of human dignity. These laws are designed to counter "slippery slope" concerns. For example, many communities have laws and standards that regulate the sale of pornography, and federal and state laws govern the employer–employee relationship.

Another way of understanding the distinction between a violation and a threat is to distinguish between harm and risk [45]. Violations of human dignity harm people, but threats to human dignity create a probability of harm. Most moral theorists agree that it is not only wrong to harm other people, but it is wrong to impose unreasonable risks on them. Many of the risks that exist in society are permitted because they are considered reasonable. The difference between a reasonable and unreasonable risk depends on the probability and magnitude of any harm, the probability and magnitude of any benefits, as well as any basic rights at stake. Likewise, threats can be understood as either reasonable (or acceptable) or unreasonable (or unacceptable).

For example, automobiles can cause significant harm (e.g., loss of life), but they also have important benefits (e.g., transportation). Moreover, they play a fundamental role in enabling people to realize their rights to education, work, and healthcare. In the final analysis, we allow automobiles to be used because the benefits of their use far outweigh the risks. However, the outcome of this cost–benefit analysis changes when we consider certain uses of automobiles – drag-racing, for instance. Drag-racing offers few benefits and creates tremendous risks; it is an unreasonable risk. Since arguments about what constitutes a reasonable vs. unreasonable risk involve an assessment of harms and benefits, they typically address the consequences of various practices and rely on empirical evidence.

Do DNA patents violate human dignity?

How might one prove that human DNA patents violate human dignity? To make this claim, one would need to prove that the very practice of human DNA patenting treats human beings as having only a market value – that DNA patenting constitutes complete commodification, not just incomplete commodification. Patenting something might not be the equivalent of ownership, but it does apply market rhetoric to an invention and treat the invention as a commodity [46]. For example, when an item is patented, one can sell rights to make, use, or commercialize the item. A patent, therefore, treats an invention as having some potential commercial or market value.

As a side note, an invention may have a non-market value as well, but a main reason for obtaining a patent is to exploit the invention's market value. If the only value of an invention is its commercial value, then the invention is a complete commodity. However, since some patented inventions may have non-market values as well, not all patents constitute complete commodification. For example, one might value a patented computer program, such as

Microsoft Word, for its economic and non-economic worth. Incidentally, other forms of intellectual property, such as copyrights and trademarks, also imply some form of commodification because they also invoke market rhetoric.

DNA patents and slavery

The analogy of DNA patenting to slavery can now be made clear: many people have claimed that DNA patenting is like slavery because it treats people as complete commodities. With slavery, people are bought and sold as pieces of property; they are treated as having only a market value. Slavery is complete commodification of a human being. DNA patenting, according to some critics, is like slavery in that it involves complete commodification of human DNA. Human DNA patenting violates human dignity because it treats people as things that can be bought and sold.

But is human DNA patenting really like slavery? A key point that we should not forget is that a patent does not imply ownership. Thus, patenting a person would not be the same thing as owning the person. Patenting only confers a right to exclude others from making, using, or marketing an invention. It does not give the patent holder positive rights to make, use, or market the invention if these practices would violate the law. Thus, someone who had a patent on a human being would not have the same rights over that person as a slave owner would.
The patented person would still be free to make many life decisions, although he or she would probably not be able to reproduce or market himself or herself without permission from the patent holder. However, this point is moot because slavery is illegal in the United States and in most other countries, and under US law a patent does not give one the right to violate the law.

. . .

DNA patents and commodification

. . .

. . . Does human DNA patenting constitute complete commodification of a human being, i.e., does it treat a human being as having only a market value? Although it is possible that a patent on a DNA sequence would treat the sequence as an incomplete commodity, I will assume, for the sake of argument, that some DNA patents would treat DNA sequences as complete commodities. Would these patents treat human beings as complete commodities? I will defend the view that human DNA patents only treat parts of human beings as complete commodities; they do not treat whole human beings as complete commodities [51].

To support this idea, consider the commodification of other objects that have parts, such as national parks, businesses, sports teams, and so on. Complete commodification of a part (or certain properties) of the thing does not imply complete commodification of the whole thing; we may treat a part (or certain properties) of a thing as having a market value without treating the whole thing as having only a market value. For example, consider Niagara Falls. Let us assume that many people value this great waterfall for its natural beauty and that its beauty cannot be measured or captured in any dollar amount. Niagara Falls is not for sale nor should it ever be for sale. Niagara Falls is not a complete commodity. Nevertheless, many people accept complete commodification of parts or properties of Niagara Falls. For example, souvenir shops market pictures and postcards depicting the falls; vendors are allowed to conduct business near the waterfall; hotels advertise honeymoon suites with a view of the falls.

I would like to suggest that human bodies are similar to Niagara Falls. We may regard whole human bodies as incomplete commodities while admitting that some parts (or properties) of human bodies are complete commodities. Human bodies contain many different parts, ranging in size from limbs, organs, and tissues, to cells, membranes, organelles, chromosomes, DNA, proteins, hormones, lipids, and even minerals and basic elements. From a purely chemical point of view, the body is composed of various elements arranged in complex molecular structures. Genes and DNA sequences are "mid-range" parts of the body in that they are much larger than atoms, such as carbon or nitrogen, but much smaller than tissues or organs.

. . .

Once we understand that human bodies are complex structures composed of many different parts with varying degrees of complexity and organization, we can see that we already treat many parts and properties of the body as marketable commodities. For hundreds of years, we have bought and sold many of the basic elements and molecules that compose the body, such as water, sodium chloride, carbon, sulfur, iron, and zinc. We have for many years patented complex molecules that occur in human bodies, such as proteins, hydrocarbons, hormones, and lipids. Most people would have no strong moral objections to these practices. Even though the human body is 70% water, we have no moral qualms about buying and selling water. We allow people to sell their hair and sperm. A person can also market properties of his or her body, such as voice, face, or figure.

If we find these practices acceptable and not a violation of human dignity, then it follows that there is nothing inherently wrong with treating a part or property of the human body as a complete commodity.

. . .

Do DNA patents threaten human dignity?

. . .

To assess a slippery slope argument, one needs to have information concerning psychosocial and economic aspects of the slope and the activity that may lead to the slide. These risks need to be weighed against any important benefits or rights that may be at stake. When assessing a slope that involves a slide toward further commodification, we need to consider questions like:

- Are there any market forces, conditions, or demands that will encourage further commodification?
- Are there any safeguards we can adopt to prevent further commodification?
- Are the benefits of commodification worth the risks?

The same slippery slope concerns also arise in discussions involving the sale of organs, human tissues, gametes, and other body parts and products [67]. Numerous writers on these subjects have addressed the harmful social and cultural consequences of commodifying the body. Using market language to describe the body, they would argue, can lead us to change our attitudes toward and beliefs about the body. As our attitudes and beliefs shift toward viewing the body as a commodity, we will find market language more acceptable, which will encourage additional changes in our attitudes and beliefs. Eventually, we (the people in society) will come to view the body as a complete commodity and will be more inclined to treat human beings as such, which may lead to exploitation, theft, manipulation, and other abuses against human beings. The only way to stop this slide toward further commodification of human beings, one might argue, is to prohibit practices that partially commodify people, such as the patenting of human DNA and cell lines, payment for tissues and organs, and so on.

Some would argue that we already have a famous court case, Moore v. Regents of the University of California (1990), that illustrates how partial commodification of the body can lead to exploitation [68]. In this case, Dr. David Golde patented a cell line developed from tissue from Moore's cancerous spleen. The cell line turned out to be a very profitable and valuable tool in cancer research, with a commercial potential of $3 billion. Golde purposely kept from Moore that he was using his cell line in research and that his cells had commercial value. Upon discovering what Golde had done, Moore sued for commercial rights to his own tissue. The California

Supreme Court ruled that although Moore did not have property rights to his own cells, Golde did violate Moore's right to informed consent [69].

Although the Moore case is a rare and sensational event, one might argue that exploitation will become more common as we encourage commodification of the body. Moreover, it only takes a few well-publicized events, like the Moore case, to create public distrust and disillusionment in medical practice and biomedical research. As patients and research subjects learn about the commercial value of the body, they may be concerned that financial incentives can cause their doctors and researchers to act unethically [70].

. . .

Conclusion

I have considered the question of whether human DNA patents violate or threaten human dignity. I have argued that only patents that constitute complete commodification of human beings – patents on the whole human genome – would violate human dignity. However, it is very unlikely that anyone will be able to patent a whole human genome since most of the human genome will soon be available in a public database. Thus, most human DNA patents will pertain to the structure or function of specific human genes, gene fragments, or genetic markers. These patents constitute incomplete commodification of human beings, and they therefore may threaten, but not violate human dignity.

. . .

Acknowledgments

I would like to thank two anonymous reviewers from The Journal of Law, Medicine & Ethics for helpful comments.

References for Resnik

30. D. Resnik, DNA patents and scientific discovery and innovation: assessing benefits and risks. Science and Engineering Ethics (forthcoming).

39. E. Gold, Body Parts (Washington DC: Georgetown University Press, 1997).

40. M. Radin, Contested Commodities (Cambridge, Massachusetts: Harvard University Press, 1996).

41. M. Hanson. Biotechnology and commodification within health care. Journal of Medicine and Philosophy, 24, no. 3 (1999): 267–287.

44. F. Berger, Pornography, Sex, and Censorship. Social Theory and Practice, 4, no. 2 (1997): 380–395.

45. J. Feinberg, Social Philosophy (Englewood Cliffs, New Jersey: Prentice-Hall, 1973).

46. Radin, supra note 40.

51. Resnik, supra note 30.

65. D. Nelkin and L. Andrews, Homo economicus: the commercialization of body tissue in the age of biotechnology. Hastings Center Report, 28, no. 5 (1998): 30–39.

67. Radin, supra note 40; Nelkin and Andrews, supra note 65; Gold, supra note 39; Hanson, supra note 41.

68. Nelkin and Andrews, supra note 65.

69. Moore v. Regents of the University of California, 793 P.2d 479 (Cal. 1990).

70. Hanson, supra note 41.

Conclusion

Intellectual property refers to a large, complicated and somewhat unwieldy set of issues. In this chapter we have been introduced to the subject. We have seen that the issues encompass discussions of rules about the ownership of data, words, and ideas; the justification of abstract concepts such as tangible and intangible property; and the truth of assertions that strong intellectual property laws encourage innovation. In the first background reading by Cureton *et al.*, we learned about four types of intellectual property law: copyright, patent, trademark and trade secrets. The case study by Resnik argued that scientists claiming patents on human DNA do not violate human rights or treat human body parts as commodities unless they claim a patent on the entire genome. Graduate students may or may not find themselves having to tease apart these various issues. But if you or your mentor suspect your research may produce results with market potential, it will be in your interest to learn about your rights and obligations in this area.

Take home lessons

- Bayh-Dole gives universities control of the intellectual property generated by researchers using federal dollars, including the right to patent, develop, and commercialize technology.
- Typically, universities own intellectual property; graduate students almost never have ownership over work they have produced as students.
- Principal investigators and graduate students leaving for other universities may not be able to take their research data with them if their funding was awarded to their first institution, which owns the data.
- Be on guard against institutional drift as Bayh-Dole increases the opportunities for universities to put the profit motive ahead of social mission and scientific discovery.

Bibliography

Aoki, K., Boyle, J. & Jenkins, J. 2008. *Bound by Law?: Tales from the Public Domain*, new expanded edn. Duke University Press Books.

Bok, D.C. 2003. *Universities in the Marketplace: The Commercialization of Higher Education.* Princeton University Press.

Resnik, D.B. 2001. DNA Patents and Human Dignity. *The Journal of Law, Medicine & Ethics*, **29**(2), 152–165.

12

Reveal conflicts

Introduction

Graduate students may find themselves working on projects involving funds from private firms. There are at least two reasons for this possibility. On the one hand, administrators encourage faculty to collaborate with industrial colleagues. On the other hand, research has become increasingly expensive, in part because today's projects often require large interdisciplinary teams. Partnerships involving researchers from the for-profit sector can lead to benefits for all parties. But they can also give rise to unforeseen problems.

To manage the relationships, universities have created Contracts and Grants office (your office may have another name, such as Sponsored Programs). These units oversee agreements in which personnel, resources, and facilities not under the university's jurisdiction are necessary. The unit is charged to protect the interests of the university. It may be permissible for faculty to receive honoraria, consulting fees, royalties, and even equity positions from outside sources, but these interests may put graduate students and postdocs into difficult positions. The mission of Contracts and Grants is to manage these relationships throughout the processes of submitting proposals, soliciting and receiving funds, conducting the research, and publishing and commercializing the results.

Collaborative arrangements have obvious advantages. For example, joint efforts can result in knowledge moving quickly from laboratories to patient care. However, they also have obvious risks. Faculty can become involved in conflicts of interests, and graduate students may consequently find themselves in the middle of competing expectations. Students have interests in publishing their research quickly, whereas private sponsors have interests in keeping the results confidential and proprietary. Sometimes these values work together for everyone's benefit. At other times, however, they pull in opposite directions.

A conflict of interest exists whenever a researcher has two or more duties that compete in a way that raises suspicions that the researcher cannot meet both interests in a professional way. Researchers' primary duties flow from their professional duty to create knowledge and to share it with students. Secondary duties may follow from this first obligation, including duties to seek stipends from training grants and salary from consulting arrangements. However, secondary duties ordinarily must yield to one's primary duties if the two conflict.

Conflicts of interest raise the specter of bias. Consider an example from medical research. A doctor involved in a clinical trial may believe that drug S is best for a given

Research Ethics: A Philosophical Guide to the Responsible Conduct of Research. Gary Comstock.
Published by Cambridge University Press. © Cambridge University Press 2013.

patient and yet be working in an experimental trial on drug T. The doctor has a primary interest in providing her patient with the best available care, a duty inclining her to choose drug S. She has a secondary interest in enrolling patients in the trial. If the doctor prescribes drug T only because she wants to increase the number of patients in the trial, questions may be raised about whether she is putting her patient's interests first.[1]

Conflicts of interest may arise, too, if the sources of a researcher's support and the results of their work coincide too neatly – when, for example, a scientist working for a tobacco company produces results that minimize the role of second-hand smoke in the epidemiology of malignant lung tumors when the data indicate otherwise (Bitton et al., 2005). In order to prevent conflicts, state statutes specify that public employees should not use their positions for personal pecuniary benefits unless those benefits are disclosed, approved, supervised, and managed. If a Principal Investigator is receiving payment in exchange for the time they spend working for a sponsor the Principal Investigator should reveal the financial arrangement in all written and oral presentations about the project.

Graduate students typically do not face potential conflicts of interest and, therefore, are not required to disclose them. However, when faculty have duties both to public and to private concerns, graduate students can be put in awkward situations. Policies generally apply to faculty, professional staff, postdoctoral associates, and visiting scholars and adjunct faculty on paid appointments; graduate students may be at a disadvantage if they do not know what these appointments entail. Conflicts of interest are most likely to arise between mentors and mentees. For example, if the senior person has stock in a company that is sponsoring the student's research, this relationship may cloud the senior person's judgment about the tasks they assign to the student.

University policies often begin by stating that conflicts cannot be eliminated but can be managed. One way to manage a potential conflict of interest is to make it known. When faculty members disclose their financial interests, they mitigate potential risks to their own objectivity and to the graduate student's interests in publication. For example, if a faculty member receives payments in exchange for the time they spend working for a company that is sponsoring their research, it might appear that they are at risk of compromising their data in favor of the company's interests. Presumably they are also giving talks and writing papers as part of their university job, and they may be paid honoraria for those activities. Is this a conflict of interest? Yes, but it is not necessarily a problem. Faculty need not refrain from giving oral presentations or writing manuscripts and receiving compensation as long as they disclose their financial relationship to the company in every presentation, verbal or written, that they make. Simply bringing the matter to the light of day can help to avoid the appearance of conflict of interest. Transparency and disclosure can go some way toward reducing the possibility of misunderstanding.

Another way to deal with conflict of interest is to pay careful attention to how the research is set up. Enlisting an independent reviewer can be helpful. So can a double-blind design in which the researchers are prevented from knowing key experimental information.

---

[1] An important note of clarification. The doctor may believe, but not know, that drug S is better than T. In this case, enrolling her patient in a trial may be a mark of epistemic humility; she is trying to find out whether her belief is correct. Conflicts of interest may arise in such cases, but they are not inevitable.

In "Objectivity in Research," the US National Institutes of Health and the US National Science Foundation required institutions to establish policies to ensure that no investigator's design, conduct, or reporting of research is biased by the investigator's financial stake in the research or in the company (National Institutes of Health, 1995). The best way to minimize irresponsible conduct of research is for the lead collaborator to describe ahead of time and in detail each person's specific roles, rights, and responsibilities. This step is especially important in two circumstances: first, when there are multiple Principal Investigators on a project, and; second, when any researcher stands to receive $10,000 or more from a company sponsoring the research, or if the researcher holds more than a 5% ownership in the company's equity (National Science Foundation, 2010). (There is nothing sacred about the number; conflicts of interest can arise when people have smaller stakes in companies, too.) A number of institutional strategies have evolved to minimize the possibility of harm. Personnel in the technology-transfer office may be trained to watch for potential trouble and faculty can be taught to avoid situations likely to be perceived as compromising their fiduciary integrity. External program reviewers and other independent consultants may also be brought in to identify potentially problematic arrangements.

How does a conflict of commitment differ from a conflict of interest? The former exists when an investigator has too much on her plate. Suppose the faculty member receives a majority of her salary from grants but also lectures regularly in classes at a medical school while directing the residency program, managing a lab full of graduate students and supervising a handful of post-doctoral fellows. If the graduate students notice that the investigator has begun to miss meetings with them and is delaying their research, the investigator may have a conflict of commitment. The solution? Simple, and evident: she must slow down and cut back. To guard against the possibility of developing conflicts of interests, principal investigators may benefit from having a group of independent external reviewers to look over their duties and warn them when they are taking on too much.

What rules of thumb should guide us in this difficult area? First, consult the NIH regulations for "interdisciplinary collaborative research." Second, understand that simply discussing a technique or data set with someone from your department is not considered interdisciplinary collaboration. When you are working with someone from a different department or university, however, difficult challenges may arise because different disciplines sometimes have different rules about matters such as authorship and data sharing. Third, when you are about to terminate a collaborative relationship, you should ensure that everyone with whom you have collaborated is on the same page about data ownership. Fourth, if working with an industrial sponsor, be aware that the sponsor may want to restrict the principal investigator's ability to publish negative results. Finally, if you have concerns in these areas, contact your technology transfer office, or the office responsible for identifying projects on campus that are candidates for patent or copyright protection. Officials there should be able to answer your questions.

There is more to be said about this area, and much of it is said in our background essay, "Shared responsibility, individual integrity." The document was composed by The Federation of American Societies for Experimental Biology, an organization of more than 80,000 research scientists. Make particular note of its 18 guiding principles.

Background essay: "Shared responsibility, individual integrity: scientists addressing conflicts of interest in biomedical research," Federation of American Societies for Experimental Biology [2]

Scope and types of academia–industry relationships in science

Relationships between academia and industry are a fundamental part of the modern life science enterprise. It is only through such relationships that the life sciences can advance most rapidly to maximize benefits to society. Collaborations between industry and academia have grown due to many factors including legislation and agency policies that encourage technology transfer and collaborative research, the increasingly complex nature of research that requires relationships across institutions and sectors, and the overall increase in the cost of doing research and development that yields therapies.

. . .

Many different types of relationships exist between industry and academia, including research contracts, research grants, and consulting or licensing arrangements. Through research contracts and grants, companies provide direct support for research projects at universities. In return, companies often receive the right to license any inventions that are developed from that research. Approximately one-quarter of academic faculty members receive research funding from industry [5], representing close to $2 billion in 2004 [4].

Companies also provide direct support of academic trainees. Of 210 life science firms surveyed in 1994, 38% supported the education of students and fellows through grants [9]. Academic investigators also transfer their knowledge to industry via consulting and advisory board membership. Approximately 80% of life science companies retain academic faculty members as consultants, the most prevalent relationship [6].

Licensing of technologies developed by academic investigators and the creation of university spin-off companies are also major types of academia–industry relationships. In FY 2004, 191 institutions reported licenses that led to the formation of 462 new companies that year [6]. Since 1980, licenses from academic institutions led to the formation of 4,543 new companies [3].

. . .

Benefits of academia–industry relationships

Many important societal benefits stem from scientific collaborations between academia and industry, including translating basic scientific findings into clinical applications, and fueling local economies. Collaboration between industry and academia has led to many important therapies and research tools, such as the gene splicing technology that initiated the biotechnology industry, diagnostic tests for breast cancer and osteoporosis, and vaccines.

Institutional licensing activities from FY 1998 to 2003 made 2,230 products commercially available, one report found [3]. Studies also reveal how academia–industry relationships make significant contributions to local economies [8]. Evidence shows academia–industry relationships are a key component of economic competitiveness and increase the future research and development spending by industry [9].

---

[2] Reprinted from Federation of American Societies for Experimental Biology, 2006, Rockville, MD. Deleted material is indicated by ellipses; the complete document is available at http://opa1.faseb.org/pdf/FASEB_COI_paper.pdf.

Academic investigators also benefit by their collaborations with industry through increased access to resources to support their ongoing projects. These collaborations enable academic investigators to participate in the application of their research, and they allow students and academic investigators to work on applied research projects. Studies show that industry funding correlates with increased faculty academic productivity (published articles) and commercial productivity (patents and licenses, products under review and on the market, and start-up companies) [5]. Academic investigators, government researchers, and industry scientists also benefit professionally by interacting with colleagues. Such interactions facilitate the bidirectional flow of knowledge and materials. Interaction with industry provides academic investigators opportunities to participate in the application of their research, and it allows students and academic investigators to work on applied research projects. Finally, industry support may help offset wage differentials between industrial and non-industrial sectors, which may assist in recruitment and retention of scientists and administrators to academia.

Challenges of academia–industry relationships and conflicts of interest

The rise in academia–industry relationships has been accompanied by increased concerns regarding conflicts of interest that are largely, but not exclusively, financial. A commonly used definition of financial conflict of interest is: a condition in which a primary interest (institutional responsibilities for research and education) is in conflict (whether real or perceived) with a secondary interest (such as financial gain) [10]. A conflict of interest is a situation, and not a behavior. The presence of a conflict of interest is not necessarily an indictment of an individual, but rather an acknowledgement of a potentially challenging situation. By focusing on relationships and not conflicts of interest in this report, we hope to direct the guidance towards smart practices and other useful tools for scientists.

The most intense scrutiny of academia–industry relations focuses on risks to human research participants. High-profile cases, such as the death of Jesse Gelsinger in a gene therapy trial at the University of Pennsylvania, highlight the need for protection of patients and research participants. The potential risk to human research participants has created a consensus within the medical and scientific community to increase attention to this issue.

Correlations between industry funding and published scientific conclusions that could be viewed as favorable to industry highlight the potential for relationships to introduce bias into research [11]. Do financial relationships with industry cause subtle or unconscious bias on the part of academic researchers [12]? Does industry funding affect the conduct of research or study design [11]? Will industry simply choose to have relationships with researchers that have predetermined favorable positions on their products? Or will they partner with those individuals who have the most expertise about the specific research area? The potential for bias remains an impassioned subject of discussion in the scientific community and the press.

There is also concern that deepening commercial ties can undermine academe's commitment to openness. For example, studies suggest that industry-funded results are less likely to be published or, when published, delayed even longer than the time necessary to file a patent [5,13].

Academia–industry relationships may impose other restrictions such as denial of access to research data or biomaterials to other investigators [13,14].

Industry relationships may impact trainees differently than principal investigators. There are concerns about specific risks, such as fewer publications or delays in publication of manuscripts and dissertations, as well as constraints in the type of research that is conducted [15,16]. From the trainee's perspective, some of these challenges may not be currently considered problematic [17]. However, similar to the protection of human research participants, protection of trainees is a fundamental responsibility of mentors, and this student–teacher relationship must be safeguarded.

For the scientific community, negative public perception and distrust of the biomedical research enterprise is perhaps one of the most worrisome challenges in academia–industry relationships. Recent public opinion research shows support for interactions between academia and industry [18]. On the other hand, lapses in judgment and reports of misconduct damage the public's faith in medical research.

. . .

Ongoing challenges for academic investigators

The vast majority of biomedical researchers are guided by the highest ethical and professional standards. The focus of the report is to discuss and provide guidance to academic investigators to address challenges that may occur due to financial relationships between academia and industry . . .

. . .

Challenges and guiding principles: how do investigators protect against research bias in industry relationships?

Public support for research is built on a foundation of trust that reported research results are credible. Therefore, the potential for academia–industry relationships to bias research and investigators is a concern shared by the scientific community and the public. A challenge for investigators is how to address the perceived or real loss of objectivity when forging a relationship with industry.

Researchers diligently strive to maintain the objectivity and integrity of their investigations [3] by their:

- intellectual honesty in proposing, performing, and reporting research;
- accuracy in representing contributions to research proposals and reports;
- fairness in peer review and collegiality of scientific interactions (including communications and sharing of resources);
- transparency in industry relationships;
- protection of human subjects and humane care of animals in research; and
- adherence to mutual responsibilities between investigators and their research teams [4].

Unfortunately, the perception of bias that results from having a financial interest can be damaging to the credibility of biomedical research. People understand money and its potential for influence. This potential for influence may cause public anxiety about financial interests in biomedical research. But the public may not understand the inherent checks and balances of scientific research designed to weed out research bias. Peer review and institutional review boards prevent investigators from obtaining or publishing any information that is not accurate or appropriately obtained. While recognizing the peer review system has limitations, ongoing review and revision is critical in minimizing individual subjectivity.

[Editor's note: consult the full report for discussions of each of the guiding principles.]

Guiding principles

1. Investigators have a responsibility and commitment to conduct scientific activities objectively and with the highest professional standards.
2. The primary responsibility of full-time investigators is to the institutions. Outside activities shall complement, not compromise, institutional responsibilities.
3. It is appropriate and beneficial for academic institutions to develop and enforce their own mechanisms of review and oversight of investigator relationships with industry.

4. The academic community can and shall monitor itself through peer review of industry relationships. Institutional committees that include peer members from the same institution are appropriate and effective in reviewing investigators' industry relationships.

5. Investigators want and need clear guidance, efficient processes, and adequate support mechanisms from their institutions during the disclosure and review process, and throughout their participation in industry relationships.

6. Investigators shall have access to and be involved in the analysis and/or interpretation of all data generated in the research.

7. Mutual understanding of constraints, principles, and policies regarding access, analysis, and dissemination of research information, data, and materials among investigators and their students and trainees, institutions, and sponsors is beneficial.

8. Investigators shall not enter into agreements with companies that prevent publication of research results. Pre-publication review by an industry sponsor to secure intellectual property rights shall occur in a timely manner (no more than 30 to 60 days) so as not to unnecessarily delay study publication.

9. Investigators shall be aware of and adhere to individual journal policies on disclosure of industry relationships

10. Consulting and advisory board relationships shall be carried out in a transparent and accountable manner and be disclosed as they are initiated.

11. When investigators have consulting relationships with investment firms related to their area of expertise, all parties shall be aware of the specific circumstances involved.

12. Investigators shall not use federal funds to the benefit of a company, unless this is the explicit purpose of the mechanism used to fund the research.

13. When investigators own significant equity in a company with which research is conducted, all parties shall be aware of the special circumstances involved.

14. When holding a significant role in a start-up company, investigators shall be guided by agreed-upon limits to the scope of the relationship.

15. Investigators shall be aware of and adhere to requirements of federal funding related to disclosure of inventions. Investigators shall adhere to patent law and institutional requirements.

16. Investigators shall not seek to influence their institution's technology transfer decisions for personal gain.

17. A mentor's outside commercial interests shall avoid impeding a trainee's timely progress toward his/her degree, restricting a trainee's right to publish his/her research in a timely manner, compromising a trainee's career progress, or restricting a trainee's freedom of inquiry.

18. Mentors and institutions should make trainees aware of their rights and responsibilities in industry relationships.

Conclusion

Academia–industry relationships ultimately have the ability to bring multiple resources to scientific advancement and the battle against disease. It is only through such relationships that advancements in the life sciences can most rapidly achieve the maximum benefit to society. Clinical and basic science investigators benefit from industry relationships through increased resources to support ongoing projects, interactions with colleagues that facilitate the bidirectional flow of knowledge and materials, and participation in the application of research.

Investigators are individually responsible for maintaining accountability in their choices to enter into relationships with industry, complying with institutional, government and journal policies, and taking responsibility to guard against bias in research. The scientific process requires scientists to work within a culture of the highest standards for research and professional conduct, and to identify and manage conflicts of interest as an inherent responsibility of their job. They must continue to make efforts to provide access to research results and disseminate findings in a timely manner. Finally, they must protect against risks to human research participants and trainees.

There are legitimate benefits to all types of academia–industry relationships. With careful disclosure and oversight, the risks can be minimized or eliminated and the benefits to the scientific community and public maximized.

References for FASEB

1. FASEB letter to the Department of Health and Human Services in response to the July 3, 2000 Federal Register notice "Human Subject Protection and Financial Conflict of Interest: Conference," http://opa.faseb.org/pdf/9x29x00ltr.pdf, Accessed January 31, 2006.

2. *Integrity in scientific research: Creating an environment that promotes responsible conduct. 2002. Institute of Medicine and the National Research Council of the National Academies.* The National Academies Press, Washington, D.C.

3. *AUTM Licensing Survey, FY 2004: A Survey Summary of Technology Licensing (and Related) Performance for U.S. and Canadian Academic and Nonprofit Institutions, and Technology Investment Firms.* Editors Ashley J. Stevens, Francis Toneguzzo, and Dana Bostrom.

4. *Science and Engineering Indicators- 2006. National Science Board. U.S.* Government Printing Office, Washington DC.

5. Blumenthal D, Causino N, Campbell EG, and Louis KS. 1996. Participation of life-science faculty in research relationships with industry. *NEJM*, **335**: 1734–1739.

6. Blumenthal D, Causino N, Campbell EG, and Louis KS. 1996. Relationships between academic institutions and industry in the life sciences – An industry survey. *NEJM*, **334**: 368–373.

7. Campbell EG, Weissman JS, Feibelmann S, Moy B, Blumenthal D. Institutional academic industry relationships: Results of case studies. *Accountability in Research* 2004; **11**(2): 103–118.

8. Zucker LG and Darby MR. 1996. Star scientists and institutional transformation: Patterns of invention and innovation in the formation of the biotechnology industry. *Proc Natl Acad Sci USA*, **93**: 12709–12716.

9. Berman EM. 1990. The economic impact of industry-funded university R&D. *Research Policy*, **19**: 349–355.

10. Thompson DF. 1993. Understanding financial conflicts of interest. *NEJM*, **329**: 573–576.

11. Bekelman JE, Li Y, and Gross CP. 2003. Scope and Impact of Financial Conflicts of Interest in Biomedical Research. *JAMA*, **289**: 454–465.

12. Kassirer JP and Angell M. 1993. Financial conflicts of interest in biomedical research. *NEJM*, **329**(8): 570–571.

13. Blumenthal D, Causino N, Campbell EG, Anderson MS, and Louis KS. 1997. Withholding of research results in academic life science: Evidence from a national survey of faculty. *JAMA*, **277**(15): 1224–28.

14. Campbell EG, Clarridge BR, Gokhale M, Birenbaum L, Hilgartner S, Holtzman NA, and Blumenthal D. 2002. Data withholding in academic genetics: Evidence from a national survey. *JAMA*, **287**(4):473–481.

15. Slaughter S, Campbell T, Holleman M, and Morgan E. 2002. The "traffic" in graduate students: Graduate students as tokens of exchange between academe and industry. *Science, Technology, & Human Values*, **27**(2):282–312.

16. Gluck ME, Blumenthal D, and Stoto MA. 1987. University-industry relationships in the life sciences: Implications for students and post-doctoral fellows. *Research Policy*, **16**:327–336.

17. Eric G. Campbell , *personal communication.*

18. Research America poll data. 2004. http://www.researchamerica.org/polldata/2004/industry_files/frame.htm.

19. *On Being a Scientist: Responsible Conduct of Research*. 1995. *The National Academy of Sciences, Committee on Science, Engineering and Public Policy*. The National Academies Press, Washington DC.

20. Ehringhaus S and Korn D. 2004. *U.S. medical school policies on individual financial conflicts of interest: Results of an AAMC survey*. Association of American Medical Colleges.

21. Krimsky S and Rothenberg LS. 2001. Conflict of interest policies in science and medical journals: Editorial practices and author disclosures. *Science and Engineering Ethics*, **7**:205–218.

22. *Recognizing and Managing Personal Financial Conflicts of Interest*. 2002. *Council on Governmental Relations*.

The FASEB statement emphasizes the trainee's right to publish (principles #8 and #17), emphasizing that industry's interest in protecting intellectual property should not result in a delay of publication of more than 1 or 2 months. It is appropriate to invoke the language of rights in this instance even though, to our knowledge, there is no law giving trainees the right to publish their results no later than 60 days after they have completed them. Such an appeal is appropriate because moral rights are the accepted way of speaking in democratic societies when a superior is in a position to exploit an inferior. In Part C we saw that moral rights may be grounded in the dignity and autonomy of each agent. Moral rights are useful, therefore, in protecting vulnerable subjects – subjects who may not in fact be protected by existing laws or contracts.

Conclusion: some reservations about rights

As we approach the end of Part C we might pause here to take stock of where we've been. We have been exploring the ways in which claims about moral rights can protect students and investigators by requiring transparency and disclosure. Rights liberate individuals by requiring respect for each person, and this is true inside and outside of the research context. Historically, rights were the philosophical foundation of the American and French revolutions of the eighteenth century. And rights were the banner for the liberation movements of the nineteenth and twentieth centuries that proclaimed the dignity of African Americans, women, and gays, lesbians, bisexuals, and transgendered individuals. Rights for nonhuman animals are now proposed and defended. Moral rights theories clearly have had powerful political applications and they provide signposts for law-makers concerned about the morality of proposed legislation. If individuals have rights, then we ought not to adopt any policy that violates them. These are all strengths of rights theories.

But two criticisms plague these theories. First, how are rights justified? Do rights rest on our autonomy, our free will? Is this why humans have rights and animals, presumably, lack them? But there is a problem here, for not all humans are autonomous (e.g., infants, the senile). But then where do rights come from? The utilitarian Jeremy Bentham famously wrote that moral rights were "nonsense on stilts," and many philosophers have complained that attempts to explain the derivation of rights invariably come up short.

Second, do moral rights undervalue the importance of the consequences of our actions? Is it really not permissible to tell a lie if by doing so you save a life? Wouldn't the world be a better place if some of the alleged rights of the current generation were curtailed in order to ensure that future generations have sufficient food and water? More generally, isn't it true that in some cases the consequences to society of a policy are so beneficial that we are justified in overriding an individual's claimed right to prevent the policy? For example, the 5th Amendment to the US Constitution allows states to seize private property under eminent domain laws, assuming just compensation is provided. It is not obvious that eminent domain laws are unethical nor is it obvious that an individual's right is absolute to dispose of private property as they wish.

To make the criticism clearer, consider another example where it seems unarguable that we ought to aggregate harms and benefits even if it means over-riding individual rights. Suppose there are five swimmers trapped by the tide on one rock, and one swimmer trapped on a second rock. You have a boat, but time enough only to visit one rock and save the swimmers there. It would seem wrong to save one when five could be rescued. However, rights theories do not allow us to draw this conclusion. The reason is that the one individual has a right equal to each of the rights of the other five. The fact that the lone swimmer is not part of a group does not render her right any less weighty than the (individual) rights of the five individuals on the other rock. To put the same point another way, the fact that the five people are members of a group does not add extra weight to their claim, and the fact that choosing to rescue the lone swimmer would harm many people "in the aggregate" does not constitute a valid reason to abandon the one and save the five. Or so rights theorists would argue.

Rights are often assumed to be inviolable. But, as the swimmer case suggests, there are many circumstances where it seems obvious that this is not true. Rights, it seems, are not absolute; they must on occasion be weighed against the consequences of our actions. Thus, the normative implications of having a right are not as clear as is often supposed by those who invoke the right.

Here is where we stand. According to moral rights theories (and contractualist theories), the lone person on the second rock will no doubt object to anyone adopting a moral principle that would require that the lone person be killed so that the five might be saved. Furthermore, no reasonable person could object to her claim that she has a right to be saved. For we can all see that anyone in the lone swimmer's position would similarly want to be saved (Taurek 1977). But this result – a result we obtain by thinking in terms of contracts and rights – does not seem acceptable to those who think, after all is said and done, that saving five people while sacrificing one is better than saving one person while sacrificing five. And that is a strike against these theories.

The motto of the Holy Roman Emperor Ferdinand I (d. 1654) was "Let justice be done, though the world perish." Really? If common sense dovetails with expert opinion on the view that the world would be much better off if one individual's right were voided, and if that opinion were then vetted and affirmed through democratic deliberative processes, then why shouldn't the good of the whole take precedence over the right of an individual?

It is important to add moral rights to our conceptual toolkit. Had we only the contractualist's reasoned agreements or – worse still – only the egoist's self-interest, we would not be equipped to understand the centrality of a person's dignity, a major feature of the moral landscape. Taken together, however, egoism, contractualism and moral rights introduce most of the central themes of normative ethics. They are not, however, exhaustive. They leave out a critical part of the moral life – the most important part, on some accounts. They leave out the consequences of our actions, and our collective, multi-generational, interest in leaving the world in better shape than we found it.

These considerations lead us to our fourth and final theory: utilitarianism.

Take home lessons

- Challenges may arise in interdisciplinary collaborations when different disciplines have different rules about authorship or data sharing.
- If you are terminating a collaborative relationship, ensure everyone with whom you have collaborated is on the same page about data ownership.
- Speaking with someone in your department about techniques or data is not considered interdisciplinary collaboration.
- Multidisciplinary research can benefit health research by translating knowledge more efficiently from the lab to the patient.
- On projects with multiple leaders, spell out each person's role to avoid misunderstanding.
- Principal Investigators should reveal financial payments from sponsors in all written and oral presentations on the project.
- Do not assume that an appeal to a moral right, even when justified, will settle a moral issue.

Bibliography

Bitton, A., *et al.* 2005. The p53 tumour suppressor gene and the tobacco industry: research, debate, and conflict of interest. *Lancet*, 365(9458), 531–540.

National Institutes of Health. 1995. Objectivity in Research. *NIH Guide*, 24(25). Available at: http://grants.nih.gov/grants/guide/notice-files/not95-179.html.

National Science Foundation. 2010. National Science Foundation Award and Administration Guide, Chapter IV – Grantee Standards. Available at: http://www.nsf.gov/pubs/policydocs/pappguide/nsf10_1/aag_4.jsp.

Taurek, J. 1977. Should the numbers count? *Philosophy and Public Affairs*, 6, 293–316.

The Federation of American Societies for Experimental Biology. 2006. *Shared Responsibility, Individual Integrity: Scientists Addressing Conflicts of Interest in Biomedical Research*. Rockville, MD: FASEB. Available at: www.faseb.org/portals/0/pdfs/opa/FASEB_COI_paper.pdf.

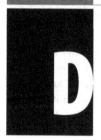

Honor all interests

In Part C, we saw that the moral circle extends beyond people in one's own group to all humans–friends and strangers, including citizens of other nations. But what about nonhuman animals? If the pains and pleasures of those outside our group hurt and please them, is it not also true that the pains and pleasures of nonhuman animals hurt and please them? Should animals count?

Utilitarianism, a theory that includes sentient animals in the circle of moral significance, has four main themes. The first theme is its identification of the fundamental good as pleasure or well-being. (Notice that pleasure and well-being differ from self-interest, keeping one's word, and human dignity.) In this view, pleasure consists of pleasant, agreeable feelings, and well-being consists of the state of living a good life, or flourishing as an autobiographical being (or some other candidate). Utilitarians do not aim primarily at ensuring that all human rights are respected, although respecting rights is an important utilitarian value since people typically do not fare well when their rights are violated. Rather, utilitarians aim at acting so as to produce a world in which as many lives as possible are as full as possible of good things, and as empty as possible of bad things.

Second, utilitarians are committed to an instrumental theory of value for everything besides pleasure or happiness. On this view, the value of an ecosystem, for example, is not intrinsic to it, but rather is dependent upon its utility to some being who can appreciate or value it: in this way, its value is instrumental. Further, this instrumental theory allows us to identify and measure something's value, even if our measurements are only very rough ones. An obvious metric is financial; one might ask with respect to the ecosystem how much money its component parts are worth. Indeed, economists can put rough price tags on, say, the value of clean water or fertile soil by figuring out what people are willing to pay for each item.

Third, the instrumental value of any item is its utility as aggregated across all of its uses by all who value, or disvalue, it. So, keeping the financial metric in mind, to decide whether an action is morally acceptable or not, add up the dollars the act will bring to any given individual, multiply by the number of individuals, and proceed similarly with the disutilities (negative values) incurred by all those harmed by the action. After comparing all the values of all possible actions, select the action that has either the highest total benefits overall, or the action with the highest average ratio of benefits to costs.

Fourth, count all values equally and calculate objectively. In most cases, one person will differ from another person in the values each derives from a given action. Consider again ecosystem services. Suppose Narek derives a thousand dollars of utility every year from the

Research Ethics: A Philosophical Guide to the Responsible Conduct of Research. Gary Comstock.
Published by Cambridge University Press. © Cambridge University Press 2013.

Neuse river by sport fishing in it and Nedra derives the same amount of value by kayaking in it. Narek's and Nedra's uses of the water are compatible; they can both enjoy the river doing what they like, and they are not competing for space on the river or for the water itself.

But suppose Nancy earns ten thousand dollars by draining off a certain amount of the river to irrigate crops on her farm. If Nancy drains off the water, then Narek and Nedra cannot use it. When agricultural uses of water compete with recreational uses, utilitarianism requires us to settle the question by favoring the use with the greatest utility. Given the assumptions and monetary values stipulated in our example, the water should be used for agriculture, because that use produces ten thousand dollars of value compared to the two thousand dollars of value from recreational use. The contribution utilitarianism has made to the debate has been to settle the issue about which is the better use of the water.

Now, one might be tempted to say that utilitarianism is not necessary to decide this case because food is more basic than sports. So, obviously, the best use of the river is farming rather than recreation. Let's modify our example now in order to assess this argument. Suppose that the revenue from the water of sport fishing and kayaking are exactly equal to the revenue from agriculture. Now we might be tempted to say we should decide in favor of farming because farming meets basic needs whereas fishing and paddling are more trivial goods. To reason in this way, however, would be to misunderstand the utilitarian doctrine of equality of interests. This doctrine holds that the relative values assigned to choices must be part of the original assessment. If we have not performed the original calculations in this way, then we have not performed them properly. If we have performed them properly, then the priority of basic food stuffs over leisure activities is already built into the assessment.

"In the second case, we have stipulated that the utility of one use of the water is exactly equal to the utility of the rival use. The agricultural use is worth, let us say, ten thousand dollars and the recreational use is worth ten thousand dollars. Here, the utilitarian concludes that the resource is worth x dollars when used to meet a fundamental human interest and x dollars when used to meet a less basic interest. Since the relative weight of the basic and less basic interests has already been calculated, the utilitarian cannot bring the same consideration back into the discussion at a later point. Assuming the values have been assigned properly, the relative value of food versus recreation has already been factored in. So the fact, if it is a fact, that Nancy's agricultural water usage has the effect of meeting a more consequential need than does Narek's and Nedra's water usage is not a new factor to be added to the equation. The point is that we are not proceeding objectively if we bring our favored preferences back into the calculation a second time after factoring those preferences into the process.

This is a point worth underscoring. Utilitarianism insists on the equality of interests and the necessity of objectivity in ethical reasoning. If everyone affected by some action has the right to have the costs and benefits to them of the action weighed equally with the costs and benefits to others, then one cannot subjectively smuggle a favorite value back into a calculation to trip the decision in one's own favor. To do so is to double-dip, like the butcher putting his finger on the scale when calculating the cost of a cut of meat for a customer.

Utilitarianism is a rigorously impartial theory in which all interests count equally. Each individual counts for one and no more – or less – than one. For contrast, compare the nineteenth century case when the US government counted each African American as three-fifths of a person for the purposes of enumeration and tax benefits. The idea then is this. Perform all calculations without personal bias, and then choose objectively whatever action will maximize good consequences. If the calculations end with a situation in which two rival courses of action both lead to a tie in which each action results in exactly the same aggregate benefits, then we must find another way to decide the matter, perhaps by flipping a coin. What we should not do in that case, however, is to settle the issue illegitimately by re-introducing considerations that have already been fully accounted for.

Research aims at a variety of good consequences

If you Google the phrase "research aims at good consequences," you will get over 500 million hits bearing headlines such as the following:

- New research aims to uncover the social consequences of online surveillance of human behavior
- Research in Rwanda aims for a good harvest of sweet potatoes
- Research shows how articular cartilage bears load and absorbs to articulating joint surfaces
- Quantitative research determines relationship of alcohol use as independent variable in divorce rate

Research is defended on consequentialist grounds more often than not. Many researchers have values and motivations similar to those of Jay, Mr. All-Scholarship whom we met in Part A. Like Jay, we pursue our projects with a self-conscious agenda to push forward the frontiers of knowledge and thereby to maximize aggregate well-being. That's not only an explicitly utilitarian justification of what we do. It is also a good reason to look at the details of this highly influential moral theory.

Naive utilitarianism requires maximizing good consequences

Utilitarians hold that persons should perform whatever actions are most likely to produce the most good. If plagiarizing will not maximize the good, the utilitarian surmises, then don't plagiarize. At one level, it's as simple as that. But difficult questions lurk. How should the good be distributed? Who should have it? And how much? What is the good? Is it one thing or many things?

Utilitarians sort themselves into two camps when they answer these questions. Monists believe there is only one intrinsically good thing, as their name implies. Some monists hold that the good is pleasure, while others argue that it is the satisfaction of desire. We'll discuss both varieties below, but first let us acknowledge the alternative to monism.

Pluralists believe the good has more than one form. Pleasure and satisfied desires are good, but so are love, friendship, justice, integrity, creative achievement, and aesthetic enjoyment. For pluralists, not only are there different goods, but they can assume more or less importance at various times during our lives, too. If you think of lives as stories, you see that part of the challenge of moving from chapter to chapter is figuring out which goods of the many goods available to us are most important at different points in the narrative. On this view, the good not only varies from person to person, but it may vary for an individual as he or she tries to form the past and future into a satisfying, integrated package. For a utilitarian who is a value pluralist, the best state of affairs is that one in which the greatest possible number of individuals are able to maximize the appropriate forms of goodness throughout their lives as they respond to new developments and challenges.

For purposes of simplicity, let us assume that pleasure is the only good. This assumption marks the following discussion as hedonistic (from *hedone*, the Greek word for pleasure). If we also assume that we should always act to produce the greatest amount of total pleasure in the world, we get naive utilitarianism.

> Naive utilitarianism: one should always act to maximize aggregate net pleasure (i.e., to maximize the sum across all individuals of pleasure minus pain).

Naive utilitarianism is intuitively plausible. It doesn't really matter whether we are monists or pluralists about value, or hedonists or preference-satisfaction utilitarians. Even non-utilitarians and anti-utilitarians agree that pleasure is good and pain is bad. The reason is simple: universally, pleasure feels good. And pain hurts – and I don't care who you are, as the comedians say. No further reasons are necessary to explain why naive utilitarianism is initially attractive.

When we think as naive utilitarians with such a hedonistic conception of the good, ethical decision-making becomes simple in one respect because we can reduce all good things to one variable: pleasure. But we can still face difficult problems, since in practice it isn't always clear how to bring about "the most" pleasure possible in the world, as the following thought experiment shows.

Imagine that Janet has an immense capacity for pleasure; she is always happy and is one of those rare people who, despite her great happiness, can always, it seems, get even happier. Devoting a few resources to her would increase the amount of pleasure in the world dramatically, given her immense capacity for happiness. Jeanette, on the other hand, is dour. For her, the glass is always half-empty. If we take the resources we are thinking of giving to Janet and give them to Jeanette instead, we'll bring about no discernible effect on world happiness. This simple case then suggests this question: does naive utilitarianism require us to give more resources to the few people who are already happy rather than try to ameliorate the sorry state of a number of unhappy people?

This is a difficult question for defenders of this theory. We can try to answer it in two steps. The first step is to decide how to weigh each person's respective units of pleasure. The second step will be to decide whether we should maximize the total amount of pleasure of all people in the world, or simply the amount of pleasure experienced by a certain subset of them.

. . . while assigning all like interests an equal weight

Naive utilitarianism weighs one unit of one person's pleasure or pain equally with one unit of every other person's pleasure or pain. According to naive utilitarianism, it would be unfair to give more weight to someone's interests simply because of that person's role in society, gender, race, or any other factor. It does not matter to this view whether an action will cause an equal amount of pain to the vice president of the United States and to an unemployed waiter. The vice president's pain isn't weighted more heavily. Each individual's pain is equally significant no matter what their role in society may be.

Of course, some people have higher tolerances for pain. Imagine that you had to administer an electric shock to an experimental subject – call him James – and then ask James to rank his pain on a scale of one (no pain) to ten (intolerable pain). Suppose you administer 32 volts and he ranks it an eight. Another subject, Jake, might have a different pain threshold; after receiving only 12 volts, Jake ranks his pain as an eight, too. The relevant measure, then, is not the scientific measure (volts), but rather the subjective experience of pain felt by each person. The appropriate scale here is each individual's. In this way, utilitarianism requires that each individual's pain as he or she reports it be counted equally alongside everyone else's. If circumstances force me to have to choose between hurting either James or Jake, and my only option is to give Jake ten units of pain or James three units, the theory requires me to shock James, since he tolerates pain better than Jake does. In short, shocking James minimizes aggregate pain. For a naive utilitarian, then, and assuming that one must either shock James or Jake, the right thing to do would be to shock James.

Notice how far away we have moved from egoism. The egoist always allows special exceptions for myself whereas the naive utilitarian never allows them. If I must choose between three units of pain for me or ten for Jake and I'm no more sensitive to pain than Jake is, I must harm myself. Unlike egoism and contractualism, naive utilitarianism doesn't allow us to make exceptions for ourselves, for loved ones, or for those with whom we have contracted. Utilitarianism is the most impartial of the four theories we have considered.

It is not only impartial between people: this impartiality extends across species. Unlike many rights theories, naive utilitarianism does not allow us to favor humans over other animals. If a nonhuman animal is sentient, its pain counts equally with respect to the pain of a human being. Naive utilitarians argue that agents must always act so as to produce the greatest amount of net pleasure in the world. Since sentient animals by definition are capable of pleasure and pain, their experiences must be taken into account too.

How would such calculations work in practice? Take this simple approach: perform action A if and only if the amount of pleasure over pain that will be in the world if you do A is greater than the balance that will be in the world if you perform any act other than A.

1. Assume that each unit of pain has a value of -1.
2. Assume that each unit of pleasure has a value of $+1$.
3. Identify all individuals including sentient animals likely to experience pain or pleasure as a consequence of each action open to you.
4. Add up all of the numbers, positive and negative.
5. Repeat steps three and four for each action open to you.
6. Choose the action with the highest value.

For example, suppose a company proposes to test a new pesticide on human research subjects. We closely examine the protocols and conclude that the trial will pose only minor inconveniences and no significant risks to the experimental subjects. We further believe that the experiment will bring substantial benefits to farmers and consumers. Now suppose that there are two different ways of conducting the experiment. Under the first design – let's call it protocol A – the consequence of the experiment will be four units of pain (or negative "utiles" or disutilities) to one research subject and six units of benefit (utiles) to each of three farmers, for a subtotal of 18 utiles. Under the second design, protocol B, the experiment would result in less pain to the research subject – only three disutilities – and the same amount of utiles (18) for the farmers.

Adding up the numbers in this scenario yields the results in Table 12.1.

Table 12.1. Calculating simple utilities

	Research subject	Farmers 1, 2, and 3	Total utility
Protocol A	-4	$+18$	$= 14$
Protocol B	-3	$+18$	$= 15$

Recall that for hedonistic utilitarians, the right action is always the action that maximizes net pleasure. Therefore, the right action in this case must be protocol B, since $15 > 14$. Of course,

Table 12.1 only represents a first crude step in what would actually be an involved and lengthy procedure. In the next step we would have to account, for example, for animal pains and pleasures. Presumably, this equation would have positive values added to it because animals would be spared the pain and suffering of research procedures if humans were being used in place of animals. Accounting for the animals would certainly complicate the picture, but no ethical calculation would be a utilitarian calculation if it excluded animals.

By now, however, you may have thought of several objections to naive utilitarianism. Here is just one of the most important.

But not all good consequences are acceptable

Some good consequences come with unacceptable price tags. You can probably complete the following headlines for yourself.

- Nazi medical experiments use Jewish boys and homosexual men to study surgical techniques without anesthesia ...
- US Public Health Service syphilis trials enroll 399 black men in "health experiment". ...
- University of Wisconsin genetics researcher duplicates photos in grant application ...
- Four-year-old orphan volunteers enrolled in industry pesticide trials ...
- Mentally incapacitated fed sugar to induce cavities in Swedish dental research ...

A Google search for "research involves human rights abuses" returns over 27 million hits.

Here's another scenario. What if the only way to maximize pleasure in the world is for a professor to require a graduate student to write another student's literature search, finish a third student's experiments, replicate a postdoc's procedures, and correct a professor's galleys? Suppose that, as a consequence of the student's sacrifices, the world gets four positive and only one negative utile, for a net gain of three utiles. Suppose further that if the student is not sacrificed, only one utile results (from her having finished her thesis), while four negative utiles result (since the others do not finish their projects). This second possible course of action will result in a suboptimal result and a net loss of three utiles.

Given our assumptions, naive utilitarianism apparently not only permits professors to take advantage of students, it requires it. For taking advantage of one student can increase maximum aggregate utility from -3 to $+3$, a gain of six points. And yet the verdict we have just reached (i.e., that professors should take advantage of graduate students) is an affront to professional judgment and common decency.

When an ethical theory leads us to endorse an action that overrides a student's rights – much less the rights of 399 farmers – as naive utilitarianism does, we have reason to think that something perhaps is wrong with the theory.[1] How do the other theories we have introduced fare on this score? Naive egoism leads to a similar conclusion; if an egoist can best achieve their interests by overriding the rights of others then the egoist ought to override those rights. Contractualism and moral rights theories do not lead to such patently unfair results, however. Contractualism can easily explain why a professor should not exploit a student. The reason is that the student may object to the professor's actions on grounds that no reasonable person could reject. Moral rights theorists can also explain why professors should not take advantage of students: such actions violate the students' rights. Of the theories considered so

---

[1] The qualification "perhaps" is important in this sentence. Strict utilitarians such as Hare and Singer do not take the fact that a moral theory leads to a counter-intuitive result to be a sufficient reason to think that the theory has an error in it.

far, only naive egoism and naive utilitarianism cannot explain why a professor should not exploit graduate students. And that is a serious strike against both theories.

Can we save utilitarianism from the objection that it leads to unjust distributions of burdens and benefits? Perhaps, but only if it has built-in a respect for rights under normal circumstances.

Two-level utilitarianism is the view that one should habitually act to respect rights but when thinking critically should maximize good consequences

Two-level utilitarianism distinguishes two ways of thinking about ethics, an ordinary and an extraordinary way. Under ordinary circumstances, according to this theory, we should decide how to act based on habits and rules we've been taught. Someone drops a ten dollar bill on the floor? Do not start surveying possible courses of action and calculating variables to see which action will produce maximum aggregate pleasure. Pick up the bill and hand it to its owner. That's the rule; that's the implicit agreement we have made with other citizens; that's the bill owner's right; and that's your duty.

In everyday life, according to the two-level theory, we should follow the common rules, carry through on the promises we've made, and act in predictable fashion because such behavior will normally produce the best consequences. As we observed in Chapter 5, we tend to face the same moral problems time and time again. In such situations we need rules of thumb to follow because we must act quickly or the moment will be lost. In such cases, stopping to assess utilities is neither possible nor advisable. Furthermore, the intuitive level rules help us to guard against our natural tendency to "cook the data" in favor of self-interest. Consequently, we must determine the right action ahead of time and then hope that we have previously cultivated the right dispositions and virtues that will help us to be good citizens – that is, to perform the right action quickly, without need for reflection.

These dispositions are captured in our beliefs that we should almost always respect peoples' rights, honor our words, keep our promises, treat others the way we would like to be treated, and be honest, responsible, courageous, and compassionate. Moral rights, according to Hare, should be regarded as the outputs of years of deliberation and reliable action-guides in situations that commonly arise. Viewed in this way, rights may not be natural or God-given, but they are nonetheless reliable underpinnings of the rules and regulations that ought to guide us most of the time. In trying to decide whether to exploit a graduate student, for example, a professor should not pause and ask herself whether exploitation in a particular instance might maximize aggregate utility. Any professors tempted to proceed in that fashion need department chairs who will remind them that graduate students have the right not to be harmed for utilitarian purposes.

Hare can be read as arguing that two-level thinking incorporates the best features of egoism, contractualism, and rights theories. If we train ourselves and our children to think that rights almost always ought to be honored we will form ourselves into individuals and societies that naturally act to produce the best consequences. According to this view, ordinary moral reasoning is based on enlightened self-interest, the virtues, and respect for the dignity of individuals. However, these rules are not always reliable, and for two reasons. First, not all of our moral intuitions are sound. Many people, Hare observes, "are completely convinced of the most deplorable moral principles" (Hare 1991). For this reason we must on occasion examine our inclinations and ask whether one of our values is prejudiced or biased. A second reason is that our intuitive-level rules may conflict, as when you have one rule telling you to sacrifice generously when a friend is lonely and depressed and another telling you to give your time and money not to your friend but to a charity that serves hungry children. In such cases, we must engage in the second kind of moral thinking, the extraordinary kind that develops overarching principles capable of settling everyday conflicts.

Hare calls this second-level kind of assessment "critical thinking," and notes that it requires us to reason as "archangels" would reason: calmly, dispassionately, comprehensively. Archangels, we imagine, have superhuman powers, including access to all of the information necessary to make the right moral choices.

Suppose you, like an archangel, know all of the possible courses of action open to you, and all of the probabilities attached to the various outcomes of those actions, and all of the facts relevant to your decision. You know, that is, how each of your possible actions will influence the future of every sentient being affected by your action. Suppose, further, that you are forced to live through all of the experiences, both positive and negative, of all the beings affected by your action. When thinking critically in this way, Hare argues, you will find yourself deliberating impartially, eventually choosing the action that will maximize the welfare of the greatest number of sentient beings while minimizing harms to them. And since you will have imagined living serially through all of the various outcomes of your action, you will choose the course of action with the smallest number of painful experiences for those negatively affected that is compatible with the largest number of pleasurable experiences for those positively affected.

But how should the pains and pleasures be apportioned between those positively and negatively affected? Here we return to the major objection to naive utilitarianism. Should we produce the greatest total amount of pleasure without regard for who has it, a decision that might well produce a world in which a few individuals have a lot of pleasure while others have little or none? Or should we produce the largest amount of pleasure for the average Joe, making it our objective to distribute goods evenly and widely? We can make the difference between these two approaches clearer by showing how each might be deployed in a public policy debate about optimal population levels.

Suppose archangels are debating policies that will affect the number of people in existence. Suppose that the amount of average and total happiness in the world will increase along with each additional person brought into existence. At some point, however, the number of people will be so great that the average person's happiness will begin to decline as the result of overcrowding. That is to say, the happiness that results from increasing the number of individuals can only be increased to a point. If there are not enough of us, the world will not have reached maximum happiness. But if there are too many of us, happiness will begin to decrease and the world will become a miserable place for all of us.

Under these assumptions, archangels will choose policies that encourage population growth when there are too few of us, and that lower population levels when there are too many of us. But where is that optimal level? The answer depends on whether archangels are "total" or "average" utilitarians. As we will now see, there are good reasons to think archangels are average utilitarians.

Consider the six target population levels in the first row of Table 12.2, a table adapted from one developed by Gary Varner (Varner 2012, section 9.5(B)). If there are 100 people whose average happiness is ten, then total happiness is 1,000. Double the population to 200, and total happiness also doubles to 2,000. In this case, the average utilitarian is indifferent to the change because the average person's happiness remains steady. The total utilitarian, however, will endorse the larger number of people because having more of us around increases total happiness.

However, consider what happens when the population doubles again to 400. As the third column indicates, a population level of 400 brings a slight decrease in average happiness. And now the views of the total and average utilitarians begin to come apart. Total utilitarians prefer 400 people to 200, because the higher population produces 3,996 units of happiness while the smaller population (200) produces only 2,000. Average utilitarians, on the other hand, prefer 200 to 400 people, because the lower population produces a slightly higher level of average happiness: a full ten instead of 9.99. Reasoning in this way, average utilitarians must call for policies to stop population growth at 200, because they cannot endorse an average happiness decline from ten to 9.99. On the other hand, total utilitarians must grow population to 1,600, at point at which total happiness reaches its zenith at 6,400.

Table 12.2. Total versus average utilitarianism, slighted modified from Varner 2012, section 9.5(B)

Greatest total vs. greatest average utility						
Population	100	200	400	800	1,600	3,200
Average happiness	10	10	9.99	7	4	1
Total happiness	1,000	2,000	3,996	5,600	6,400	3,200

Comparing the results of the 200 and 1,600 population levels points to a potential shortcoming of total utilitarianism. Total utilitarianism does not seem to care about what egoists call the distinctness of persons. Rather, it treats all of us as "receptacles of value" (Regan 1983), as if each of us were a pitcher carrying water (the stand-in for value). We (the pitchers) don't matter – what matters is the total amount of water that we carry in the aggregate. Total utilitarianism only weighs the total amount of water contained in the pitchers; it has no regard for the pitchers themselves, or whether some pitchers have more water than do others. For this reason, total utilitarianism prefers 1,600 pitchers with water levels at four to 800 pitchers with water levels at seven.

To make the problem easier to grasp, let's add one more assumption, namely that one's quality of life is not pegged to an absolute number such as 7.0 or 9.99, but rather falls within a certain range. For example, we can easily imagine that a life falling within the range 0–4 is a life that is miserable, barely worth living at all. A life falling within the range 5–7, however, is increasingly tolerable, and one in the 8–10 range is increasingly joyful and rewarding. Now, assuming – as we are – that few people can tolerate life below the threshold of 4.0, we can understand the reason archangels will be average utilitarians. For if one had to live sequentially through the lives of 1,600 unhappy people and then through the lives of 800 happy people, one would choose to act to bring about the second option. Average utilitarianism coheres with egoism, contractualism, and rights theories in its insistence on the separateness and integrity of persons, a point on which total utilitarianism falters.

Average utilitarianism is the better theory, and yet it, too, has a problem. Compare the results of the 200 and 400 population levels. Even though we could double the number of happy people in the world with only a miniscule drop in average happiness (of 0.01), average utilitarianism will not allow us to add 200 happy people, since the extra people come at the cost of a (very slightly) decrease in average happiness. But to object to the existence of 200 people simply because their lives will cost everyone a tiny unit of happiness seems miserly at best. We can correct the problem by acknowledging the imprecision of our figures and adopting the range, or threshold, solution proposed in the preceding paragraph. Rather than comparing absolute numbers to each other – for example, 7 to 9.9 – we ought to compare ranges of numbers instead – for example, 0–4 to 8–10.

If we interpret average utilitarianism according to this view, we'll have a theory that gives plausible answers to our original question: how do we maximize overall aggregate pleasure? The answer is this: choose policies that increase the number of people whenever population falls below 200, and choose policies that decrease the number whenever population is above 800.

Two-level utilitarianism is attractive for many reasons. It gives intuitively appealing answers and is easy to use. It draws on tools policy-makers use in making decisions (or, at least, tools that policy-makers like to claim that they use in making decisions). It's useful for identifying impartial and disinterested policies that can be justified in terms of cost–benefit analyses. It combines the strengths of egoism, contractualism, and rights theory. It insists, as egoists do, that we try to achieve our categorical interests. It insists, as contractualists do, that we observe our professional codes. And it insists, as rights theorists do, that we ordinarily treat all persons as distinct and free beings worthy of respect. The two-level theory encourages us to pursue the good of all and to try to make the world a better place by training ourselves to think of others as possessing rights. And it provides a method by which we can resolve conflicts that may arise between rights.

The claims in the previous paragraph are consistent with our discussions of egoism, contractualism, and rights theories in Parts A, B, and C. For example, in discussing rights theories we concluded that both of the following claims can be true at the same time:

(a) In the normal course of things, we have the moral right we called *Do no harm*, that is, the right not to be harmed for utilitarian reasons.
(b) In extraordinary circumstances, such as our imagined case of benign human pesticide toxicity testing, we may override this right to promote the greatest good.

As we have seen, two-level thinking approves of overriding the no harm principle in the case of pesticide testing under the specific assumptions made in Part C. Still, the theory would permit overriding the no harm principle only if we can ensure that doing so will not weaken general belief in the principle. For if the effectiveness and usefulness of the right were to be undermined by testing pesticides on people, then we would also undermine our ability to make the right decision in ordinary cases when we should unreflectively honor the no harm principle. That, in turn, would have bad consequences, since people generally would come to think that they could no longer rely on the no harm principle in everyday circumstances. If the weakening of the principle were an indirect side effect of overriding it in the specific case of human pesticide testing, then utilitarian archangels would prohibit human pesticide testing and come down with moral rights theorists against the testing.

A further feature of two-level thinking is that those taking this stance care about what we teach our children and they insist that social institutions be formed so that people have workable methods of making ethical choices and a reasonable assurance that their rights will be respected. If a decision reached at the level of critical thinking will seriously undermine one reached by intuitive-level thinking, then the two-level theory may well side with the lower-level decision against the higher-level decision. Moral rights can only be effective in maximizing aggregate good if people believe that rights have, as Varner puts it, "deontological flavor" (Varner 2012, section 1.5 and ch. 3).

. . . including good consequences for sentient animals

Two-level utilitarianism holds that the pleasures and pains of all sentient animals must be taken into account in our moral calculations. After all, animals, like children, have the capacity to suffer and to form desires and preferences, even if they lack the capacity to form categorical interests or enter into contracts. For they have, nonetheless, an interior life. It feels like something to be one of them. They have emotions, can form alliances, deceive mates, and make tools to use as instruments to achieve their short- and medium-range goals. And they're capable of making choices and exercising self-control.

When we describe animals in this way, do we mean to include all animals? That is a contentious issue and one we must explore in detail in a later chapter. For the moment, consider a quick answer: we're talking about sentient animals. Dogs and cats, for example, have the same neural apparatus that supports our pain reception, nociception, processing, and expression, so they're included. Viruses and microrganisms lack those structures, so they aren't. All mammals are sentient, and, in addition, most if not all of them seem capable of being happy or sad.

Now, if someone objects and says that this claim about the mental and emotional lives of animals – attributing to animals cognitive states that are only available to humans – is unjustified anthropocentrism, we can appeal to an argument from analogy (Allen 1995). If when hurt, nonhuman mammals exhibit the pain behaviors humans exhibit when humans are hurt, and if, when happy, mammals exhibit the pleasure behaviors humans exhibit when humans are happy, then the argument from analogy suggests nonhuman animals really do feel the kind of depression and frustration, joy and anticipation that we feel. If the argument from analogy works – and we have not seen a reason that it shouldn't – then our moral decisions must take the interests of mammals (at least) into account.[2]

But where is the limit of the expanding moral circle? Just where do we stop attributing moral standing? If we include mice and rats as well as cows and pigs, why not include viruses and pathogens? It is an important question. How far can the circle expand before it strains credulity? Must we learn to care about plants, rocks, and wind currents? Cell phones and old computer terminals? Aren't some things in the world not entitled to moral protections?

Varner provides a powerful argument to extend the line of moral significance to encompass not only animals that are mammals, but all vertebrates. Yet the line of moral significance goes no farther for Varner. Invertebrates (with a few exceptions, such as cuttlefish) lack the neural apparatus necessary to support the capacity for pleasure and pain. If a certain animal cannot feel pain or pleasure, how can it contribute to (or subtract from) the amount of happiness in the world? Like plants, animals without the hardware needed to feel hurt cannot be hurt – at least not in the morally relevant sense. In short (and begging a multitude of important philosophical and empirical questions), it seems that microorganisms, molds, sponges, clams, oysters, and the like do not have moral standing for two-level thinkers.

For two-level utilitarians, things have intrinsic value only if they are sentient, and so we have no reason to worry about our treatment of viruses and weeds, even though they are living. Nor do we need to care, morally speaking, about the interests of inert objects such as sand, water, and chemical structures. These things do not have feelings and do not have a good of their own. There's no one "there" capable of taking an interest of its own in anything.

---

[2] For an overview of the arguments by analogy regarding sentience in the animal kingdom, see Varner 2012, ch. 5.

While on first glance the metaphor of the expanding circle might suggest that expansion has no limits, we now see that the implication is not true. If literally everything counted morally – even the basic constituents of matter, say, bosons and fermions – we would never be able to make the required calculations, never be able to make a moral decision at all. In such a sorry state, the infinitely expanding circle would hamstring us rather than free us. Fortunately, we need not worry about reaching such an impasse because, according to the two-level theory, the moral circle stops expanding once it includes all sentient animals. When we move beyond sentient beings, things have instrumental value only. It follows that we may rightly use such things as means to our ends.

It should be clear by now that the two-level theory offers a clear stopping point for our enlightened concern; we stop at sentience. Inanimate objects and living things that are insentient lie outside the moral circle. And yet some philosophers argue for expanding the circle still farther, as we will see at the end of chapter fifteen.

Conclusion: how to proceed as a utilitarian

Faced with moral decisions, two-level utilitarians proceed initially in the way egoists do. Both ask: which decision will lead to the satisfaction of my best interests? Unlike egoists, however, utilitarians go on to ask: which decision will lead to the satisfaction of the best interests of everyone affected? Answering this question requires that we carefully weigh the happiness and unhappiness the decision will produce. For example, if facing the choice to plagiarize or not plagiarize, the universalizability requirement – at least on this reading – requires you not to plagiarize. Why? Because, on consideration, you would recognize the general unhappiness that plagiarizing would cause; you would sincerely regret having to live through the experiences of everyone involved if you were to plagiarize and you would sincerely prefer to live through their experiences if you did not plagiarize.

Insofar as morality is "universalized prudence," two-level utilitarianism has a parallel with egoism. The two levels require that we understand who we are and what experiences we value most, so that we can imaginatively and vividly entertain the consequences of our actions on ourselves – and then the consequences on others. For if I had to live through everyone else's experiences in turn rather than simply to live through my own experiences, then I would choose, Hare argues, to maximize aggregate goodness. The reason is that I would have to enjoy or suffer all of the costs and benefits following my decision sooner or later. The two-level theory asks us to think of morality as a kind of prudence writ large. When we think about the value of our future experiences, we should not discount them just because they are not on the immediate horizon. Similarly, when we think about the value of others' experiences, we should not discount them just because they are the experiences of others. The parallels between two-level utilitarianism and egoism make the golden rule a useful tool for helping children learn to see their actions from a moral point of view.

But the two-level theorist does not stop where the egoist stops. The two-level theorist insists that we each consider the effects of our behavior on others. Here, in everyday practice, we assume that moral rules of thumb and individual rights are sound guides to conduct. When we face novel situations, however, we must make time, gather resources, and reflect like archangels: objectively and disinterestedly. It is possible here that the results of our deliberations might lead us to act on a principle contrary to a rule found in our professional code – or even, on the rarest of occasions, to override, for example, a moral right found in the UN's Declaration of Human Rights. But such results had better be infrequent, and we should probably only act on them after consulting with other archangels.

Thinking in terms of two levels also provides a method for policy-makers. The method, risk–benefit analysis, has long been the preferred decision-making tool among regulators in contemporary market-driven economies. The method invokes concepts and procedures that are familiar to many citizens having to make important decisions on behalf of institutions such as corporations and governmental regulatory bodies. For this reason, utilitarianism may represent the most powerful contribution of moral philosophy to social practice. We will learn in the rest of Part D how two-level utilitarianism may guide reflection on the use of animals in research and decision-making in environmental policy.

When followed conscientiously, utilitarianism encourages us to make the world a better place for everyone, no matter their race, gender, religion, age – or species.

Bibliography

Allen, C. 1995. *Animal Consciousness*. Available at: http://plato.stanford.edu/entries/consciousness-animal/#4.3 [Accessed June 22, 2008].

Hare, R.M. 1991. A philosophical self-portrait. In T. Mautner, ed. *The Penguin Dictonary of Philosophy*. London: Penguin Books, pp. 234–235.

Regan, T. 1983. *The Case for Animal Rights*. Berkeley: University of California Press.

Varner, G.E. 2012. *Personhood, Ethics, and Animal Cognition: Situating Animals in Hare's Two-Level Utilitarianism*. Oxford: Oxford University Press.

Treat humanely

If you work in a discipline such as toxicology, psychology, or neurology, you may well find yourself in the position of having to decide whether you will harm animals in research. Those who decide to perform harmful animal research are either doing it for the benefit of the actual animals used, as in veterinary work with sick or injured animals, or have been able to find for themselves an answer to the question: what gives us the right to inflict pain and suffering on innocent creatures? The justifications offered for harming animals are almost always consequentialist in form; by harming a small number of animals in as limited a way as possible, goes the argument, we can produce great benefits for humans and other animals. In this chapter we will explore this utilitarian way of thinking.

According to the US Department of Agriculture, 1,134,693 vertebrate animals were used in research in the USA in 2010 (Animal and Plant Health Inspection Service 2011). Of that number, 71,317 were nonhuman primates and roughly 85,000 were cats or dogs. More than 300,000 animals were used in experiments involving pain that was treated with drugs, and almost 100,000 were caused pain with no drugs administered.

By all accounts, these figures vastly underestimate the actual numbers of animals used because the Animal Welfare Act does not require researchers to report figures on the most commonly used species: rats, mice, birds, fish, and frogs. According to Larry Carbone, the number of rodents alone used in 2001 was 80 million (Carbone 2004). (The numbers are also a fraction of the total numbers of animals killed for food and fiber in the USA, which the US Department of Agriculture estimates at 35 million cows, 110 million hogs, and 8.8 billion chickens (United States Department of Agriculture 2011).) The commonly accepted rationale for using animals in biomedical research is to advance basic knowledge of human disease and function and so to improve human life without having to subject humans to the experiments being run on the animals.[1]

Everyday rules for treating animals humanely in research

Two-level utilitarians should look first for the rules widely used by people thinking in ordinary ways about the use of animals in research. As background, they might note that between 92% and 97% of US consumers are meat-eaters even though the US Department of

---

[1] This chapter does not address issues that arise in other research endeavors involving animals, such as companion animal research or observational field studies of wild animals.

Research Ethics: A Philosophical Guide to the Responsible Conduct of Research. Gary Comstock.
Published by Cambridge University Press. © Cambridge University Press 2013.

Agriculture (USDA) claims that vegetarianism is a healthy and nutritious alternative to meat-eating. A safe, assumption, therefore, is that vegetarianism is not one of the everyday rules of thumb in this culture. If one allows the killing of nine billion mammals for food, it is unlikely that one would object to the killing of animals for scientific research. So, research involving animals is probably justifiable in ordinary moral thinking. For while modern humans could replace meat with tofu in our diets and down and wool with synthetic materials in our winter jackets, the use of animals in research is not so easily replaced. And the consequences of animal research, common wisdom has it, have produced many of the life-saving pharmaceuticals and other advanced healthcare technologies of the modern world. In cultures dominated by meat-eaters, therefore, the two-level utilitarian is going to expect to find widespread intuitive support for animal research.

The previous paragraph summarizes the attitude out of which emerged the Animal Welfare Act (AWA), the federal US law passed in 1966 and amended on several occasions (United States Code, edition 2009). It requires the USDA's Animal and Plant Health Inspection Service (APHIS) to establish and enforce minimum care standards including regulations concerning how much space must be allotted per research animal, and how animals should be housed, handled, fed and watered. APHIS requires, for example, veterinary care, nutritious food and ample water unless an Institutional Animal Care and Use Committee (IACUC) has approved an exemption. The *Guide for the Care and Use of Laboratory Animals* spells out protections for all vertebrate research animals, including rodents and birds. The Office of Laboratory Animal Welfare (OLAW) enforces the Guide's regulations, and the IACUC on each campus enforces the regulations at the local level. An IACUC must have at least five members: the university's attending veterinarian, a practicing scientist experienced in research involving animals; a member whose primary concerns are in a nonscientific area; and an individual not affiliated with the institution to represent community interests and concerns. At NC State the committee consists of 17 members: ten faculty, five non-faculty professionals, and two individuals not associated with the university.

If you are filling out an application for IACUC approval of your research proposals, you will have to supply a fair amount of information. The committee will want to know, among other things, how many animals and of what species you will use. How will you house, feed, and care for them? How will you acquire them? If you intend to deprive them of food and water or subject them to noxious stimuli or physical restraint, what is your scientific rationale for doing so? How many procedures will be performed on each animal? How often? How long will each procedure last? How will you provide veterinary care for the animals and what will you do if one becomes sick or injured?

The IACUC rules, as we say, have been developed on the basis of widely accepted beliefs, including the idea that mammals are conscious, can experience pain and pleasure, and have a welfare. How these beliefs are translated into practice differs from institution to institution. Each institution's IACUC is charged with ensuring that the welfare of all experimental animals is protected against unjustified harm. The IACUC need not disapprove research protocols in which an animal's welfare is to be compromised, because the members of the IACUC may decide that the cost to the animal's welfare is outweighed by the scientific benefits. Along these lines, the Research Animal Resource page of the University of Minnesota's IACUC states that, with regard to the use of vertebrate animals, all researchers must assume that:

any procedures that would be expected to cause more than slight or momentary pain or distress in a human being will cause similar pain or distress in an animal, unless scientifically demonstrated otherwise.

Distress is defined as a maladaptive response to a stressor. It is recognized that some stress is normal, but if animals react in such a way that their health is being compromised (e.g. anorexia in response to induced disease or self-aggression in response to psychological stress) this is considered distress. (University of Minnesota Research Animal Resources 2000)

The regulations also indicate that whenever an animal is subjected to certain procedures that would cause stress in a human being researchers must assume that the animal is being caused pain or distress as well. The procedures include surgery, post-surgical recovery, physical restraint for more than an hour, tail snipping, being deprived of food or water for a long period, electrical shock, inflammatory disease, skin lesions, and high doses of irradiation. In some experiments animals are subject to procedures that will "require the animal to reach a moribund state or die spontaneously as the endpoint of the study" (Office of Responsible Research Practices 2010). In such cases, the animal must be euthanized at the earliest point possible. Whenever it is compatible with the scientific aims of the researcher, an animal's pain must be relieved with appropriate veterinary care, including analgesia or anesthesia.

How can one tell when an animal is in pain? The University of Minnesota document lists a number of possible signs: decreased activity; abnormal postures, such as a hunched back; poor grooming; loss of appetite; weight loss; dehydration; decrease or increase in pulse or respiratory rate; unusual physical response to touch, such as withdrawal, lameness, abnormal aggression, vocalizing; teeth grinding; vomiting or diarrhea. How should researchers respond to such indicators? With empathy and professional action; the university veterinarian must be consulted and a plan developed to relieve the pain. If relief is not possible and the pain is not necessary to test the experimental hypothesis, then the animal must be euthanized.

As noted, most people in the United States are not opposed to the rearing and killing of animals for food, and yet they are opposed to needless animal suffering. This attitude is sometimes called the "animal welfare" position to distinguish it from the more strict, and vegetarian, "animal rights" view (Regan 1983). Animal rights defenders categorically oppose almost all uses of animals in research. But animal welfarists also oppose some uses, such as research that causes significant suffering to animals but results in trivial or useless knowledge, or research based on scientifically invalid methods in which, for example, the results of a procedure do not transate into any useful knowledge for humans.

An animal welfare approach led biologists Russell and Burch in 1959 to formulate three principles – the "Three R's" – to guide research. Whenever any one of the three principles can be used without interfering with one's scientific goal, one should adopt it.

1. Replace animals with methods and models that do not involve live or sentient animals.
2. Reduce the number of animals used to the lowest number possible to obtain the data at which the protocol aims.
3. Refine one's scientific procedures to eliminate or minimize potential pain or distress to the animal and to enhance the animal's well-being (Russell and Burch 1959).

For example, one way to replace an animal in an experiment is to use an in vitro cell culture rather than the live animal. Another way is to use computer modeling simulations of the problem under investigation.

Critical thinking about using animals in research

We have been summarizing the rules of thumb that guide us as we think about the humane treatment of animals. But a problem arises in trying to satisfy the rules insofar as they contain an implicit contradiction. Here, for example, are two statements found in the North Carolina State University Animal Care and Use Policy. The Preamble proclaims that

> *The use of animals is essential to the teaching, extension, and research missions of North Carolina State University* [emphasis added]. Significant benefits to the health and welfare of both animals and humans have resulted from animal use in research, and continued use is crucial to future advancements. Without the use of animals, adequate instruction of students in many programs such as agriculture, the biological sciences, and veterinary medicine would be impossible. However, those who utilize animals are morally and legally obligated to care for them properly and use them humanely. Each faculty member, staff member, or student involved in the use of animals is directly responsible for promoting and protecting their welfare within the instructional, extension, and research programs of the University (Sponsored Programs and Regulatory Compliance).

The paragraph contains two claims. The first is that using animals in research is necessary – "essential ... crucial" – to the mission of the university and that adequate instruction of students would be "impossible" without it. The second is that those using animals are morally obligated to care for animals humanely. But how is it possible to be humane when, for example, confining a vertebrate mammal to a cage? Recognizing the insult to an animal's welfare that confinement brings, the list of specific policies tries to mediate the conflict. The first policy, for example, expresses limits on the use of animals and requires that alternative means must be used whenever feasible.

Policy:

1. *Animals should be used in teaching, research, and extension programs only as required to demonstrate principles, to obtain new information, and achieve results which will ultimately benefit society* [emphasis added]. Whenever feasible, mathematical models, in vitro biological systems, demonstrations, and computer and audiovisual aids should augment, complement, or possibly replace animal use entirely, thereby reducing the number of animals needed (Sponsored Programs and Regulatory Compliance).

Here the intuitive-level system rules give rise to conflicts that critical thinking must resolve. For if an animal's pain counts in our moral calculations, as it clearly does for utilitarians, why doesn't an animal's death count? To address this question, two-level utilitarians must move from following ordinary rules to thinking critically in the way that a certain kind of utilitarian, specifically, an act-utilitarian, would think. The following two articles can help us along this path by providing arguments for and against consequentialist justifications of animal experimentation.

In the first article, Carl Cohen argues that animal death does not count because animals are not contractors and therefore cannot be the kinds of beings that are part of our moral community. Animals, in sum, lack rights altogether, including a right to life. It is, on Cohen's view, permissible both to eat animals and to use them in research because doing so violates no one's rights and maximizes aggregate utility. Utilitarians who think animal research must be stopped are simply mistaken in their calculations, argues Cohen.

Background essay: "The case for the use of animals in biomedical research," by Carl Cohen[2]

Using animals as research subjects in medical investigations is widely condemned on two grounds: first, because it wrongly violates the rights of animals, and second, because it wrongly imposes on sentient creatures much avoidable suffering. Neither of these arguments is sound. The first relies on a mistaken understanding of rights; the second relies on a mistaken calculation of consequences. Both deserve definitive dismissal.

Why animals have no rights

A right, properly understood, is a claim, or potential claim, that one party may exercise against another. The target against whom such a claim may be registered can be a single person, a group, a community, or (perhaps) all humankind. The content of rights claims also varies greatly: repayment of loans, nondiscrimination by employers, noninterference by the state, and so on. To comprehend any genuine right fully, therefore, we must know who holds the right, against whom it is held, and to what it is a right.

Alternative sources of rights add complexity. Some rights are grounded in constitution and law (e.g., the right of an accused to trial by jury); some rights are moral but give no legal claims (e.g., my right to your keeping the promise you gave me); and some rights (e.g., against theft or assault) are rooted both in morals and in law.

The differing targets, contents, and sources of rights, and their inevitable conflict, together weave a tangled web. Notwithstanding all such complications, this much is clear about rights in general: they are in every case claims, or potential claims, within a community of moral agents. Rights arise, and can be intelligibly defended, only among beings who actually do, or can, make moral claims against one another. Whatever else rights may be, therefore, they are necessarily human; their possessors are persons, human beings.

The attributes of human beings from which this moral capability arises have been described variously by philosophers, both ancient and modern: the inner consciousness of a free will (Saint Augustine); the grasp, by human reason, of the binding character of moral law (Saint Thomas); the self-conscious participation of human beings in an objective ethical order (Hegel); human membership in an organic moral community (Bradley); the development of the human self through the consciousness of other moral selves (Mead); and the underivative, intuitive cognition of the rightness of an action (Prichard). Most influential has been Immanuel Kant's emphasis on the universal human possession of a uniquely moral will and the autonomy its use entails. Humans confront choices that are purely moral; humans – but certainly not dogs or mice – lay down moral laws, for others and for themselves. Human beings are self-legislative, morally autonomous.

Animals (that is, nonhuman animals, the ordinary sense of that word) lack this capacity for free moral judgment. They are not beings of a kind capable of exercising or responding to moral claims. Animals therefore have no rights, and they can have none. This is the core of the argument about the alleged rights of animals. The holders of rights must have the capacity to comprehend rules of duty, governing all including themselves. In applying such rules, the holders of rights must recognize possible conflicts between what is in their own interest and what is just. Only in a community of beings capable of self-restricting moral judgments can the concept of a right be correctly invoked.

Humans have such moral capacities. They are in this sense self-legislative, are members of communities governed by moral rules, and do possess rights. Animals do not have such moral capacities. They are not morally self-legislative, cannot possibly be members of a truly moral

[2] Reprinted from *New England Journal of Medicine*, 1986, 315, pp. 866–869. Carl Cohen is Professor of Philosophy, University of Michigan, ccohen@umich.edu.

community, and therefore cannot possess rights. In conducting research on animal subjects, therefore, we do not violate their rights, because they have none to violate.

To animate life, even in its simplest forms, we give a certain natural reverence. But the possession of rights presupposes a moral status not attained by the vast majority of living things. We must not infer, therefore, that a live being has, simply in being alive, a "right" to its life. The assertion that all animals, only because they are alive and have interests, also possess the "right to life" is an abuse of that phrase, and wholly without warrant.

It does not follow from this, however, that we are morally free to do anything we please to animals. Certainly not. In our dealings with animals, as in our dealings with other human beings, we have obligations that do not arise from claims against us based on rights. Rights entail obligations, but many of the things one ought to do are in no way tied to another's entitlement. Rights and obligations are not reciprocals of one another, and it is a serious mistake to suppose that they are.

Illustrations are helpful. Obligations may arise from internal commitments made: physicians have obligations to their patients not grounded merely in their patients' rights. Teachers have such obligations to their students, shepherds to their dogs, and cowboys to their horses. Obligations may arise from differences of status: adults owe special care when playing with young children, and children owe special care when playing with young pets. Obligations may arise from special relationships: the payment of my son's college tuition is something to which he may have no right, although it may be my obligation to bear the burden if I reasonably can; my dog has no right to daily exercise and veterinary care, but I do have the obligation to provide these things for her.

Obligations may arise from particular acts or circumstances: one may be obliged to another for a special kindness done, or obliged to put an animal out of its misery in view of its condition – although neither the human benefactor nor the dying animal may have had a claim of right.

Plainly, the grounds of our obligations to humans and to animals are manifold and cannot be formulated simply. Some hold that there is a general obligation to do no gratuitous harm to sentient creatures (the principle of nonmaleficence); some hold that there is a general obligation to do good to sentient creatures when that is reasonably within one's power (the principle of beneficence). In our dealings with animals, few will deny that we are at least obliged to act humanely – that is, to treat them with the decency and concern that we owe, as sensitive human beings, to other sentient creatures. To treat animals humanely, however, is not to treat them as humans or as the holders of rights.

A common objection, which deserves a response, may be paraphrased as follows:

> If having rights requires being able to make moral claims, to grasp and apply moral laws, then many humans – the brain-damaged, the comatose, the senile – who plainly lack those capacities must be without rights. But that is absurd. This proves [the critic concludes] that rights do not depend on the presence of moral capacities.

This objection fails; it mistakenly treats an essential feature of humanity as though it were a screen for sorting humans. The capacity for moral judgment that distinguishes humans from animals is not a test to be administered to human beings one by one. Persons who are unable, because of some disability, to perform the full moral functions natural to human beings are certainly not for that reason ejected from the moral community. The issue is one of kind. Humans are of such a kind that they may be the subject of experiments only with their voluntary consent. The choices they make freely must be respected. Animals are of such a kind that it is impossible for them, in principle, to give or withhold voluntary consent or to make a moral choice. What humans retain when disabled, animals have never had.

A second objection, also often made, may be paraphrased as follows:

> Capacities will not succeed in distinguishing humans from the other animals. Animals also reason; animals also communicate with one another; animals also care passionately for their young; animals also exhibit

desires and preferences. Features of moral relevance – raionality, interdependence, and love – are not exhibited uniquely by human beings. Therefore [this critic concludesl, there can be no solid moral distinction between humans and other animals.

This criticism misses the central point. It is not the ability to communicate or to reason, or dependence on one another, or care for the young, or the exhibition of preference, or any such behavior that marks the critical divide. Analogies between human families and those of monkeys, or between human communities and those of wolves, and the like, are entirely beside the point. Patterns of conduct are not at issue. Animals do indeed exhibit remarkable behavior at times. Conditioning, fear, instinct, and intelligence all contribute to species survival. Membership in a community of moral agents nevertheless remains impossible for them. Actors subject to moral judgment must be capable of grasping the generality of an ethical premise in a practical syllogism. Humans act immorally often enough, but only they – never wolves or monkeys – can discern, by applying some moral rule to the facts of a case, that a given act ought or ought not to he performed. The moral restraints imposed by humans on themselves are thus highly abstract and are often in conflict with the self-interest of the agent. Communal behavior among animals, even when most intelligent and most endearing, does not approach autonomous morality in this fundamental sense.

Genuinely moral acts have an internal as well as an external dimension. Thus, in law, an act can be criminal only when the guilty deed, the *actus reus*, is done with a guilty mind, *mens rea*. No animal can ever commit a crime; bringing animals to criminal trial is the mark of primitive ignorance. The claims of moral right are similarly inapplicable to them. Does a lion have a right to eat a baby zebra? Does a baby zebra have a right not to be eaten? Such questions, mistakenly invoking the concept of right where it does not belong, do not make good sense. Those who condemn biomedical research because it violates "animal rights" commit the same blunder.

In defense of "speciesism"

Abandoning reliance on animal rights, some critics resort instead to animal sentience – their feelings of pain and distress. We ought to desist from the imposition of pain insofar as we can. Since all or nearly all experimentation on animals does impose pain and could be readily forgone, say these critics, it should be stopped. The ends sought may be worthy, but those ends do not justify imposing agonies on humans, and by animals the agonies are felt no less. The laboratory use of animals (these critics conclude) must therefore be ended or at least very sharply curtailed.

Argument of this variety is essentially utilitarian, often expressly so; it is based on the calculation of the net product, in pains and pleasures, resulting from experiments on animals. Jeremy Bentham, comparing horses and dogs with other sentient creatures, is thus commonly quoted: "The question is not, Can they reason? nor Can they talk? but, Can they suffer?"

Animals certainly can suffer and surely ought not to be made to suffer needlessly. But in inferring, from these uncontroversial premises, that biomedical research causing animal distress is largely (or wholly) wrong, the critic commits two serious errors.

The first error is the assumption, often explicitly defended, that all sentient animals have equal moral standing. Between a dog and a human being, according to this view, there is no moral difference; hence the pains suffered by dogs must be weighed no differently from the pains suffered by humans. To deny such equality, according to this critic, is to give unjust preference to one species over another; it is "speciesism." The most influential statement of this moral equality of species was made by Peter Singer:

> The racist violates the principle of equality by giving greater weight to the interests of members of his own race when there is a clash between their interests and the interests of those of another race. The sexist violates the principle of equality by favoring the interests of his own sex. Similarly the speciesist allows the interests of his own species to override the greater interests of members of other species. The pattern is identical in each case.

This argument is worse than unsound; it is atrocious. It draws an offensive moral conclusion from a deliberately devised verbal parallelism that is utterly specious. Racism has no rational ground whatever. Differing degrees of respect or concern for humans for no other reason than that they are members of different races is an injustice totally without foundation in the nature of the races themselves. Racists, even if acting on the basis of mistaken factual beliefs, do grave moral wrong precisely because there is no morally relevant distinction among the races. The supposition of such differences has led to outright horror. The same is true of the sexes, neither sex being entitled by right to greater respect or concern than the other. No dispute here.

Between species of animate life, however – between (for example) humans on the one hand and cats or rats on the other – the morally relevant differences are enormous, and almost universally appreciated. Humans engage in moral reflection; humans are morally autonomous; humans are members of moral communities, recognizing just claims against their own interest. Human beings do have rights; theirs is a moral status very different from that of cats or rats.

I am a speciesist. Speciesism is not merely plausible; it is essential for right conduct, because those who will not make the morally relevant distinctions among species are almost certain, in consequence, to misapprehend their true obligations. The analogy between speciesism and racism is insidious. Every sensitive moral judgment requires that the differing natures of the beings to whom obligations are owed be considered. If all forms of animate life – or vertebrate animal life? – must be treated equally, and if therefore in evaluating a research program the pains of a rodent count equally with the pains of a human, we are forced to conclude (1) that neither humans nor rodents possess rights, or (2) that rodents possess all the rights that humans possess. Both alternatives are absurd. Yet one or the other must be swallowed if the moral equality of all species is to be defended.

Humans owe to other humans a degree of moral regard that cannot be owed to animals. Some humans take on the obligation to support and heal others, both humans and animals, as a principal duty in their lives; the fulfillment of that duty may require the sacrifice of many animals. If biomedical investigators abandon the effective pursuit of their professional objectives because they are convinced that they may not do to animals what the service of humans requires, they will fail, objectively, to do their duty. Refusing to recognize the moral differences among species is a sure path to calamity. (The largest animal rights group in the country is People for the Ethical Treatment of Animals; its co-director, Ingrid Newkirk, calls research using animal subjects "fascism" and "supremacism." "Animal liberationists do not separate out the human animal," she says, "so there is no rational basis for saying that a human being has special rights. A rat is a pig is a dog is a boy. They're all mammals.")

Those who claim to base their objection to the use of animals in biomedical research on their reckoning of the net pleasures and pains produced make a second error, equally grave. Even if it were true – as it is surely not – that the pains of all animate beings must be counted equally, a cogent utilitarian calculation requires that we weigh all the consequences of the use, and of the non-use, of animals in laboratory research. Critics relying (however mistakenly) on animal rights may claim to ignore the beneficial results of such research, rights being trump cards to which interest and advantage must give way. But an argument that is explicitly framed in terms of interest and benefit for all over the long run must attend also to the disadvantageous consequences of not using animals in research, and to all the achievements attained and attainable only through their use.

The sum of the benefits of their use is utterly beyond quantification. The elimination of horrible disease, the increase of longevity, the avoidance of great pain, the saving of lives, and the improvement of the quality of lives (for humans and for animals) achieved through research using animals is so incalculably great that the argument of these critics, systematically pursued, establishes not their conclusion but its reverse: to refrain from using animals in biomedical research is, on utilitarian grounds, morally wrong.

When balancing the pleasures and pains resulting from the use of animals in research, we must not fail to place on the scales the terrible pains that would have resulted, would be suffered now, and would long continue had animals not been used. Every disease eliminated, every vaccine developed, every method of pain relief devised, every surgical procedure invented, every prosthetic device implanted – indeed, virtually every modern medical therapy – is due, in part or in whole, to experimentation using animals. Nor may we ignore, in the balancing process, the predictable gains in human (and animal) well-being that are probably achievable in the future but that will not be achieved if the decision is made now to desist from such research or to curtail it.

Medical investigators are seldom insensitive to the distress their work may cause animal subjects. Opponents of research using animals are frequently insensitive to the cruelty of the results of the restrictions they would impose. Untold numbers of human beings – real persons, although not now identifiable – would suffer grievously as the consequence of this well-meaning but short-sighted tenderness. If the morally relevant differences between humans and animals are borne in mind, and if all relevant considerations are weighed, the calculation of long-term consequences must give overwhelming support for biomedical research using animals.

Concluding remarks
Substitution

The humane treatment of animals requires that we desist from experimenting on them if we can accomplish the same result using alternative methods – in vitro experimentation, computer simulation, or others. Critics of some experiments using animals rightly make this point.

It would be a serious error to suppose, however, that alternative techniques could soon be used in most research now using live animal subjects. No other methods now on the horizon or perhaps ever to be available can fully replace the testing of a drug, a procedure, or a vaccine, in live organisms. The flood of new medical possibilities being opened by the successes of recombinant DNA technology will turn to a trickle if testing on live animals is forbidden. When initial trials entail great risks, there may be no forward movement whatever without the use of live animal subjects. In seeking knowledge that may prove critical in later clinical applications, the unavailability of animals for inquiry may spell complete stymie. In the United States, federal regulations require the testing of new drugs and other products on animals, for efficacy and safety, before human beings are exposed to them. We would not want it otherwise.

Every advance in medicine – every new drug, new operation, new therapy of any kind – must sooner or later be tried on a living being for the first time. That trial, controlled or uncontrolled, will be an experiment. The subject of that experiment, if it is not an animal, will be a human being. Prohibiting the use of live animals in biomedical research, therefore, or sharply restricting it, must result either in the blockage of much valuable research or in the replacement of animal subjects with human subjects. These are the consequences – unacceptable to most reasonable persons – of not using animals in research.

Reduction

Should we not at least reduce the use of animals in biomedical research? No, we should increase it to avoid when feasible the use of humans as experimental subjects. Medical investigations putting human subjects at some risk are numerous and greatly varied. The risks run in such experiments are usually unavoidable, and (thanks to earlier experiments on animals) most such risks are minimal or moderate. But some experimental risks are substantial.

When an experimental protocol that entails substantial risk to humans comes before an Institutional review board, what response is appropriate? The investigation, we may suppose, is promising and deserves support, so long as its human subjects are protected against unnecessary dangers. May not the investigators be fairly asked: have you done all that you can to eliminate risk to humans by the extensive testing of that drug, that procedure, or that device on animals? To achieve maximal safety for humans we are right to require thorough experimentation on animal subjects before humans are involved.

Opportunities to increase human safety in this way are commonly missed, trials in which risks may be shifted from humans to animals are often not devised, sometimes not even considered. Why? For the investigator, the use of animals as subjects is often more expensive, in money and time, than the use of human subjects. Access to suitable human subjects is often quick and convenient, whereas access to appropriate animal subjects may be awkward, costly, and burdened with red tape. Physician-investigators have often had more experience working with human beings and know precisely where the needed pool of subjects is to be found and how they may be enlisted. Animals, and the procedures for their use, are often less familiar to these investigators. Moreover, the use of animals in place of humans is now more likely to be the target of zealous protests from without. The upshot is that humans are sometimes subjected to risks that animals could have borne, and should have borne, in their place. To maximize the protection of human subjects, I conclude, the wide and imaginative use of live animal subjects should be encouraged rather than discouraged. This enlargement in the use of animals is our obligation.

Consistency

Finally, inconsistency between the profession and the practice of many who oppose research using animals deserves comment. This frankly ad hominem observation aims chiefly to show that a coherent position rejecting the use of animals in medical research imposes costs so high as to be intolerable even to the critics themselves.

One cannot coherently object to the killing of animals in biomedical investigations while continuing to eat them. Anesthetics and thoughtful animal husbandry render the level of actual animal distress in the laboratory generally lower than that in the abattoir. So long as death and discomfort do not substantially differ in the two contexts, the consistent objector must not only refrain from all eating of animals but also protest as vehemently against others eating them as against others experimenting on them. No less vigorously must the critic object to the wearing of animal hides in coats and shoes, to employment in any industrial enterprise that uses animal parts, and to any commercial development that will cause death or distress to animals.

Killing animals to meet human needs for food, clothing, and shelter is judged entirely reasonable by most persons. The ubiquity of these uses and the virtual universality of moral support for them confront the opponent of research using animals with an inescapable difficulty. How can the many common uses of animals be judged morally worthy, while their use in scientific investigation is judged unworthy?

The number of animals used in research is but the tiniest fraction of the total used to satisfy assorted human appetites. That these appetites, often base and satisfiable in other ways, morally justify the far larger consumption of animals, whereas the quest for improved human health and understanding cannot justify the far smaller, is wholly implausible. Aside from the numbers of animals involved, the distinction in terms of worthiness of use, drawn with regard to any single animal, is not defensible. A given sheep is surely not more justifiably used to put lamb chops on the supermarket counter than to serve in testing a new contraceptive or a new prosthetic device. The needless killing of animals is wrong; if the common killing of them for our food or convenience is right, the less common but more humane uses of animals in the service of medical science are certainly not less right.

Scrupulous vegetarianism, in matters of food, clothing, shelter, commerce, and recreation, and in all other spheres, is the only fully coherent position the critic may adopt.

At great human cost, the lives of fish and crustaceans must also be protected, with equal vigor, if speciesism has been forsworn. A very few consistent critics adopt this position.

It is the *reductio ad absurdum* of the rejection of moral distinctions between animals and human beings.

Opposition to the use of animals in research is based on arguments of two different kinds – those relying on the alleged rights of animals and those relying on the consequences for animals.

I have argued that arguments of both kinds must fail. We surely do have obligations to animals, but they have, and can have, no rights against us on which research can infringe. In calculating the consequences of animal research, we must weigh all the long-term benefits of the results achieved – to animals and to humans – and in that calculation we must not assume the moral equality of all animate species.

Cohen argues against the claim that ending animal research would lead to the best overall consequences. Furthermore, he argues that since animals cannot contract with us, they are not the sorts of beings that we are. Animals are not part of the moral community.

The next reading takes issue with each of Cohen's arguments. LaFollette and Shanks argue that Cohen's view is internally inconsistent and systematically underestimates the suffering of animals in research.

For example, LaFollette and Shanks think Cohen's position unfairly trades on ambiguities in the way it deploys the argument from analogy. The argument from analogy is this. Humans and mice share many properties in common: for example, both are mammals, share many genes, and have homologous neural structures. Therefore, the effects of a drug on the one will be the same as on the other. LaFollette and Shanks take issue with this argument. They claim that the argument ignores basic biochemical, anatomical, and physiological differences between species. Consequently, we should not be surprised if the same drug has different effects in different animals, or one effect in mice, a different effect in rats, a third effect in monkeys, and a fourth effect in humans. A problem with Cohen's argument, argue LaFollette and Shanks, is that it illegitimately plays both sides of the fence. On the one hand, it minimizes differences between humans and experimental animals when minimizing will serve the purpose of validating the extrapolation of data from animals to humans. On the other hand, it maximizes differences between humans and animals when maximizing serves the purpose of denying rights to animals. Can we have it both ways? If the gulf is as wide as Cohen alleges, are extrapolations from data acquired from other species valid when applied to humans?

LaFollette and Shanks think utilitarian calculations will generally not lead to the conclusion that we are justified in using animals in research. As you read, ask yourself whether their arguments seem stronger than Cohen's.

Background essay: "Util-izing animals" by Hugh LaFollette and Niall Shanks (Deceased)[3]

Biomedical experimentation on animals is justified, researchers say, because of its enormous benefits to human beings. Sure animals die and suffer, but that is morally insignificant when compared to experimentation's spectacular payoffs. As Carl Cohen, a leading philosophical apologist for vivisection, writes:

> When balancing the pleasures and pains resulting from the use of animals in research, we must not fail to place on the scales the terrible pains that would have resulted, would be suffered now, and would long continue had animals not been used. Every disease eliminated, every vaccine developed, . . . indeed, virtually every modern medical therapy is due, in part or in whole, to experimentation using animals.[4]

---

[3] Reprinted from *Journal of Applied Philosophy* 12, no. 1 (April 1995): 13–25. Hugh LaFollette is Cole Chair in Ethics, University of South Florida, hughlafollette@tampabay.rr.com. Niall Shanks (deceased) was Curtis D. Gridley Distinguished Professor of History and Philosophy of Science, Wichita State University.
[4] Cohen, C. (1986): "The Case for the Use of Animals in Biomedical Research", *New England Journal of Medicine*, vol. 315, pp. 868.

The moral worth of animals

Researchers would need to demonstrate the success of animal experimentation even if animals had no moral worth. For if animal experimentation were invaluable (or just marginally valuable), it would be a waste of scarce public resources. However, this proffered justification of research openly acknowledges the moral worth of animals. Unless animals had moral worth, it would make no sense to say that we must include their deaths and suffering "on the scales." If they are devoid of value – or their value were morally negligible – the impact of experimentation on them would never enter the moral equation. In short, even defenders of research acknowledge that the interests of non-human animals can outweigh the interests of humans if, in some particular case, the animals' interests are sufficiently greater than the interests of humans.

Not that this is much of an acknowledgement. Some philosophers have argued that non-humans animals have considerable moral worth – even if not as much as do humans.[5] However, many utilitarians assume humans have a far greater moral worth than animals. That is, they adopt speciesism; they believe humans have more moral worth than any animals simply because they are members of our species. Such an assumption should ultimately be challenged – but not here. For present purposes, we shall assume that non-human animals have non-negligible moral worth, albeit considerably less worth than humans. As it turns out, the recognition of even this minimal claim sets the stage for potent moral objections to animal experimentation.[6] And, if arguments against research are plausible on this minimalistic assumption, then defenders of research will be wholly vulnerable to any view which holds that the moral worth of animals is similar to, or at least not substantially less than, the worth of humans.

Exactly what it means for a utilitarian to say that animals have less moral worth than humans is debatable. Historically utilitarian arguments have been used to evaluate actions involving creatures of the same moral worth. How do we extend these arguments to cases involving creatures of different worth? Consider, for instance, "cruelty to animal" statutes on the books in most developed countries. Although what counts as "cruelty to animals" varies from government to government, at least this much is true of all such laws: it is wrong to inflict excruciating pain on an animal merely to bring a human some tinge of pleasure. For instance, most people think it wrong to kill a gorilla to make an ashtray from its hand or to kill an elephant to use its tusks for a paperweight.

To state this generally, even if creatures$_A$ have less moral worth than creatures$_H$, as long as creatures$_A$ have non-negligible worth – of the sort specified by "cruelty to animal" statutes – then there must be circumstances under which morality demands that we favor creatures$_A$ over creatures$_H$. For instance, even if creatures$_H$ are more valuable, if the harm to creatures$_A$ is considerably greater than the harm to creatures$_H$ – or if there are considerably greater numbers of creatures$_A$ who must suffer that harm – then morality demands that we favor creatures$_A$ over creatures$_H$ in those circumstances. Were that not so, it would make no sense to say that creatures$_A$ had any moral worth.

Thus, a utilitarian would hold that the moral worth of an action would be the product of a) the moral worth of the creature which suffers (benefits), b) the seriousness of the wrong it suffers (the significance of its benefit), and c) the number of such creatures which suffer (benefit). This would

---

[5] Clark, S.R.L. (1977) *The Moral Status of Animals*. Oxford: University Press; Regan, T. (1983) *The Case for Animal Rights*. Berkeley: University of California; Rachels, J. (1990) *Created From Animals*. Oxford: University Press; and Singer, P. (1990) *Animal Liberation*, 2nd edition. New York: Avon Books.

[6] Most defenders of research acknowledge the moral value of animals. Cohen, for instance, states that we are not "morally free to do anything we please to animals." (p. 866) But even those who do not explicitly recognize the value of animals are committed to their having a value by engaging in such utilitarian calculations.

give us a fairly straightforward way of making utilitarian judgements involving creatures of different moral worth.

But not entirely straightforward. For instance, the Cohenesque defense of animal experimentation frequently gets cast, at least in the public debate, as if the choice to pursue or forbid animal experimentation is the choice between "your baby or your dog." But this way of framing the question is misleading. Doubtless there are choices to be made. Perhaps experimentation is justified. But the choice has not been nor will it ever be between "your baby and your dog." It couldn't be.

Single experiments (and certainly not single experiments on single animals) will never lead to any medical discovery. Only coordinated sequences of experiments can lead to discovery. Animal experiments are part of a pattern of activity – an institutional practice – and that *practice* or *institution* may significantly benefit humans. But no isolated experiment can. Thus, we must reformulate the moral question: should we continue the *practice* of animal experimentation? Apologists of research will say yes: they claim the practice will save innumerable human lives.

Three moral asymmetries

According to Cohen the benefits of research *"incalculably* outweigh the evils."[7] (emphasis ours) Other defenders of research obviously agree. Although this utilitarian claim appears straightforward and relatively uncontroversial, it is neither straightforward nor uncontroversial. As the previous comments showed, apologists must demonstrate that the practice of animal experimentation yields greater benefits than any alternative practices. Likely they can demonstrate this only by rejecting three widely held moral presumptions.

a) Acts vrs. omissions

The researchers' calculation will be implausible unless we reject the widely held belief that there is a significant moral distinction between evil we do and evil we do not prevent. Most people assume that we are more responsible for what we do than for what we do not prevent. For instance, most people assume it is morally worse to kill someone than to let them die; it is morally worse to steal than to fail to prevent someone else from stealing; and that it is morally worse to tell a lie than to fail to correct someone else's lie. Those who hold this view do not necessarily claim the failure to prevent evil is morally innocent (although some theorists say just that). They do hold, however, that it is not *as* wrong to permit an evil as to perpetrate one.[8]

Moreover, most theorists and lay people think it is not merely worse to perpetrate an evil than to permit it; they think it is *much* worse. For instance, most people would be aghast if Ralph failed to save a drowning child, particularly if he could have done so with little effort. But aghast as they might be, they would not think Ralph as bad as his neighbor Bob who held a child's head under water until she drowned. So, although we need not specify what "much worse" means, it means minimally this: the person who drowns the child should be imprisoned for a long time (if not executed) while the person who allowed the child to drown should not be punished at all – although perhaps he should be morally censured for his callousness.[9] Even in European cultures which have "Good Samaritan" laws,

---

[7] Cohen, C. (1990) "Animal Experimentation Defended," in *The Importance of Animal Experimentation for Safety and Biomedical Research*, ed. S. Garattini Amsterdam: Kluwer Academic Publishers, p. 8.

[8] Several points in our paper were anticipated by Stephen R.L. Clark in "How to Calculate the Greater Good," 1977) *Animals' Rights: A Symposium*, ed. Patterson, D. and Ryder, R. (Centaur Press: London) pp. 96–105.

[9] Obviously if the person had some special duties to the child, for instance, it she were a lifeguard at the pond, then she could be held liable for the child's death. But in this case, her obligation would be explained by her special status: she has assumed the responsibility for people swimming in her pond.

someone who violates such laws (say, by not saving a drowning child) may be punished, but far less severely than someone who killed a child. And *that* most assuredly indicates a profound moral difference.

How is this applicable to the experimenters' position? Like this: the experimenter wants to knowingly kill – and often inflict pain and suffering on – creatures with non-negligible moral worth to prevent future harm to humans. That is, they are *doing* an evil act as a means of *preventing* other evil acts. Experimenters, would likely contend that this asymmetry is applicable only if the wrong perpetrated is morally equal to the wrong not prevented. And, since animals are not *as* valuable as humans, then the wrong not prevented is morally much more weighty than the wrong perpetrated.

For the purposes of argument we agreed that humans are more valuable than animals. Even so, this does not free the experimenter from the force of the asymmetry. This asymmetry has moral bite even if the evil not prevented is worse than the evil perpetrated. For instance, it is worse for a child to die than for a child to be spanked for inappropriate reasons (say, because the parent had a bad day at the office). But this difference in moral weight can be outweighed by the moral asymmetry between what we do and what we do not prevent. For instance, most people will think an adult worse for spanking his child (or worse still, a strange child in a nearby ghetto) for inappropriate reasons than for not feeding that ghetto child.

A defender of research might further respond that this example is irrelevant since both cases involve children – creatures of the same moral worth. However, for reasons given earlier in the paper, this objection fails. That one creature has less moral worth than another certainly enters the moral equation, but it is not the only factor. We must also include the seriousness of the harm (significance of the benefit) and the number of creatures subjected to that harm (recipients of the benefit). We now offer a particular case to illustrate this asymmetry at work despite the putative difference in moral worth.

Ralph fails to go to a nearby ghetto to feed a starving child. His next door neighbor, Bob, drives to the same ghetto, picks up a stray puppy, takes it home and kills it slowly, causing it great pain – although no more pain than the starving child feels. The law would do nothing whatsoever to Ralph; Bob could be arrested and charged with cruelty to animals. Moreover, the community would not condemn Ralph – after all, few of their number would feed the starving child. But most people in the community would roundly condemn Bob for his cruelty and callousness. They would not want to live next door to Bob, nor have him as their son-in-law.[10]

Consequently, if this asymmetry is morally relevant, it is relevant even given the presumed difference in moral worth. The benefits to humans must be *substantially* greater than the costs to animals, else the moral benefits will not outweigh the immorality of perpetrating an evil as compared to preventing one. How much greater we cannot specify numerically. However, unless the defenders of animal research are disingenuous when they assert that animals have some non-negligible moral worth – or lower that worth in an *ad hoc* manner so that vivisection is always

---

In the cases in question, however, we are asking about the role this asymmetry plays when the people in question have not assumed any special responsibility for the children.

[10] Some researcher might argue that they have special obligations to people – obligations that override the force of this asymmetry. But it is not entirely clear why a researcher would say this or what it would mean. Lifeguards are hired *to save people from drowning*. Researchers are not hired *to save people from kidney disease*. Moreover, special obligations are just that – special. They are owed to specific people. But to which specific people do researchers owe these obligations? You, me, Aunt Joan? Finally, if sense could be made of the claim that researchers have special obligations to humans who might benefit from their research, even greater sense could be made of the claim that they have special obligations to their lab animals. After all, the law *requires* them to care for their lab animals; it does not require them to benefit specific humans beings.

justified come what may – experiments which kill numerous animals and yield only slight benefits to humans will not cut the moral mustard.

Some theorists do not accept this moral distinction; they think there is no moral difference between what we do and what we permit. For them, this asymmetry provides no objection to animal experimentation. But, as we argue later, rejecting this asymmetry – even if we should reject it – has consequences unacceptable to most researchers. Moreover, although this first asymmetry is rejected by a few theorists, the next two are almost held universally.

b) Definite harms vrs. possible benefits

The utilitarian defense of experimentation becomes still more problematic once we note that the real trade off is not merely between what we do and what we permit, but what we do – inflicting suffering on animals in the name of biomedicine – is *definite*, while preventing the suffering of humans is possible – and the probability of success is likely unknown. For the moment, however, let us assume that we know the probability that a coordinated sequences of animal experiments will benefit humans. We can illustrate the animal experimenter's quandary using game theoretical reasoning for decisions under risk. It is sometimes legitimate to give up some definite benefit B in the hope of obtaining a greater benefit B_i – if B_i is sufficiently great. For instance, you might give up $10 to obtain a 10% chance of gaining $200. Generally speaking, game theoretic reasoning indicates it is legitimate to give up a definite benefit B for some other benefit B_i, if the product of the utility and probability of B_i occurring is much greater than the utility of B (being definite, its probability is 1). Thus, even if researchers could ignore the first asymmetry, they would still have to *show* – and not merely assume – that the product of the probability and utility of benefits to humans is greater than the product of the certain suffering of laboratory animals (adjusted for the diminished value of the animals) and the number of animals who suffer. That is easier said than done.

In the actual experimental situation, the probability of any sequence of coordinated animal experiments being successful is usually unknown at the time of experimentation. Thus, the experimenter's predicament seems closer to game-theoretic scenarios of decisions under uncertainty, where the various outcomes of actions are (roughly) known, but the probabilities of those outcomes are not. In this case, while the harm to animals is definite, the probability that humans will benefit from experiments is unknown.[11]

Consequently unless researchers can quantify the success of the institution. they will be hard put to justify that institution given the definite evil to animals. Moreover, it will be argued below that assessing the utility of the institution of animal experimentation may likewise be difficult, if not practically impossible. Since both the utility and the probability of the benefits of animal experimentation are unknown, and the harm to animals substantial and definite, it is difficult to know how researchers will morally defend their practice.

c) The creatures which suffer vrs. the creatures which benefit

The creatures who pay the costs of experimentation are not the one's reaping the benefits.[12] This clashes with the moral presumption against inflicting suffering on one creature with moral value in

---

[11] Even this may be too generous – for properly speaking, the various outcomes of a coordinated series of experiments will be unknown prior to experimentation, while the harm to animals is nevertheless definite.

[12] Of course researchers are prone to say that animal experimentation benefits animals too. We find this claim questionable and more than a little disingenuous. The experiments are not done to benefit animals. If animals benefit it is frequently an accidental consequence of experimentation, not its goal. Moreover, even if true, the creatures which suffer will not be the ones who benefit from that suffering. *Some* dog may benefit, but not the dog who was "sacrificed."

order to benefit some other creature. Although it is noble for someone to undergo a painful bone marrow transplant to save the life of a stranger, we think it would be wrong to *require* them to undergo that procedure. We assume people should not be required to sacrifice for others. Or, even if we think people should be required to make some sacrifices, most people would think it inappropriate to require the ultimate sacrifice. Yet each year in the United States nearly 70 million mammals – creatures of acknowledged moral worth – are expected to make the ultimate sacrifice to benefit other creatures, namely humans.[13]

As before, a defender of research might respond that this case is irrelevant since both examples involve humans, creatures of the same moral worth. Again, as we argued earlier, for utilitarians the overall moral worth of an action is a product of the moral worth of the creature which suffers (benefits), the seriousness of the wrong it suffers (the importance of the benefit), and the number of creatures which must suffer (benefit). Thus, the third asymmetry is relevant to an assessment of the utilitarian calculation, even though we have admitted, for purposes of argument, that animals have less moral worth than humans.

For instance, even if we assume that non-human animals have less moral worth than do humans, most people think there are some sacrifices animals should not have to make to benefit us. Most people think it wrong for people to kill a gorilla so they can make an ashtray out of its hand or to kill an elephant so they can use its tusks for a paperweight. That is, although most people think neither the gorilla nor the elephant has the same moral worth as a person, they assume these animals cannot be asked to give up their lives so humans can obtain some relatively insignificant benefits. The defenders of research agree. That is why they claim that the benefits of research are direct and substantial. They want to show that its benefits outweigh the costs to the lab animals.

This cluster of asymmetries drives homes the fact that researchers must identify overwhelming gains if they are to have any hope of morally justifying their practice. Of course they could just reject these widely held moral views. It seems Cohen rejects them. And other respectable ethical theorists have rejected at least one of them (usually the first one). But the rejection comes at considerable cost. Not only would rejecting these asymmetries clash with widely held moral beliefs, each rejection has consequences which many researchers would find most morally unpalatable.

Consequences of rejecting these asymmetries

Consider what follows from a rejection of the first asymmetry. If acts and omissions were of equal moral weight, then animal experimenters could not *categorically* rule out non-consensual experiments on humans – even though they claim they are so opposed. Here's why. If defenders of animal experimentation deny the act/omission distinction, then they are committed to the claim that we should pursue any activity which yields greater goods than the goods sacrificed by the activity. Consequently, they can never say that any activity is, in principle, morally impermissible: there might always be some greater moral good which is achievable only through that activity.

Hence, if certain biomedical benefits could only be achieved through non-consensual experiments on humans, then, if the benefits are greater than the costs, such experiments would be morally justified. This is a most unwelcomed consequence for animal experimenters. For two reasons. First, most experimenters want to *categorically* deny the permissibility of non-consensual biomedical experiments on humans.[14] That they cannot do. At most they can say that such experimentation could be justified only if the benefits were substantial – it is just that such conditions are rarely satisfied, and thus, experimentation on humans is rarely justified.

---

[13] Rowan, A. (1984) *Mice, Models, and Men.* (New York: State University of New York Press), p. 70.
[14] See, Cohen (1986) p. 866. See also *AMA White Paper* (1986), pp. 1, 7.

Second, this line of defense will be difficult to hold. It is implausible to think that experiments on non-consenting humans would never yield substantial biomedical benefits to a far larger number of humans. Certainly some commentators on Nazi war crimes claim that some German experimentation yielded biomedical benefits for other humans. Experiments on prisoners – although presumably consensual – have also yielded significant results, especially clinical trials of new drugs. Finally, all new compounds are tested (consensually) on small numbers of humans before being widely used in the human population. Humans make good test subjects. Consequently, if non-consensual experiments on humans are justified *if* the benefits are great enough, it seems likely that experiments will sometimes be justified.

On the other hand, if researchers want to rule out such experiments in principle, then it must be that they believe that it is *categorically* worse to commit an evil than to fail to prevent one. But, as we have already argued, researchers adopting that position will have a difficult time defending animal experimentation. Perhaps, this defense would work if the benefits of experimentation are demonstrably overwhelming. Perhaps.

Rejecting the second asymmetry likewise comes at considerable cost. The second asymmetry seems incontestable. It would be the height of foolishness to give up any good G_1 for the mere chance of obtaining some other good G_2 if G_2 were not greater than G_1.[15] Abandoning this asymmetry would be to abandon rationality itself: it would be to license sacrificing any good in the mere hope that some other good will possibly be achieved.

Abandoning the third asymmetry would require abandoning the idea of the moral separateness of creatures, a view central to all Western conceptions of morality. Some theorists interpret this asymmetry absolutely – that we can never, under any circumstances require one creature of moral worth to suffer to benefit another one. This strong interpretation of this asymmetry is at the core of libertarianism.[16] Were this interpretation applied to the issue of animal experimentation, animal experiments could never be justified, no matter how great the benefit.

Most theorists, though, interpret this asymmetry more weakly to indicate that one creature of moral worth can never be required to suffer for the benefit of another creature unless the sacrifice is small and benefits substantial. Even on this weaker version, the benefits of experimentation would have to be overwhelming to justify the practice. For instance, most laypeople assume it would be inappropriate to *require* people to undergo a bone marrow transplant to save someone else's life, even though the benefit relative to the pain is considerable. Moreover, virtually everyone would be opposed to *requiring* people to give up one of their good kidneys to save someone else's life. Thus, even if we assume animals have less value than humans, this asymmetry – like the two before – implies that researchers must show staggering benefits of experimentation to morally justify the practice.

What really goes on the scales?

Cohen's accounting of what goes on the moral scales is incomplete. For instance, when determining the gains relative to the cost of animal experimentation we must include not only the costs to animals (which are direct and substantial), but also the costs to humans (and animals) of misleading experiments. For instance, the pre-occupation with misleading animal models likely delayed for twenty years the development of effective preventative measures for polio.[17] How many lives were lost or ruined because of this delay? Such losses must be placed on the scales.

---

[15] As before, the value of G will be a product of the value of the creature suffering (benefitting), the nature of the suffering (benefit), the number of creatures suffering (benefitting) – and now, the probability that the suffering (benefit) will occur.

[16] Nozick, R. (1974) *Anarchy, State, and Utopia* (New York: Basic Books).

[17] Paul, J.R. (1971) *A History of Poliomyelitis*, New Haven: Yale University Press, pp. 384–385.

Moreover, since we should include *possible* benefits (since no benefits are certain) on the scales, we must also include *possible* costs. For instance, some people have speculated that AIDS was transferred to the human population through an inadequately screened oral polio vaccine given to 250,000 Africans in the late 1950s. Such a claim has not been established; it may well be false.[18] But even if it is not true, something like it might well be true. We know, for instance, that one simian virus (SV_{40}) entered the human population through inadequately screened vaccine.[19] Moreover, we know that animal experiments have mislead us on more than one occasion (e.g., determining the dangers or smoking). Therefore it is difficult to know how researchers could plausibly claim that there would be no substantial ill-effects of future animal experimentation. These possible ill-effects must be counted.

Finally – and perhaps most importantly – what is crucial for the moral calculation is not the benefits animal experimentation has produced and will produce, but the benefits which *only* animal research could produce. To determine this utility we must ascertain a) the role that medical intervention played in lengthening life and improving health, b) the contribution of animal experimentation to medical intervention, and c) the benefits of animal experimentation *relative to* those of non-animal research programmes.[20] Since even the AMA recognizes the value of non-animal research programmes, then what goes on the moral scales are not all the purported benefits of animal experimentation, but only the *increase* in benefits relative to alternative programmes.[21] Since we do not know what these other programmes would have yielded, determining the increase in benefits would be exceedingly difficult to establish, even if we could easily determine the contributions of animal experimentation. But, as it turns out, determining even these benefits is difficult – if not impossible.

Difficulties of calculation

What our argument shows is that if a utilitarian defense of animal experimentation is to be plausible, apologists must demonstrate that the *increase* in benefits of animal experimentation relative to non-animal research programmes clearly outweighs its costs – including the moral costs identified earlier. And that, of course, is exactly what experimenters claim.

> "In fact, virtually every advance in medical science in the 20th century, from antibiotics and vaccines to antidepressant drugs and organ transplants, has been achieved either directly or indirectly through the use of animals in laboratory experiments."[22]

The result of these advances is significant. "A longer life span has been achieved, decreased infant mortality has occurred, effective treatments have been developed for many diseases, and the quality of life has been enhanced for mankind in general." All these benefits are attributable, we are told, to experiments on animals. As the *White Paper* asserts:

---

18 Some physicians thought the claim was plausible. See, for example, the letter to the editor by B.F. Elswood and R.B. Striker (1993) *in Research in Virology* vol. 144, pp. 175–6.

19 Hayflick, L. (1972) "Human Virus Vaccines: Why Monkey Cells?", *Science*, May 19, pp. 813–814. Several hundred thousand people have been exposed to SV40 through vaccines. In vitro the virus mutates normal human cells into cancerous cells.

20 Strictly speaking we should also determine the benefits of "mixed research programs," i.e., those which rely on reduced levels of animal experimentation in conjunction with some non-animal-based experiments and research methodologies.

21 The AMA specifically recognizes the benefits of cell culture studies, computer simulations, clinical studies and epidemiological investigation. *AMA White Paper*, p. 27.

22 Ibid. p. 16.

... [H]ad scientific research been restrained ... as antivivisectionists and activists were ... urging, many millions of Americans alive and healthy today would never have been born or would have suffered a premature death.[23]

This is a gross exaggeration. There is considerable evidence that interventionist medicine has played only a relatively small role in lengthening life and improving human health. As an editorial in *Lancet* summarizes the evidence: "public health legislation and related measures have probably done more than all the advances of scientific medicine to promote the well-being of the community in Britain and in most other countries."[24]

Or, as medical historians McKinlay and McKinlay explain it:

> In general medical measures (both chemotherapeutic and prophylactic) appear to have contributed little to the overall decline in mortality in the United State since 1900 – having in many instances been introduced several decades after a marked decline has already set in and having no detectable influence in most instances. More specifically, with reference to these five conditions (influenza, pneumonia, diphtheria, whopping cough and poliomyelitis) for which the decline in mortality appears substantially after the point of intervention – and on the unlikely assumption that all this decline is attributable to intervention – it is estimated that at most 3.5 per cent of the total decline in mortality since 1900 could be ascribed to medical measures introduced for the diseases mentioned here.[25]

The related point is vividly shown by a close examination of U.S. health statistics. The life expectancy in the U.S. increased 43% from 1900 to 1950 – before the advent of many medical treatments and vaccines. Since 1950 life span has increased only 7.4%. Since the rate of mortality from motor vehicle accidents has decreased by more than 20% since 1950, that decline in mortality accounts for most of the increase in life expectancy.[26] Hence, medical intervention has not single-handedly conquered disease and illness. Thus, medical intervention prompted by animal experimentation has not been the panacea described by the AMA.

There are theoretical reasons which explain the limitations of animal experimentation. Biomedical researchers claim that by observing the effects of various stimuli in non-human animals, they can form legitimate expectations about the likely reactions of humans subjected to similar stimuli. In earlier papers we argued that inferences from animal models to humans are highly questionable, both from standpoint of the logic of analogical reasoning and from evolutionary biology.[27]

There is also ample empirical evidence of the limitations of animal experimentation. Even when species are phylogenetically close we cannot assume they will react similarly to similar stimuli. Tests for cancer in rats and mice yield the same results only 70% of the time.[28] Moreover, the concordance between rats and mice drops to 50% for cancers which are

---

23 Ibid. p. 17.

24 *Lancet* (1978) August, pp. 354–5.

25 McKinlay, J.B. and McKinlay, S. [1977]: "The Questionable Contribution of Medical Measures to the Decline of Mortality in the United States in the Twentieth Century," *Health and Society*, 55: 405–28.

26 *Health United States* (1988) Publication of the Department of Health and Human Services, pp. 53, 72.

27 LaFollette, H. and Shanks, N. 1995: "Two Models of Models in Biomedical Research," *Philosophical Quarterly*; 1994a: "Chaos Theory: Analogical Reasoning in Biomedical Research". *Idealistic Studies*; 1994b: "Animal Experimentation: The Legacy of Claude Bernard," *International Studies in the Philosophy of Science*; 1993a "Animal Modelling in Psycho-pharmacological Contexts" *Behavioral and Brain Sciences*, (commentary), pp. 653–4; 1993b: "The Intact Systems Argument: Problems with the Standard Defense of Animal Experimentation," *Southern Journal of Philosophy*, pp. 323–33; 1993c: "Animal Models in Biomedical Research: Some Epistemological Worries" *Public Affairs Quarterly*, pp. 113–30.

28 Lave, L.B. *et. al.* (1988) "Information Value of the Rodent Bioassay", *Nature*, vol. 336, pp. 631–633.

site-specific.[29] Some regulatory agencies, e.g., the FDA, require by fiat that the human-rat concordance be equal to the rat-mouse concordance. But as Lave *et. al.*, and Gold *at. al.*, point out, this is an implausible assumption.

Similar disanalogies were evident in the study of teratogens. Our "closest" biological relatives – the primates – show biological effects which are significantly disanalogous from those in humans.

> Nonhuman primates offer the closest approximation to human teratological conditions because of phylogenetic similarities ... However, a review of the literature indicates that except for a few teratogens (sex hormones, thalidomide, radiation, etc) the results in non-human primates are not comparable to those in humans.[30]

Other researchers reach the same conclusion.

> It is the actual results of teratogenicity testing in primates which have been most disappointing in consideration of these animals' possible use as a predictive model. While some nine subhuman primates (all but the bushbaby) have demonstrated the characteristic limb defects observed in humans when administered thalidomide, the results with 83 other agents with which primates have been tested are less than perfect. Of the 15 listed putative human teratogens tested in nonhuman primates, only eight were also teratogenic in one or more of the various species ... The data with respect to the "suspect" or "likely" teratogens in humans under certain circumstances were equally divergent. Three of the eight suspect teratogens were also not suspect in monkeys or did not induce some developmental toxicity.[31]

Researchers themselves acknowledge the differences between non-human animals and humans. That is why they choose test subjects based on non-causal (economic) criteria.

> In practice, such selection seems to be dominated by factors based on practicality. Animal models are selected on the basis of how many criteria they possess, such as: ready availability, low cost, ease of handling, high fertility, ease of breeding, large litters, short gestation length, ease of mating time determination, low rates of spontaneous deaths and developmental abnormalities, ease with which their fetuses can be examined, and the amount of information available on their reproduction, development, and response to developmental toxicants ... The rationale for using such criteria is that none of the animal models tested is an obvious counterpart of humans in response to developmental toxicants. This leaves the issue of practicality foremost in the selection process.[32]

This point has also been made by other prominent researchers:

> A great deal of time and effort has been expended discussing the most suitable species for teratology studies, and it is time that a few fallacies were laid to rest. First, there is no such thing as an ideal test species, particularly if the intent is to extrapolate the results to man. The ideal is approximated only when testing veterinary products or new food materials in the domestic species for which they are intended ... [33]

Selecting animal models on the basis of non-causal criteria is part and parcel of the instrumentalist's strategy which pervades the institution of biomedical research. Researchers claim that the practice of animal experimentation is valuable, notwithstanding demonstrative causal

---

[29] Gold, L., Slone, T., Manley, N. and Bernstein, L. (1991) "Target Organs in Chronic Bioassays of 533 Chemical Carcinogens," *Experimental Health Perspectives* 93, p. 243, 245.

[30] Mitruka, B.M. *et. al.* (1976) *Animals for Medical Research: Models for the Study of Human Disease,* New York: Wiley, p. 467.

[31] Schardein, J.L. (1985) *Chemically Induced Birth Defects,* New York: Marcel Dekker, pp. 20, 23.

[32] Hood, R.D. (1990) "Animal Models of Effects of Prenatal Insult" in *Developmental Toxicology: Risk Assessment and the Future* (ed) R.D. Hood, New York: van Nostrand, pp. 184–185.

[33] Palmer, A.K. (1978) "Design of Subprimate Animal studies", in *The Handbook of Teratology,* (eds) J.G. Wilson and F.C. Fraser, vol. 4, New York: Plenum Press, p. 219.

disanalogy between test species and humans.[34] They think the contribution of animal research to biomedical advancement can still be ascertained from surveys of primary research literature and histories of medicine.

Not so. Both sources of information *underreport* manifest dissimilarities between animals and humans.[35] If a researcher is trying to discover the nature of human AIDS and conducts a series of experiments on rats only to find that they cannot develop AIDS, these findings may well not be reported. And, even if negative findings are reported, they are less likely to be read and discussed by professionals – especially if the negative results are not thought to have uncovered an explanation for the failure. Consequently, we cannot assess the value of the institution of animal experimentation simply by tallying successes – or even ratios of successes to failures – in the extant research literature. Some animal researchers recognize just this problem:

> One of the reasons that many contributors have missed the point is that they have drawn conclusions from published data, which represent only a small sample of the many screening tests performed. Moreover, these represent a biased sample because of the generally greater interest in positive results and the tendency of editors, whether of a sensational newspaper or an erudite journal, to cater to the tastes of their readers. Consequently, lessons gained from the high proportion of negative results and borderline cases that occur in practice are lost, as are also the occasional positive responses which regrettably never see the light of day, for commercial or political reasons.[36]

Many standard "histories" of biomedical research amplify the distorted picture of the success of animal research found in the primary literature. When historians of medicine discuss some biomedical advance, they likely omit failed experiments – even when those experiments appear in the primary research literature. "In science, as in everyday life, one tends to remember the winners. The losers are usually forgotten."[37] Historians typically report events thought to be crucial to understanding the current state of the science. Failures do not typically play a role in that understanding. Finally many biomedical historians are members of the disciplines about which they are reporting. They understandably write histories which articulate their understanding of the discipline. Since vivisection is integral to these disciplines, we should not be surprised that these histories often emphasize its "successes." In summary, There is no simple or straightforward way to find the evidence required to substantiate the contribution of animal experimentation. More is required than counting "successes" reported in the literature.

Finally, since we have never systematically tried non-animal experimentation, it is difficult to know how anyone could be confident that the benefits of animal experimentation are sufficiently greater than those of non-animal research programmes. In the past researchers have used the "intact systems argument" to give reason why, *in principle*, only animal experimentation could yield significant biomedical phenomena about humans. But, in our 1993b, we showed that defense is flawed.

Conclusion

None of this shows that animal experimentation has been worthless. None of this shows that abandoning animal experimentation will not hinder some biomedical advances. What it does

---

[34] In all candor, however, the value of much animal experimentation may be economic rather than biomedical. Animal research is a multi-billion dollar industry. With such fiscal momentum, it is not hard to see how an institution could become insensitive to the real limitations of animal research.

[35] Of course, both the primary research literature and histories of biomedical research will report some failures of research. The issue here is whether biomedically significant dissimilarities between humans and non-human animals will be given "equal reporting" by researchers working under the umbrella of a fundamentally vivisectionist paradigm.

[36] Palmer, *op.cit.* p. 216.

[37] R.N. Giere (1991) *Understanding Scientific Reasoning*, 3rd edition (Ft. Worth: Harcourt, Brace, Jovanovich), p. 74.

show is that animal experimentation has been less valuable than researchers have led us to believe. In addition, it has shown that researchers will be hard pressed to give a precise accounting of its value. Thus it seems doubtful that researchers can plausibly claim that the benefits of animal experimentation are overwhelming. Yet given the arguments earlier in the paper, that is exactly what they need to show to morally justify the practice.

Perhaps researchers might respond that it is we who must demonstrate that research is not valuable, that it is we who must show that the evils of experimentation outweigh it benefits. Not so. For the moral onus always rests on anyone who wishes to perpetrate what is, all things being equal, a moral wrong. Since people on both sides of this debate – researchers included – acknowledge the moral status of non-human animals, then they must provide clear and demonstrable evidence that the value of the institution of research exceeds its moral costs. That they had not done. Given the arguments in this paper, it is difficult to know how they could.

References for LaFollette and Shanks

1. Cohen, C. (1986). The case for the use of animals in biomedical research. *New England Journal of Medicine* **315**: 868.

2. Clark, S.R.L. (1977) *The Moral Status of Animals*. Oxford: University Press.

3. Regan, T. (1983) *The Case for Animal Rights*. Berkeley: University of California.

4. Rachels, J. (1990) *Created From Animals*. Oxford: University Press.

5. Singer, P. (1990) *Animal Liberation*, 2nd edn. New York: Avon Books.

6. Cohen, C. (1990) Animal experimentation defended. In *The Importance of Animal Experimentation for Safety and Biomedical Research*, ed. S. Garattini. Amsterdam: Kluwer Academic Publishers, p. 8.

7. Rowan, A. (1984) *Mice, Models, and Men*. New York: State University of New York Press, p. 70.

8. Nozick, R. (1974) *Anarchy, State, and Utopia*. New York: Basic Books.

9. Paul, J.R. (1971) *A History of Poliomyelitis*. New Haven: Yale University Press, pp. 384–385.

10. Hayflick, L. (1972) Human virus vaccines: why monkey cells? *Science*, May 19, pp. 813–814.

11. *Lancet* (1978) August, pp. 354–5.

12. McKinlay, J.B. and McKinlay, S. (1977) The questionable contribution of medical measures to the decline of mortality in the United States in the twentieth century. *Health and Society* **55**: 405–428.

13. Lave, L.B., *et al.* (1988) Information value of the rodent bioassay. *Nature* **336**: 631–633.

14. Gold, L., Slone, T., Manley, N. and Bernstein, L. (1991) Target organs in chronic bioassays of 533 chemical carcinogens. *Experimental Health Perspectives* 93: 243, 245.

15. Mitruka, B.M., *et al.* (1976) *Animals for Medical Research: Models for the Study of Human Disease*. New York: Wiley, p. 467.

LaFollette and Shanks respond to Cohen by denying outright his claim that the value of animal research far outweighs whatever disvalue it has for animals. If one makes judgments about animal experimentation using ordinary rules of thumb, one is likely to find LaFollette and Shanks's argument unconvincing. But when one moves to a second level and begins to think critically, one realizes that the claims of LaFollette and Shanks demand answers. How much pain is actually being caused to research animals? How much benefit is actually being realized by humans? For two-level utilitarians, justifications of animal experiments rest on how the facts turn out. The authors of both of our readings make empirical claims. And both Cohen and LaFollette and Shanks assume that the facts support their view. But do we actually know how to make trans-species evaluations? Can we validly place a number on the pain and suffering an animal endures? Should we discount animal pain in a way that we do not discount human pain?

These are difficult questions, and answers to them are not readily available. In concluding, it may be worth observing that a 2007 literature review of clinical trials in which drugs were first tested on animals found that only half of the drugs produced results in humans corresponding to the results obtained in the animal models (Perel *et al.* 2007). The authors of the study emphasize the fact that they have a small sample size (six studies), and they caution against drawing general conclusions from their work. But they go on to wonder whether their findings don't suggest that "[d]iscordance between animal and human studies may be due to bias or to the failure of animal models to mimic disease adequately."

Critical thinkers will not take the Perel study as the final word on the subject. We will have additional questions to answer. What do we know about the journal in which the Perel study was published? (Is it peer-reviewed? Does it have a reputation as an organ for studies with an animal liberationist bias?) Have other studies been conducted? Do they support Perel? (What, for example, should we make of the literature review published in the *Journal of the American Medical Association* of 2000 highly cited animal studies that finds that only 37% of animal studies "translate into successful human research" (Hackam & Redelmeier 2006)?) These are urgent questions and those using animals in research will want to have answers to them.

Conclusion

If you are using or will use animals in your research, your institution's IACUC will probably require you to complete an online tutorial that explains their policies. If your institution does not have a tutorial, you will find an extensive guide to the subject on the website of the IACUC at the University of Minnesota. But don't stop there. Go on to become a critical thinker. Ask yourself whether you can justify your use of animals in light of the issues raised by LaFollette and Shanks.

Take home lessons

- Do not handle animals unless you have been properly trained.
- Only use animals in research when it is required.
- Follow all guidelines regarding housing and behavioral needs of the animals.
- Whenever feasible replace animals with mathematical models or in vitro biological systems.
- Restrict the number of animals used to the minimum necessary to attain one's scientific goals.
- Know how to determine when the animal is in pain or distress.
- Use anesthetics and analgesics whenever necessary.
- Provide species-appropriate care after procedures.
- Euthanize animals using approved methods.
- Know why the benefits to humans of using an animal will outweigh the costs to that animal.

Bibliography

Animal and Plant Health Inspection Service. 2011. Annual Report Animal Usage by Fiscal Year. Available at: http://www.aphis.usda.gov/animal_welfare/efoia/downloads/2010_Animals_Used_In_Research.pdf.

Carbone, L. 2004. *What Animals Want: Expertise and Advocacy in Laboratory Animal Welfare Policy*, 1st edn. New York: Oxford University Press.

Hackam, D.G. & Redelmeier, D.A. 2006. Translation of research evidence from animals to humans. *JAMA: The Journal of* the *American Medical Association*, **296**(14), 1731–1732.

LaFollette, H. & Shanks, N. 1995. Util-izing animals. *Journal of Applied Philosophy*, **12**(1), 13–25.

Office of Responsible Research Practices, I.A.C. and U.C. 2010. *Pain and Distress in Laboratory Animals*. Available at: http://orrp. osu.edu/iacuc/osupolicies/guidelines/ PainandDistressinLaboratoryAnimals.cfm [Accessed March 3, 2012].

Perel, P. *et al.* 2007. Comparison of treatment effects between animal experiments and clinical trials: systematic review. *BMJ: British Medical Journal*, **334**(7586), 197–200.

Regan, T. 1983. *The Case for Animal Rights*. Berkeley: University of California Press.

Russell, W.M.S. & Burch, R.L. 1959. *The Principles of Humane Experimental Technique*. London: Methuen. Available at:

http://www2.lib.ncsu.edu/catalog/record/ NCSU491931.

Sponsored Programs and Regulatory Compliance. n.d. *Animal Care and Use Policy*. Available at: http://www.ncsu.edu/ sparcs/iacuc/lab1.php.

United States Code, 2009 edition. 2009. *Title 7 – Agriculture, Chapter 54 – Transportation, Sale, and Handling of Certain Animals*. Available at: http://www.gpo.gov/fdsys/pkg/ USCODE-2009-title7/html/USCODE-2009- title7-chap54.htm.

United States Department of Agriculture. 2011. *Poultry Slaughter – 2010 Summary*.

University of Minnesota Research Animal Resources. 2000. Experiment Guidelines for the Prevention, *Assessment and Relief of Pain and Distress in Laboratory Animals*. Available at: http://www.ahc.umn.edu/rar/ pain&distress.html.

Chapter 14

Preserve environments

Utilitarianism requires respect for all sentient beings, and this is the reason that two-level utilitarians insist on including animals' pains and pleasures in their calculations. But prominent environmentalists think utilitarians do not go far enough. They want to see the moral circle expanded to include non-sentient entities such as ecosystems, natural processes, plants, rocks, and rivers. How might a two-level theorist address the concerns of environmentalists to preserve all of nature? This chapter addresses this question in terms of the effects of environmental policies on current humans, animals, and future generations of humans and animals.

Aldo Leopold, an eloquent critic of utilitarian valuations of nature, held that nature not only has intrinsic value but that, in addition, its intrinsic value must ground practical environmental management decisions. On such a view, the value of wilderness is not its utilitarian value because nature untouched by human hands does not, cannot, have a price tag. The desire of policy-makers to assign utility values to environmental goods is an indicator for Leopold of our lack of understanding of what he calls "the biotic community."

Leopold is not alone in regarding the plant and animal worlds as having primarily non-utilitarian value. Some defend their views with philosophical arguments, and others defend it with religious, cultural, or spiritual claims. Others seem convinced of the view because they have particular, and particularly strong, attachments to specific mountains, valleys, streams, beaches, or marine areas. If one's sense of identity is inseparable from a particular place, that place may have acquired for us a value that we cannot measure on a monetary scale.

For example, every major religion, it seems, has at least one prominent representative who construes nature as intrinsically valuable (e.g., St. Francis of Assisi, the Buddha, Meher Baba, Jain monks). The Bible, for example, depicts nature as the creation of a good God who declares all plants and animals and all the heavens and the earth "good." Some American Indian cosmologies construe the earth as a mother, the sky as a father, the birds as brothers, the moon as sister. It comes as no surprise that on such views, nature is thought to be sacred, for it has a value on par with the value of the people we most love and revere. To reduce the value of one's relative to a monetary value would be a sacrilege.

Leopold, as we say, was perhaps America's most eloquent environmental writer along these lines. He wrote that a land ethic "changes the role of Homo sapiens from conqueror of the land-community to plain member and citizen of it" (Leopold 1949). He urged his readers to learn to live in "a state of harmony between men and land." His basic moral principle was drawn from his observations of the balances of nature and from the conviction that we must

Research Ethics: A Philosophical Guide to the Responsible Conduct of Research. Gary Comstock.
Published by Cambridge University Press. © Cambridge University Press 2013.

have respect for the earth: "a thing is right when it tends to preserve the integrity, stability and beauty of the biotic community. It is wrong when it tends otherwise" (Leopold 1949).

Some ecologists, many of them inspired by Leopold, now argue that humans have already exceeded the limits nature needs to maintain its equilibrium and homeostasis. The catastrophic effects of population explosion, industrial change, and international market economies have undercut the stability of ecological systems. Global climate change is but one example; others include loss of biodiversity, extinction of species, and ozone depletion.

If Leopold is right, we ought to change the modern, industrial, way of life because it fails to show respect for nature's intrinsic value.

Ecosystems have utility for future people and animals

Contrast Leopold's view with a utilitarian approach. Utilitarians are skeptical about the claim that nature is sacred in its own right. Let us grant that individual humans have intrinsic value because they are autonomous persons. But how, the skeptics ask, can groups of individuals have it – much less groups of individuals that do not (yet) exist?

Two-level utilitarians typically think nature is important but they do not want to try to justify its value in terms of notions they find mysterious or unclear. Insensate processes, such as weather patterns and estuary ecosystems, have value for utilitarians because of the benefits these processes bring to individuals. Consequentialist thinkers may also be wary of appeals to mystical notions and allegorical interpretations of nature because they fear that these strategies will not be effective rhetorically in convincing people to change their lifestyles in environmentally friendly ways.

The background essay illustrates a utilitarian approach to these questions. In "The Ethics of Climate Change," John Broome is especially interested to explain the proper role of scientific experts who use economic valuations to advise policy-makers. Broome's point is that anyone who tries to set a value on an environmental good must account for the fact that some goods are renewable and some are not. Renewable goods, such as crops and forests, may be renewable for many years into the future if they are used in a sustainable manner.

However, other goods, such as coal and oil, are non-renewable. These goods cannot be used in the future if they are used up today. Therefore, economists must choose a discount rate when assessing present and future value. If our actions today pollute the environment in such a way that we warm the globe for future generations, then we must take the costs to future generations into account when assessing the present value of the good. Broome challenges his reader to balance the books honestly. When weighing our attempts to increase our own prosperity we must also weigh the chances that taking any particular action may harm the welfare of our great grandchildren. If you choose a high discount rate, then you value the interests of the current generation more highly than the interests of future generations. If you choose a low discount rate – or a zero per cent discount rate – then you value the preferences and needs of future generations equally to ours.

Broome's point is that social scientists in general, and economists in particular, make ethical judgments even as they deny doing so. He gives this following defense of this claim. Consider the selection of a high discount rate. An economist may claim that she has adopted this rate not on the basis of moral values but simply on the preferences of citizens. She may further accuse the low- or the zero-discounters, such as Broome himself, of substituting their own philosophical commitments for the actual values of current citizens. To proceed in this way in economics would be a cardinal sin.

Broome rebuts this argument by alleging that the high-discounters have it backwards. The high-discounters are substituting their philosophical commitment to current citizens for objectivity regarding the interests of all citizens, present and future. In a democracy, argues Broome, this is unfair and potentially destructive. The role of experts in such societies should be to marshal the best arguments they can, clearly identify their assumptions, and submit their arguments to the public for scrutiny. The experts should not be making the decisions; the decisions should be made in public forums and by legislative representative bodies. As Broome points out, in no other area would we expect expert advisers simply to record their clients' preferences, run some calculations, and think that the result was the correct answer to a policy issue. The role of the utilitarian calculator in environmental policy, argues Broome, is to inform public debate with sound data and solid reasoning.

Background essay: "The ethics of climate change", by John Broome[1]

What should we do about climate change? The question is an ethical one. Science, including the science of economics, can help discover the causes and effects of climate change. It can also help work out what we can do about climate change. But what we should do is an ethical question.

Not all "should" questions are ethical. "How should you hold a golf club?" is not, for instance. The climate question is ethical, however, because any thoughtful answer must weigh conflicting interests among different people. If the world is to do something about climate change, some people – chiefly the better-off among the current generation – will have to reduce their emissions of greenhouse gases to save future generations from the possibility of a bleak existence in a hotter world. When interests conflict, "should" questions are always ethical.

Climate change raises a number of ethical questions. How should we – all of us living today – evaluate the well-being of future generations, given that they are likely to have more material goods than we do? Many people, some living, others yet to be born, will die from the effects of climate change. Is each death equally bad? How bad are those deaths collectively? Many people will die before they bear children, so climate change will prevent the existence of children who would otherwise have been born. Is their nonexistence a bad thing? By emitting greenhouse gases, are the rich perpetrating an injustice on the world's poor? How should we respond to the small but real chance that climate change could lead to worldwide catastrophe?

Many ethical questions can be settled by common sense. Sophisticated philosophy is rarely needed. All of us are to some extent equipped to face up to the ethical questions raised by climate change. For example, almost everyone recognizes the elementary moral principle that (with some exceptions) you should not do something for your own benefit if it harms another person. True, sometimes you cannot avoid harming someone, and sometimes you may do it accidentally without realizing it. But whenever you cause harm, you should normally compensate the victim.

Climate change will cause harm. Heat waves, storms and floods will kill many people and harm many others. Tropical diseases, which will increase their range as the climate warms, will exact their toll in human lives. Changing patterns of rainfall will lead to local shortages of food and safe drinking water. Large-scale human migrations in response to rising sea levels and other climate-induced stresses will impoverish many people. As yet, few experts have predicted specific numbers, but some statistics suggest the scale of the harm that climate change will cause. The European heat wave of 2003 is estimated to have killed 35,000 people. In 1998 floods in China

---

[1] Reprinted from *Scientific American*, 298(6), pp. 96–102. John Broome is White's Professor of Moral Philosophy and Fellow of Corpus Christi College, University of Oxford, john.broome@philosophy. ox.ac.uk.

adversely affected 240 million. The World Health Organization estimates that as long ago as 2000 the annual death toll from climate change had already reached more than 150,000.

In going about our daily lives, each of us causes greenhouse gases to be emitted. Driving a car, using electric power, buying anything whose manufacture or transport consumes energy – all those activities generate greenhouse gases that contribute to climate change. In that way, what we each do for our own benefit harms others. Perhaps at the moment we cannot help it, and in the past we did not realize we were doing it. But the elementary moral principle I mentioned tells us we should try to stop doing it and compensate the people we harm.

This same principle also tells us that what we should do about climate change is not just a matter of weighing benefits against costs – although it is partly that. Suppose you calculate that the benefit to you and your friends of partying until dawn exceeds the harm done to your neighbor by keeping her awake all night. It does not follow that you should hold your party. Similarly, think of an industrial project that brings benefits in the near future but emits greenhouse gases that will harm people decades hence. Again suppose the benefits exceed the costs. It does not follow that the project should go ahead; indeed it may be morally wrong. Those who benefit from it should not impose its costs on others who do not.

Ethics of costs and benefits

But even if weighing costs against benefits does not entirely answer the question of what should be done about climate change, it is an essential part of the answer. The costs of mitigating climate change are the sacrifices the present generation will have to make to reduce greenhouse gases. We will have to travel less and insulate our homes better. We will have to eat less meat. We will have to live less lavishly. The benefits are the better lives that future people will lead: they will not suffer so much from the spread of deserts, from the loss of their homes to the rising sea, or from floods, famines and the general impoverishment of nature.

Weighing benefits to some people against costs to others is an ethical matter. But many of the costs and benefits of mitigating climate change present themselves in economic terms, and economics has useful methods of weighing benefits against costs in complex cases. So here economics can work in the service of ethics.

The ethical basis of cost–benefit economics was recognized recently in a major report, the Stern Review on the Economics of Climate Change, by Nicholas Stern and his colleagues at the UK Treasury. The Stern Review concentrates mainly on comparing costs and benefits, and it concludes that the benefit that would be gained by reducing emissions of greenhouse gases would be far greater than the cost of reducing them. Stern's work has provoked a strong reaction from other economists for two reasons. First, some economists think economic conclusions should not be based on ethical premises. Second, the review favors strong and immediate action to control emissions, whereas other economic studies, such as one by William Nordhaus of Yale University, have concluded that the need to act is not so urgent.

Those two issues are connected. Stern's conclusion differs from Nordhaus's principally because, on ethical grounds, Stern uses a lower "discount rate." Economists generally value future goods less than present ones: they discount future goods. Furthermore, the more distant the future time when goods become available, the more the goods are discounted. The discount rate measures how fast the value of goods diminishes with time. Nordhaus discounts at roughly 6% a year; Stern discounts at 1.4%. The effect is that Stern gives a present value of $247 billion to having, say, a trillion dollars' worth of goods a century from now. Nordhaus values having those same goods in 2108 at just $2.5 billion today. Thus, Stern attaches nearly 100 times as much value as Nordhaus does to having any given level of costs and benefits 100 years from now.

The difference between the two economists' discount rates is enough to explain the difference between their conclusions. Most of the costs of controlling climate change must be borne in the near future, when the present generation must sacrifice some of its consumption. The benefits will mostly come a century or two from now. Because Stern judges the present value of those benefits to be higher than Nordhaus does, Stern can justify spending more today on mitigating climate change than Nordhaus can.

The richer future

Why discount future goods at all? The goods in question are the material goods and services that people consume – bicycles, food, banking services and so on. In most of the scenarios predicted for climate change, the world economy will continue to grow. Hence, future people will on average possess more goods than present people do. The more goods you already have, the less valuable are further goods, and so there is good reason to discount them. To have one bathroom in your house is a huge improvement to your life; a second bathroom is nice but not so life-changing. Goods have "diminishing marginal value," as economists put it.

There may be a second, purely ethical reason for discounting goods that come to relatively rich people. According to an ethical theory known as "prioritarianism," a benefit – by which I mean an increase in an individual's well-being – that comes to a rich person should be assigned less social value than the same benefit would have if it had come to a poor person. Prioritarianism gives priority to the less well off. According to an alternative ethical theory known as "utilitarianism," however, a benefit has the same value no matter who receives it. Society should simply aim to maximize the total of people's well-being, no matter how that total is distributed across the population.

What should the discount rate be? What determines how fast the value of having goods in the future diminishes as the future time in question becomes more remote? That depends, first, on some nonethical factors. Among them is the economy's rate of growth, which measures how much better off, on average, people will be in the future than they are today. Consequently, it determines how much less benefit future people will derive from additional material goods than people would derive now from those same goods. A fast growth rate makes for a high discount rate.

The discount rate also depends on an ethical factor. How should benefits to those future, richer people be valued in comparison to our own? If prioritarianism is right, the value attached to future people's benefits should be less than the value of our benefits, because future people will be better off than we are. If utilitarianism is right, future people's benefits should be valued equally with ours. Prioritarianism therefore makes for a relatively high discount rate; utilitarianism makes for a lower one.

The debate between prioritarians and utilitarians takes a curious, even poignant turn in this context. Most debates about inequality take place among the relatively rich, when they consider what sacrifices they should make for the relatively poor. But when we think about future people, we are considering what sacrifices we, the relatively poor, should make for the later relatively rich. Usually prioritarianism demands more of the developed countries than utilitarianism does. In this case, it demands less.

Temporal distance

Another ethical consideration also affects the discount rate. Some philosophers think we should care more about people who live close to us in time than about those who live in the more distant future, just because of their temporal distance from us. If those philosophers are right, future well-being should be discounted just because it comes in the future. This position is called "pure discounting." It implies we should give less importance to the death of a 10-year-old 100 years in the future than to the death of a 10-year-old now. An opposing view is that we should be temporally impartial, insisting that the mere date on which a harm occurs makes no difference to its value. Pure discounting makes for a relatively high discount rate; temporal impartiality makes for a lower one.

To determine the right discount rate, therefore, the economist must answer at least two ethical questions. Which should we accept: prioritarianism or utilitarianism? And should we adopt pure discounting or be temporally impartial?

These questions are not matters of elementary morality; they raise difficult issues in moral philosophy. Moral philosophers approach such questions by combining tight analytical argument with sensitivity to ethical intuitions. Arguments in moral philosophy are rarely conclusive, partly because we each have mutually inconsistent intuitions. All I can do as a philosopher is judge the truth as well as I can and present my best arguments in support of my judgments. Space prevents me from setting out my arguments here, but I have concluded that prioritarianism is mistaken and that we should be temporally impartial. For more detail, see Chapter 10 of my book *Weighing Goods* (1991) and section 4.3 of my book *Weighing Lives* (2004).

Market discount rates?

Stern reaches those same ethical conclusions. Since both tend toward low discounting, they – together with Stern's economic modeling – lead him to his 1.4% rate. His practical conclusion follows: the world urgently needs to take strong measures to control climate change.

Economists who oppose Stern do not deny that his practical conclusion follows from his ethical stance. They object to his ethical stance. Yet most of them decline to take any ethical position of their own, even though they favor an interest rate higher than Stern's. As I have explained, the correct discount rate depends on ethical considerations. So how can economists justify a discount rate without taking an ethical position?

They do so by taking their higher discount rate from the money market, where people exchange future money for present money, and vice versa. They adopt the money-market interest rate as their discount rate. How can that be justified?

Some values are determined by people's tastes, which markets reveal. The relative value of apples and oranges is determined by the tastes revealed in the fruit market. But the value that should be attached to the well-being of future generations is not determined by tastes. It is a matter of ethical judgment.

So does the money market reveal people's ethical judgments about the value of future well-being? I doubt it. The evidence shows that, when people borrow and lend, they often give less weight to their own future well-being than to their present well-being. Most of us are probably not so foolish as to judge that our own well-being is somehow less valuable in old age than in youth. Instead our behavior simply reflects our impatience to enjoy a present benefit, overwhelming whatever judgment we might make about the value of our own future. Inevitably, impatience will also overwhelm whatever high-minded arguments we might make in favor of the well-being of future generations.

But for the sake of argument, suppose people's market behavior genuinely reflected their judgments of value. How could economists then justify proclaiming an ethically neutral stance and taking the discount rate from the market? They do so, purportedly, on democratic grounds – leaving ethical judgments to the public rather than making them for themselves. The economists who criticize Stern claim the democratic high ground and accuse him of arrogantly trying to impose his own ethical beliefs on others.

They misunderstand democracy. Democracy requires debate and deliberation as well as voting. Economists – even Stern – cannot impose their beliefs on anyone. They can only make recommendations and argue for them. Determining the correct discount rate requires sophisticated theory, and we members of the public cannot do it without advice from experts. The role of economists in the democratic process is to work out that theory. They should offer their best recommendations, supported by their best arguments. They should be willing to engage in debate with one another about the ethical bases of their conclusions. Then we members of the public must reach our own decisions with the experts' help. Without their help, our choices will be uninformed and almost worthless.

Once we have made our decisions society can act through the democratic process. That is not the job of economists. Their recommendations are inputs to the process, not the output of it. The true arrogance is imagining that you are the final arbiter of the democratic process.

Ethical considerations cannot be avoided in determining the discount rate. Climate change raises many other ethical issues, too; one crucial one [is] the problem of catastrophic outcomes. . . . It will require serious work in ethics to decide what sacrifices we should make to moderate climate change. Like the science of climate change, the ethics of climate change is hard. So far it leaves much to be resolved. We face ethical as well as scientific problems, and we must work to solve them.

Conclusion

Broome argues that the policies we adopt in the face of climate change and species extinction must be based on sound economic calculations. And he argues that economists must appeal to controversial ethical positions to defend their views. If setting discount rates significantly affects consumer behavior, then what is the best discount rate in a democratic society that cares about the interests of future generations?

These questions loom before us and they bring us full circle. By exploring a range of initial ethical questions we have discovered that many more questions await us. More research, as they say, is needed, especially in climatology and econometrics. To develop sound environmental policies we must develop new knowledge in those disciplines and the disciplines related to them.

We need capable new question-askers to push outward the boundaries of the sciences, engineering, and social sciences. We also need capable new question-askers to analyze arguments, explain the meaning and implications of moral claims, and figure out which ethical theory, or combination of ethical theories – if any – is best. How we ought to select a discount rate for future valuations of environmental goods is a question fraught with scientific uncertainty. It is also loaded with philosophical uncertainty. Broome has underlined a central contention of this book: the study of ethics must be a central part of every researcher's advanced education. The welfare of future generations may hinge as much on our making progress in humanities scholarship as it does on progress in the earth and physical sciences.

Take home lessons

- Understand the long-term consequences of your impact on the environment.
- Assess for yourself the extent to which your consumption of goods today might constrain your ability to consume in the future.
- Figure out what you think about Broome's contention that we should not discount for the future.
- Ask yourself what you can do now to help your lab minimize its environmental footprint.
- Don't overlook the ethical assumptions of your research, especially when doing work in the social sciences.

Bibliography

Broome, J. 2008. The ethics of climate change. *Scientific American*, **298**(6), 96–102.

Leopold, A. 1949. *A Sand County Almanac.* Oxford University Press.

Chapter 5

Cultivate responsibility

University researchers have a special obligation to pursue the common good, an obligation that has not always been part and parcel of the university mission. Medieval universities (Al-Azhar University in Cairo, Egypt, established in the tenth century, may be the oldest) were constructed for the scholastic guilds, the members of which were the sons of land-owning families. The curriculum, or *magistrorum*, was designed around religious knowledge, and the main subjects included theology, law, the arts, and medicine. Furthering the good of commoners or of the wider society was not a part of the mission. Nor was this part of the mission of European universities established during the Renaissance's eleventh to fourteenth centuries. Again, only young men of the wealthy elite classes were allowed to study, and they had to know Latin to pursue scholarship. One of the central purposes of a higher degree was to continue the *universitas scholarium*, reviving it with a new generation of humanistic scholars steeped in classical languages and values. Improving the state of the working classes was not part of this aim.

On this score, little had changed by the seventeenth century when the first US universities were created. Modeled on British institutions such as Oxford and Cambridge, private institutions such as Harvard, Yale, and Princeton set out to train the sons of the leaders of the New World. The students learned Greek, Latin, and other ancient languages, and their instructors preserved and promoted the study of classical texts. Students pursued research in the sciences in addition to their humanistic studies in theology, history, and philosophy.

A major shift occurred in the nineteenth century with the creation of the US land-grant universities. Civic-minded educators committed to ideals of democracy and justice realized that US higher education was not serving the majority of US citizens. In 1870, over half of all Americans in the work force were farmers. Furthermore, most of them, as well as three-quarters of all African American farmers, did not own the land they tilled (Mintz 2007). As one might expect, agricultural and industrial workers typically did not believe that their sons and especially their daughters needed a classical education. And they looked to Congress for assistance in creating a system of higher education to meet their needs.

They received it. Legislators created the land-grant universities and tasked them not with repopulating themselves with a small class of privileged men, but rather with providing practical knowledge to large numbers of commoners and farmers. Land grant universities were established under a congressional mandate sponsored by Justin Morrill in 1862. The Morrill Act levied taxes on citizens in every state to establish institutions specializing in higher education in "agriculture and mechanical arts." Campuses were intended to be open

Research Ethics: A Philosophical Guide to the Responsible Conduct of Research. Gary Comstock.
Published by Cambridge University Press. © Cambridge University Press 2013.

to all who wanted to study, regardless of income level or class and, eventually, race or gender. As James Bonnen puts it, the idea of the land grant grew out of Americans' increasing "frustration with an unresponsive set of mostly private colleges providing a classical or 'literary' education for a wealthy elite of less than 1% of the population." For, as Bonnen notes, few US colleges at that time were willing "to sully their hands addressing society's common but real needs" (Bonnen 1998), namely the needs of farmers and "mechanics," that is, industrial workers.

The mission of the land grant university was in step with the vision of nineteenth-century utilitarians such as John Stuart Mill and others who argued for public education. From the day that the first land grant opened its doors, members of the industrial and rural classes have been welcome. Admissions policies emphasized equality of opportunity, and the curricula created entirely new fields of study (such as animal husbandry, agricultural education, and industrial engineering) to address the needs of working people. Nor should it have been otherwise, because the taxpayers of each state funded land grants, itself a novel American experiment. That is: in return for the support of the taxpayers, land grant students and faculty came under a special obligation to expend their research efforts in ways consistent with the interests of those supporting them.

With this noble history of land grant universities as background, we must immediately register two qualifications. First, land grants did not initially live up to the ideal. In Southern states, these institutions were not hospitable places for African Americans, denying them admission (Williams and Williamson 1988). In response, Congress passed the Second Morrill Act in 1890 to set up a group of land grants in every state that was denying minorities access. These institutions are now known as historically black colleges and universities or, more recently, as historically minority-serving institutions. However, the 1890 schools, as one might expect, never enjoyed as much funding and resources as were provided to land grants. To what extent has research overcome discriminatory practices toward African Americans? While much progress has been made, a great deal of ground remains to be made up. For more discussion of this point, compare the number of research awards made by the US National Institutes of Health to African Americans compared to the percentage of grant submissions by African Americans (Ginther et al. 2011).

Second proviso: throughout the twentieth century, as land grant universities successfully pursued their missions, they invented new machines, bred new species of plants and animals, and gave seeds away free to farmers through their extension systems. This vast output of practical knowledge dramatically improved not only the technologies available to farmers, merchants, and industrialists, but also their working conditions. In the last two decades of the twentieth century, however, as tax burdens increased on the general population, citizens began to urge land grants to do more to support themselves. Accordingly, a smaller percentage of the land grant university budget was supplied by state taxes (Dillon 2005) and more of it began to come from student tuition, federal research grants, and private sector support for research, especially research resulting in patentable products. Some observers argue that land grants are, in fact, on a path toward privatization. Some speculate that land grants are losing public support because they are slowly abandoning their historical mission of promoting the well-being of all of the people in their respective states (Anon 2001).

We might speculate about other aspects of land grants. Is the traditional mission compromised by faculty members doing research for the tobacco or computer or oil industries? When a faculty member's salary is paid entirely by the taxpayers, it is clear to whom researchers owe primary allegiance. But whose interests does a faculty member serve when a corporation provides 40% to 80% of their research dollars? Obviously, serious ethical questions arise when private corporations provide substantial research dollars to public universities.

In fact, conflicts of interest as well as commitment may arise as a result of the increasing dependence of land grants on private sector support. Questions of ownership of data and about a researcher's freedom to publish his or her results may arise when a company funding research wants to commercialize any and all practical results.

Of course, not everyone is convinced that land grants are under the sort of pressure just described. Some argue that current stresses on land grant budgets are the expected results of typical business cycles. During recessions, state governments cut funding to higher education. But the funds will be restored, argue these observers, when the economy begins to pick up again.

Perhaps land grants will have to behave more like private universities in the future. Or perhaps not; perhaps they are now simply experiencing the pangs of a temporary economic downturn and will eventually return to business as usual, receiving greater public funding during brighter financial times to come. In either case, the purpose of the institution will remain largely unchanged: to pursue practical education and research resulting in generalizable knowledge of value to working people.

Here we have been concentrating on the public mission of land grants because it so clearly reflects a utilitarian and consequentialist spirit. Land grant universities were created to promote democracy, provide open access, and to pursue research that would promote the public good. But land grants are not alone in these commitments. All research universities include in their mission statements commitments to the advancement of science and the service of society. The Wingspread Declaration summons American institutions to refocus on these values and redouble efforts to promote them.

Background essay: "Wingspread declaration on renewing the civic mission of the American research university," by Harry Boyte and Elizabeth Hollander[1]

. . .

The civic responsibilities of research universities[2]

Civic engagement is essential to a democratic society, but far too many Americans have withdrawn from participation in public affairs. Higher education can contribute to civic engagement, but most research universities do not perceive themselves as part of the problem or

---

[1] Abridged and reprinted from the complete document which is at http://www.compact.org/ initiatives/civic-engagement-at-research-universities/wingspread-declaration-on-the-civic-responsibilities-of-research-universities/. Deleted material is indicated by ellipses. Harry Boyte is Co-director, Center for Democracy and Citizenship, Minneapolis, MN, boyte001@umn.edu. Elizabeth Hollander is Senior Fellow, Tisch College, Tufts University, elizabeth.Hollander@tufts.edu.

[2] On behalf of participants in a Wingspread conference. We are indebted to Barry Checkoway of the University of Michigan, Elizabeth Hollander of Campus Compact, and Stanley Ikenberry of the American Council on Education for preparing an initial draft, and to Harry Boyte of the University of Minnesota and Elizabeth Hollander for their leadership roles in preparing the final statement. The Prelude reads:

of its solution. Whereas universities were once centrally concerned with "education for democracy" and "knowledge for society," today's institutions have often drifted away from their civic mission.

At the same time, however, there are new stirrings of democracy in American higher education. From one campus to another, there is increasing interest in efforts to better prepare people for active citizenship in a diverse democracy, to develop knowledge for the improvement of communities and society, and to think about and act upon the public dimensions of our educational work.

What are some strategies for renewing the civic mission of the American research university? This question was the focus of a conference of higher education leaders at Wingspread that produced the following declaration about the renewal process.

> At bottom, most of the American institutions of higher education are filled with the democratic spirit. Teachers and students alike are profoundly moved by the desire to serve the democratic community.
>
> Charles Eliot, President, Harvard, 1908

Across the country a historic debate is under way over the future of America's great public and research universities. From many sources, including state legislatures, governing boards, public constituencies, and the mass media, research institutions are challenged to justify what they do and how they do it. The beliefs and practices that universities have espoused, affecting research, teaching, and outreach, are under review, spurred by calls for accountability, efficiency, and utility as well as by questions about the theories of knowledge embedded in prevailing reward and evaluation systems. The controversies of this debate also reflect trends and questions in higher education as a whole.

At their broadest and most engaged, research institutions of higher education in America have been, in Charles Eliot's words, "filled with the democratic spirit." Such spirit took many different forms. Columbia University, according to Seth Low, breathed the air of the city of New York, its working class population, its problems, and its opportunities. At the University of Chicago, America's pragmatic philosophy and world-renowned sociology department emerged, in part, from vital partnerships between the Hull House settlement and scholars. At land grant institutions,

---

This document is the result of collaboration by participants at a Wingspread conference involving university presidents, provosts, deans, and faculty members with extensive experience in higher education as well as representatives of professional associations, private foundations, and civic organizations. The purpose of the conference was to formulate strategies for renewing the civic mission of the research university, both by preparing students for responsible citizenship in a diverse democracy, and also by engaging faculty members to develop and utilize knowledge for the improvement of society.

The Wingspread conference was held December 11–13, 1998. At the end of the conference, participants formed working groups and committed themselves to action strategies for renewing the civic mission. They reconvened for a second conference on July 19–21, 1999.

The conference was coordinated by the University of Michigan Center for Community Service and Learning, with sponsorship by the Association of American Universities, American Association for Higher Education, American Council on Education, Association of American Colleges and Universities, Campus Compact, New England Resource Center for Higher Education, University of Pennsylvania Center for University Partnerships, and the Johnson Foundation, with support from the W.K. Kellogg Foundation.

Wingspread is an international educational conference center designed by Frank Lloyd Wright and maintained by the Johnson Foundation in Racine, Wisconsin.

Printing and distribution of the Wingspread Declaration are made possible primarily by Campus Compact with support from the Ford Foundation, and by the University of Michigan Center for Community Service and Learning with support from the Johnson Foundation and the W.K. Kellogg Foundation.

the cooperative extension system of county agents saw itself as "building rural democracy" and helping to develop communities' capacities for cooperative action. As late as 1947, the President's Commission on Higher Education titled its report *Education for Democracy*.

In the post-war years, American research universities have seen an explosion in numbers of students, in fields of study, and in international prestige. Questions of diversity and justice, issues of whom universities choose to admit and serve are central to the democratic spirit. On these grounds our schools have made clear advances. Today, research universities are more richly varied in the cultures, economic backgrounds, and outlooks of our students. Our curricula are more inclusive of diverse cultures, traditions, and ways of knowing. Fields of research and scholarship have proliferated, and path-breaking advances have been made in areas scarcely imagined a generation or two ago. Research universities today evidence renewed engagements with communities. Many have joined the service-learning movement that involves students in real world problems and issues.

Though incomplete, such changes nonetheless represent substantial progress toward a more inclusive and a more just system of higher education. Yet despite such gains, few leaders in research universities today would make Eliot's claim that their fundamental mission is to serve democracy or that they are filled with the democratic spirit.

Today, higher education mirrors the democratic discontents of the larger society. Nowhere is this truer than in our great research universities. T.S. Eliot's haunting question in his 1937 poem *The Rock* – "where is the wisdom we have lost in knowledge, where is the knowledge we have lost in information?" – has become a question for our age.

Research institutions are subject to the same forces in the society that focus on "efficiency of means" and neglect continuing discussion about civic purposes and public meanings of our individual and collective work. Ends are regarded as fixed. Even when debated they are separated from the larger tasks of democracy.

Such dynamics take the form of proposals to make colleges more responsive to the demands of students redefined as customers. Allocations of resources are pushed toward their most remunerative uses with a slighting of other institutional values. A powerful new trend is the "virtual university." Public service today often has a commercial cast. All of these developments can have value as parts of a larger whole. But they cannot be taken for the whole. Students are far more than "customers"; they need to be understood as co-creators of their learning. Universities are far more than data banks for distance learning; they are places where students, faculty, and staff interact in multi-dimensional ways and, at best, learn and develop together. And communities are far more than sites of economic growth; they are places where a variety of public and private values need articulation, recognition, and cultivation.

As agents of the democracy, colleges and universities will consciously prepare a next generation of involved citizens reflecting the full and immensely varied cultural and economic mix of America, by creating innumerable opportunities for them to be in college and to do the work of citizenship. This means conceiving of institutions of higher learning as vital, living cultures, not simply an aggregation of discrete units in competition with each other. The public dimensions of our common cultures require intense and self-conscious attention. Opportunities for students, faculty, staff, administrators to use their many talents for the greater good must once again pervade every aspect of our work.

Yet today, many students feel that college is out of their grasp and those who are in college often feel disengaged and powerless. They find few opportunities for civic participation. Every department, every discipline, every unit of our research universities experiences pressures to draw back from connection to the whole. Cultures of research-oriented schools have become increasingly competitive, individualist, and characterized by the "star system." Faculty identities are drawn away from the local civic community and toward national and international disciplinary and sub-disciplinary reference groups. Moreover, faculties are socialized throughout their graduate school preparation to think in highly individualized and privatized terms about their work in ways that make it difficult to believe in the possibilities for effective cooperative action for change.

Despite these trends and pressures, many faculty devote themselves to the pressing tasks of our commonwealth and seek out colleagues, inside and outside their disciplines, to work with in their efforts. We need a far-ranging examination of our purposes and practices so that such work is honored, celebrated, and built upon.

The challenge

Against this background, we issue this Wingspread Declaration based on the conviction that now is the time to boldly claim the authority and ability to focus our energy on the civic purposes of higher education. Those of us in higher education can change its directions and commitments. We can mobilize support for change from outside constituencies by making alliances with those constituencies. We can shape our cultures, renew our civic missions, and guide our destinies.

The challenges facing higher education go beyond the need to add more service-learning experiences or to reward faculty for community-oriented research. As important as these objectives are, the more fundamental task is to renew our great mission as the agents of democracy. This task points to deep strategic challenges: how to tap and free the powers and talents of all elements of our schools – our faculty, our students, our staff, our administrators – for public engagement? How to break down the artificial and arbitrary "silo cultures" that now stifle creativity, connection, and community? How to renew throughout our institutional life and cultures a robust sense that our work contributes to the commonwealth of our communities, our nation and the world?

How might this vision of public engagement be made manifest? It will take many different forms in different universities. Here we suggest some ways that an engaged university will embody its mission.

1. Students: what will it mean for our student bodies to be filled once again with the democratic spirit?
    1. A core element in the mission of the research university is to prepare students for engaged citizenship through multiple opportunities to do the work of citizenship. Such work involves real projects of impact and relevance, through which students learn the skills, develop the habits and identities, and acquire the knowledge to contribute to the general welfare.
    2. The university curricula and courses challenge students' imaginations, draw on student experiences and interests, and cultivate students' talents and public identities. This means sustained attention to how our curricula help to develop civic competencies and civic habits. These include the arts of public argument, civic imagination, the ability to critically evaluate arguments and information, the capacities and curiosity to listen constantly, interest in and knowledge of public affairs, capacities for intergroup dialogue, and the ability to work with others different from themselves on common projects and problem solving in ways that deepen appreciation of others' talents.
    3. Campus co-curricular activities on and off campus offer multiple opportunities for students to get engaged in community projects that enhance the civic welfare and common good, to register to vote, and to participate actively in political campaigns and other change-oriented activities. Further, such activities create space for constant reflection about how such experiences might shape their future careers and life work.
    4. Students help build and sustain genuinely public cultures full of conversation, argument, and discussion about the meaning of their learning, their work, and their institutions as a whole. Students encounter and learn from others different from themselves in experience, culture, racial background, ideologies and views.
    5. Students have multiple opportunities to help create knowledge and do scholarship relevant to and grounded in the public problems of society, while learning rigorous methodologies and the demanding crafts of fine scholarship.

2. Faculty (including teaching staff): what will it mean for the faculty to be filled with the democratic spirit?
   1. Faculty help create, participate in, and take responsibility for a vibrant public culture at their institutions. Such a public culture values their moral and civic imaginations and their judgments, insights, and passions, while it recognizes and rewards their publicly engaged scholarship, lively teaching, and their contributions through public work.
   2. Faculty members have opportunities and rewards for socially engaged scholarship through genuine civic partnerships, based on respect and recognition of different ways of knowing and different kinds of contributions, in which expertise is "on tap, not on top."
   3. Faculty teaching includes community-based learning and undergraduate action research that develops substantive knowledge, cultivates practical skills, and strengthens social responsibility and public identity for citizenship in a diverse democratic society.
   4. Faculties' professional service is conceived of and valued as public work in which disciplinary and professional knowledge and expertise contribute to the welfare of society, and also can occasion the public work of many other citizens.
   5. Faculty members are encouraged and prepared when they desire to pursue "public scholarship," relating their work to the pressing problems of society, providing consultations and expertise, and creating opportunities to work with community and civic partners in co-creating things of public value.
   6. Faculty members engage in diverse cross-disciplinary work projects that improve the university and create things of lasting value and significance.
   7. Faculty are encouraged to mentor students, providing out-of-classroom opportunities to build communities of learning on and off campus. These opportunities have the potential to expose students to the public work of faculty whose own moral imaginations and public talents are vitally engaged in relevant scholarship and work of social significance.

   . . .

3. The institution: what will it mean for our institutions, composed of faculty, students, staff, and administrators and guided by the deliberations of trustees, to be filled with the democratic spirit as whole institutions?
   1. This will mean that our institutions develop admissions policies and financial arrangements that are shaped by the imperative to create diverse "publics" within our institutions. This imperative understands economic, ethnic, racial, religious, and ideological diversity to be a crucial ingredient in learning cultures for the world that is emerging.
   2. Trustees, like administrators, think of themselves as public philosophers as well as stewards and promoters of institutional resources, seeking to articulate and to advance the public and democratic purposes of higher education.
   3. Stakeholders in our universities define institutional work as a whole in ways that highlight civic mission broadly, that tie work to large public questions and issues, and that unearth distinctive civic histories, cultures, and contributions. In this context, part of the challenge is for leaders, at all levels, to develop a variety of infrastructures of support, including multidimensional understandings of "scholarship" in promotion and tenure procedures for faculty work that serves its civic mission. Such support includes creating high standards, demanding expectations, and rigorous methods of evaluation of engaged scholarship, teaching, and public work.
   4. The university creates and sustains long-term partnerships with communities, with K-12 schools in an integrated system of democratic education and education for democracy, and with a range of civic bodies. These will be framed in ways that reflect the university's commitments to and self-interests in community building and civic vitality, that integrate

community experience into the learning of students and the professional service opportunities for staff, and that fully reflect the public dimensions of scholarly work.

5. The university promotes public understanding of its work as an essential part of its mission, recognizing an institutional responsibility for publicly useable knowledge, developing formal structures to sustain such uses.

6. The university similarly creates structures that generate a more porous and interactive flow of knowledge between university and communities. These aim at making the university's knowledge more accessible to communities, and constantly informing university scholarship with the experiences, knowledge, and public issues that arise from the life of communities. Such structures might include public forums co-created with community partners that enliven public cultures and conversations in locales; infrastructures of support for public scholarship based on a partnership model between university and community and civic groups; and efforts to disseminate exciting scholarship and findings.

Making democracy come alive

Research universities and leaders from all levels of our institutions need to rise to the occasion of our challenge as a democracy on the edge of a new millennium. We need to help catalyze and lead a national campaign or movement that reinvigorates the public purposes and civic mission of our great research universities and higher education broadly. We need to renew for the next century the idea that our institutions of higher education are, in a vital sense, both agents and architects of a flourishing democracy, bridges between individuals' work and the larger world.

In this spirit and to these ends, we call upon all associations, professions, disciplines, faculty bodies, employee associations, and student organizations related to research universities and higher education to consider these questions, to debate, revise, and expand these propositions, and to join with us in renewing the civic mission of American higher education. Our challenge in a time of change is to transform knowledge into wisdom and to make democracy come alive, for ourselves and for those who follow after us.

The Wingspread Declaration urges all researchers, whatever their field, to nurture democracy, encourage public service, and reinvigorate the university's civic mission. Historically, reform movements – whether they are in the area of public accountability for war, racial discrimination, or income maldistribution – have been propelled and guided by students at universities. What can you do to help your university renew its commitment to democratic values and open access? One answer: encourage your department to sponsor seminars on these topics.

Conclusion: some reservations about two-level utilitarianism

At the end of each part of this book, we have surveyed a few of the most important weaknesses of the theories under consideration. Here we note two major difficulties with two-level utilitarianism.

First, the theory gives us little direction for deciding when to rely on intuitive thinking and when to slow down to think critically. Clearly, we must, on this theory, value the interests of all humans and all sentient animals potentially affected by our actions, including those making up future generations. But intuitive thinking typically does not take all of those interests into account – the calculations are too complicated, time is too short – and critical thinking may be necessary. But how do we know when to think critically and when to act automatically?

As a practical matter, few of us can gather even a tenth of the amount of the data necessary to make any of the required judgments when critical thinking is required. So, critical thinking bumps up against the cognitive resource limits of human psychology. But if our rules of thumb are not trustworthy on a particular occasion, and if we lack the information and time required to proceed as archangels, how then shall we proceed? If we never think critically we will not maximize the aggregate good but if we are expected to make most decisions like an archangel then the theory seems to ask too much of us. Thus the theory seems to confront us with an irresolvable moral paradox.

The weakness identified here in two-level utilitarianism is not that it overestimates our ability to take all relevant facts into account within the time span we have for making decisions. The theory does have that unhappy feature and it anticipates and resolves that problem by permitting us to act on familiar rules of thumb in most instances. The problem identified here is deeper. Two-level thinking seems to give us contradictory guidance about which action we ought to perform in situations of conflict between ordinary moral thinking and critical thinking. Which of these methods should guide our decisions when we have some time and resources – but not infinite time or resources – to reflect on a perplexing matter?

Here is another way to put a related concern. The concern has to do with the psychological plausibility of utilitarianism. We did not evolve to care for strangers, so most of us seem to lack significant motivation to maximize the good when doing so involves caring for people we do not know. We simply don't care about such people; we certainly don't care about them in the same way or to the same extent that we care for ourselves and our family members. We love ourselves and our relatives more than we love others. Hungry children in distant lands have lives that could be greatly improved by even a minimal amount of sacrifice on our part. We know this, and yet we are rarely moved to act charitably. Two-level thinking might tell us that we ought to sacrifice for people whose names we can't pronounce; but how can it honestly expect us to act habitually on that expectation?

A second reservation is related to the first. Two-level utilitarianism imposes extraordinarily demanding duties on us. Thinking critically, we are responsible for the welfare of everyone on the face of the planet. And not only for strangers residing now in states with which our country has no diplomatic ties or political agreements, but for future – including distant-future – strangers, too: strangers whose identities and attitudes about us and our grandchildren we cannot possibly know. Utilitarianism seems to overestimate our ability to live up to exceedingly demanding obligations. And it certainly saddles us with counterintuitive obligations, obligations to care as much about the happiness of strangers-yet-to-come-into-being as the happiness of our daughters and grandfathers. But shouldn't my daughter's happiness matter more?

This second problem is a version of a more general question faced by this theory. How does two-level utilitarianism distribute benefits? Who gets the goodies, so to speak – and who gets saddled with the losses? Anyone who cares about justice seeks to respect persons and their moral rights – perhaps even future persons and their rights. And yet utilitarianism does not seem to take as seriously the feature of persons we called their distinctness as contractualism and moral rights theories do. In seeking only the maximization of happiness across individuals and irrespective of the fact that one person may get all the pleasure while another innocent person suffers all the pain, two-level theories seem not to respect the fact that persons are separate beings whose individual welfare matters to them.

The expanding circle model of moral decision-making, at least as described by Hare and Singer, comes to a rest at utilitarianism. And thinking along the lines suggested by this book's outline, you might be tempted to conclude that two-level theory is the one best, all-encompassing theory. I think there is some truth in this idea, and yet I hasten to add (without contradicting myself) that you and others who read this book should train yourself to think and act most often and for all practical purposes as a moral rights theorist who honors contractual agreements while also egoistically protecting yourself. That is, when all is said and done, in ordinary circumstances it is in each person's best interests to act on the rules we have been taught, keeping our promises and respecting others' rights.

In sum, while the outline of our topics suggests that two-level theory is the "correct" theory, it's important to see that the other traditions play a vital role, too. We needn't think as two-level utilitarians all the time, or even most of the time. For we'll all be better off in general if we heed our egoistic concerns and protect our reputations; if we mostly act automatically to observe the terms of the covenants we have entered; and if we acknowledge the dignity and claims of strangers on us. In most decisions we do not need to calculate all of the costs and all of the benefits. We ignore the central lessons of egoism, contractualism, and moral rights theories at our peril. Two-level utilitarianism, in fact, insists that we generally use the resources of all four theories – relying on considerations about my interests to get started, moving on to consider the interests of our group, nation, and other sentient animals, and only then onto the claims of all beings, including future generations. Even though the two-level theory comes last in our presentation of ethical theories, we must remember the importance it accords each of the other views.

If in the future you find yourself confronting a novel ethical dilemma or difficult moral decision, take advantage of the counsel provided in the moral theories we've discussed. But rely, too, on the folks who surround you, the community members we saluted at the beginning of this work. With the wisdom of trustworthy peers and colleagues on the one hand, and the wisdom accumulated in the judgments of ethical experts on the other, you'll have the best chance to make the right decision.

Take home lessons

- Encourage your lab leader to conduct discussions of research ethics and participate actively in them.
- Work within your professional association to sponsor debates on the civic mission of the group.
- Explore for yourself what effect your choice of research topics has on society at large.

Bibliography

Anon. 2001. Land-grant universities: An old dream in trouble. *The Economist*. Available at: http://www.economist.com/node/638824 [Accessed October 6, 2011].

Bonnen, J.T. 1998. The land grant idea and the evolving outreach university. In R.M. Lerner & L.A. Simon, eds. *University-Community Collaborations for the Twenty-First Century: Outreach to Scholarship for Youth and Families*. New York: Garland. Available at: http://www.adec.edu/clemson/papers/bonnen2.html.

Boyte, H. & Hollander, E. 1999. *Wingspread Declaration on the Civic Responsibilities of Research Universities*. Available at: http://www.compact.org/initiatives/civic-engagement-at-research-universities/wingspread-declaration-on-the-civic-responsibilities-of-research-universities/.

Dillon, S. 2005. At public universities, warnings of privatization. *The New York Times*. Available at: http://www.nytimes.com/2005/10/16/education/16college.html?_r=1 [Accessed September 23, 2011].

Ginther, D.K. *et al.* 2011. Race, ethnicity, and NIH research awards. *Science*, 333(6045), 1015–1019.

Mintz, S. 2007. *The Farmers' Plight, Period: 1890s*. Available at: http://www.digitalhistory. uh.edu/database/article_display.cfm? HHID=156.

Williams, T.T. & Williamson, H. 1988. Teaching, research, and extension programs at historically black (1890) land-grant institutions. *Agricultural History*, 62(2), 244–257.

Conclusion

Let us take stock. We've emphasized in this book the centrality of the research community and we have taken a philosophical approach to the traditional RCR topics. We've also stressed the idea that researchers, even as they watch out for hidden dangers, must persist in asking new questions. We have placed some red flags around areas where pitfalls lurk. And we've introduced the expanding moral circle as a heuristic device to guide our decisions when we are confronted with a difficult moral decision.

As the circle makes clear, we have not exhausted our responsibilities once we have followed our profession's rules. For research exists to benefit all of society and a researcher's obligations reach beyond his or her circle of friends, loved ones, and other researchers. We must respect the rights of strangers even though they are beyond the reach of our explicit contracts, take seriously the interests of all animals we conscript into our studies, and consider the interests as well of future generations. For their pains and sufferings will matter just as much to them as ours do to us. When deciding how to act, we respect human rights, but we also use our professional training to make the world as attractive and rewarding as possible for as many as possible.

The moral circle is grounded in four ethical theories. The theories are briefly summarized in Table 1.

Given that each theory has some weakness or other, how should we proceed in making decisions? The expanding circle heuristic does not invite us to choose theories randomly, as if we were selecting dessert from a menu. Instead, it requires that we take all of the considerations on the chart into account and seek the well-being of all individuals potentially affected by our actions. Table 1 reminds us that ethical decision-making may be difficult and that we must use our moral imaginations and challenge ourselves to ensure that we are thinking in a truly comprehensive way. Table 2 builds on Table 1 to suggest questions we should ask as we think critically about issues in practical ethics.

The questions provide a road map, but they are suggestive rather than exhaustive; they do not settle all questions about ethical duties in research but should rather stimulate more questions. As the number of questions increases, they may become increasingly complex. When ethical questions become particularly difficult, do not face them alone. Consult with your friends, colleagues, and mentors. These websites are also sources of good information.

- Ethics CORE (Collaborative Online Resource Environment)
- Association for Practical and Professional Ethics
- Bioethics Resources on the Net, National Institutes of Health
- Columbia University Responsible Conduct of Research website

As we come to the end of this book it may be instructive to return to Max Weber. In 1918, he wrote that, "In science, each of us knows that what he has accomplished will be antiquated in ten, twenty, fifty years. That is the fate to which science is subjected; it is

Research Ethics: A Philosophical Guide to the Responsible Conduct of Research. Gary Comstock. Published by Cambridge University Press. © Cambridge University Press 2013.

Table 1. Four ethical theories

Ethical theory	Principle	Practical advice	Research ethics case	Weakness
1. Egoism	I ought to do what is in *my* best interests	Focus on my ultimate goal	Research misconduct	Seems to be arbitrarily prejudiced toward one person's interests (mine)
2. Contractualism	I ought to do what is in *our* best interests, honoring our *agreements*, explicit and implicit	Observe my profession's rules; be honest, fair, law-abiding, and responsible	Professional codes, cooperative authorship, use of statistics	Seems to make it impossible to criticize the group's rules
3. Rights	I ought to respect each individual's moral *rights*	Never harm an individual in order to secure benefits for others	Use of humans in research, informed consent	Seems to have a difficult time justifying natural rights
4. Utilitarianism	I ought to do what is in the best interests of *all*, optimizing overall best consequences for *sentient beings*	Consider equally the like interests of all individuals affected by my actions	Use of animals in research, and global climate change	Seems to undervalue the weight of our attachments to those nearest and dearest to us

the very meaning of scientific work. Every scientific 'fulfillment' raises new 'questions'; it asks to be 'surpassed' and outdated." As we have considered various topics in these pages, we have celebrated the resources of our community, encouraging junior scholars to be in close dialog with senior researchers. But we must be careful not to claim too much for our group. For we know that our work will be accumulating dust on library shelves before long, and we know that our own fallible judgments and moral values must remain subject to revision.

"Fellow students!" Weber declared,

> You come to our lectures and demand from us the qualities of leadership, and you fail to realize in advance that of a hundred professors at least ninety-nine do not and must not claim to be football masters in the vital problems of life, or even to be "leaders" in matters of conduct.

None of us are football masters in the vital problems of life. That is why we, at our best, constantly engage each other about matters of conduct. That is why we, at our best, constantly seek to expand our community to include the most diverse range of question-askers possible. At our best, we listen to all reasonable opinions, challenge those we find mistaken, and change our own opinions when we are presented with good reasons to do so. For "after all," as Weber concluded, "it is somewhat too convenient to demonstrate one's courage in taking a stand where the audience and possible opponents are condemned to silence" (Weber 1946).

Table 2. An expanding circle method of making ethical decisions

1. Egoism
   a. What are the facts of the case? How might the case affect my welfare?
   b. What courses of action are open to me? What decisions could I make in response to the facts?
   c. What threats, if any, does the case present to my short- and long-term interests? Of the decisions I could make, which one will best serve my categorical interests?

2. Contractualism
   a. Have I entered into any prior agreements that bind me in this situation? What course of conduct does my professional code of ethics recommend?
   b. If the professional rule is to do x, or if a counselor advises doing y, can I articulate a good reason that I ought to do x (or y)?
   c. Could any free and reasonable person object to the course of action I am about to take?

3. Rights
   a. Is there any danger of violating someone's moral rights?
   b. How do I respect the integrity and dignity of each person involved? How do I honor the fact that each person potentially affected by my action is a free, distinct, and autonomous question-asker and reason-giver?
   c. What decision is recommended by our community's intuitive moral rules? Given our traditional cultural, religious, and educational values of fairness and justice, what rule of thumb guides decisions in cases like these?

4. Utilitarianism
   a. What aggregate consequences – good and bad – for all concerned are likely to follow if I act on the decision I am contemplating?
   b. What would I do in this situation if I had perfect information about the pains and pleasures, happinesses and unhappinesses, that my decision would cause in every current and future sentient being potentially affected by my action?
   c. If I had to live serially through the experiences of all beings affected by my action – both the good and the bad experiences – which set of those experiences would I choose?

We end where we began. We are delighted that you may want to join us. We trust that you have received a proper introduction to the community. We look forward to discussing with you questions others may not want voiced. And we promise that among us you will find others, many others, who will support you in what you are trying to accomplish.

Bibliography

Weber, M. 1946. Science as a vocation. In C.W. Mills & H.H. Gerth, eds. *From Max Weber: Essays in Sociology.* New York: Oxford University Press, pp. 129–156.

Index

academia-industry relationships, 221, 224–225, *See also* conflicts of interest
   benefits of, 221–222
   challenges, 222–223
   guiding principles, 223–224
   protection against research bias, 223
acts versus omissions, 255
Allen, Mary, 25, 29
alternative dispute resolution (ADR), 207
Alzheimer's disease, 210
American Society of Civil Engineers (ASCE), 112
American Veterinary Medical Association (AVMA), 115
Anderson, Melissa, 49
Animal and Plant Health Inspection Service (APHIS), 244
Animal Welfare Act (AWA), 244
animals
   moral rights of, 157, 249–250
      case against, 247–249
   sentient animals, 114, 157, 233, 238–240
   use in research, 243, 264–265
      case for, 247–253
      critical thinking about, 246
      difficulties in calculating benefits, 253
      misleading results, 259
      moral asymmetries, 255
      pain identification and management, 245
      reduction, 251–252
      rules for humane treatment, 243–245
      substitution, 251
      utilitarianism and, 229, 238–240
      welfare approach, 245
   ecologists, 114–115

Arandt, Hannah, 172
Ariely, Dan, 4, 44, 54
assassins, 137
Association for Computing Machinery (ACM), 112
Association for Women in Science, 190
assumption of existing preferences, 179–180
attribution, 60
authorship issues, 118–124
   case study, 124–129
   coauthor acknowledgement, 121–124
   guidelines, 130–131
   primary author, 123–124
average, 150–151

Bailar, John, 200–201
Baltimore, David, 5
Batlogg, Bertram, 122
Bayh-Dole Act, 1980, 202
beneficence, 171
Berne Convention for the Protection of Artistic Property, 205
bias
   in surveys, 148–149
   observation bias, 68–69
   publication bias, 77, 137
blots, image manipulation, 80–84
Bok, Derek, 202
Bonnen, James, 275
breast cancer example, 179
Briggs, S. P., 62
Bronson, Charlotte, 61
Brown, J. H., 139
Burger, Jerry, 176

Campbell, Keith, 120
Carley, John, 166
cause and effect, 147
cheating, 39–40, *See also* research misconduct
   detectors of cheaters, 47–53
   egoism and, 41–56

faculty responsibilities, 54–55
   getting away with, 43
   internal filters, 44–47
   punishment of, 51–53
   reasons not to cheat, 43–44
   reasons to cheat, 41–43
   students' responsibilities, 55
   tolerance of, 46–47
Chubin, D. E., 139
citation, 60
climate change ethics, 269–273
   costs and benefits analysis, 270–271
   harms caused by climate change, 270
coauthor acknowledgement, 121–124
codes of conduct.
      See professional codes of conduct
coincidence, 149
Collaborative Institutional Training Initiative (CITI), 171
collaborative relationships.
      See academia-industry relationships
Collins, Francis, 199
commodification, DNA patents and, 214–215
confidentiality of data, 145–146
conflict of commitment, 220
conflicts of interest, 136, 218–225
   guiding principles, 223–224
   protection against research bias, 223
confusion of the inverse, 149–150
consent. *See* informed consent
conservation biology, 113
contracts, 92–93
   unwritten agreements, 93–95
contractualism, 13, 99, 102–103, 234, 286
   narrow contractualism (NC), 92

problems with, 94–95,
152–153
reason-giving contractualism,
100–102
strengths of, 152
utilitarianism relationship,
110–111
copyright, 204–206, 210,
See also intellectual
property rights
Creative Commons movement,
212
Crick, Francis, 119
critical inquiry, 7
critical thinking, 110, 236,
281–282
about animal use in research,
246
Cronin, Blaise, 119

Darsee, John R., 134
data collection, 144–145
data management, 86
confidentiality, 145–146
data ownership, 202–203
Davis, J. I., 139
De Vries, Raymond, 49
decision-making, external
influences, 71–72
demoters, 137
Dennett, Daniel, 48
departure from accepted
practice, 79, *See also*
research misconduct
image manipulation,
79–86
descriptive ethics, 10
design patents, 206
digital image manipulation.
See image manipulation
dignity
DNA patents and, 213–216
respect for, 162–163, 171
violations of, 213
discount rates, 268–269, 271
market discount rates,
272–273
temporal distance and, 272
diverse interests of students,
21–22
DNA patents, 212–216
commodification and, 214–215
human dignity and, 213–216
slavery and, 214
Do no harm right, 164
Dolly the sheep, 120

Doris, John, 71
duplicate publication, 60–61

Ecological Society of America
Code of Ethics, 108–115
ecosystem utility, 268–269
Eddy, D. M., 149
egoism, 12–13, 35–36, 234, 286
categorical interests and,
34–35
cheating and, 41–56
detectors of cheaters, 47–53
internal filters, 44–47
reasons not to cheat,
43–44
reasons to cheat, 41–43
problems with, 68, 87–89, 99
rational egoism, 34–35
simple egoism, 30–31, 35
strengths of, 87
whistle blowing and, 30–32,
41–43
Ekman, Paul, 97
Emanuel, Linda, 122, 124
engagement with fellow
researchers, 76–77
environmental issues, 267–268
climate change ethics,
269–273
costs and benefits analysis,
270–271
discount rates, 268–269, 271
market discount rates,
272–273
temporal distance and, 272
ecosystem utility, 268–269
ethics, 10–14
descriptive, 10
ethical theories, 11–14, 286
introduction to ethical
thinking, 7–8
mentoring on, 187–188
metaethics, 10
normative, 10–11
of climate change, 269–273
of mentoring, 188–189
expanding moral circle, 14–16,
239–240, 282, 287

fabrication, 23
fairness, 12
falsification, 23
female scientists. *See* women in
science
Fischer, Frank, 59
Fleischmann, Martin, 121, 135

Forscher, Bernard, 138
Fox, Mary Frank, 189
framing effect, 70, 179–181
Franklin, Benjamin, 209
Franklin, Rosalind, 119
Friedman, Paul J., 123

Gawrylewski, Andrea, 55
gels, image manipulation,
80–84
Gelsinger, Jesse, 222
Ginther, Donna, 199
giving reasons for actions,
94–97, 99–100
reason-giving contractualism,
100–102
Gleser, Leon, 137–138
Golde, David, 215
Goldman, Irwin, 24, 28
Goodstein, D., 136
Goodwin, Elizabeth, 24–30, 34
grant proposal peer review,
139–140
Grosberg, R. K., 139
Gunsalus, C. K., 53

Hackam, D. G., 124
Hall, Monty, 72–75
Hardy, G. H., 137
Hare, R. M., 13, 110, 116, 235
harm, 10–11
climate change effects, 270
definite harm versus possible
benefit, 257
Hauser, Marc, 3
Hawkins, Marvin, 121
Helsinki Declaration, 172
heuristics, 69–71
Hildreth, James, 200
Houk, V. N., 123
Hrabowski, Freeman, 201
Hubert, Amy, 24
Hulbert, S. H., 62
human dignity. *See* dignity
human pesticide toxicity
testing case study,
163–167
human rights. *See* moral rights
Hwang Woo Suk, 120
Hyde, Lewis, 209

ideas, theft of, 49–50, 66
image manipulation, 79–80
blots and gels, 80–84
brightness/contrast
adjustments, 81–83

image manipulation (cont.)
  cleaning up background, 83
  gross misrepresentation, 81
  splicing lanes together, 84
guidelines, 80
micrographs, 84–86
  enhancing a specific
    feature, 84
  linear vs. nonlinear
    adjustments, 84–85
  misrepresentation of
    microscope field, 85
  resolution, 85–86
implicit agreements, 93–95
industry relationships.
    See academia–industry
    relationships
informed consent, 170,
    177–181
  assumption of existing
    preferences, 179–180
  complications with,
    170–172
  deliberative model, 181
  difficulty obtaining,
    172–176
  freedom promotion, 178
  importance of, 176–177
  physician–patient relationship
    and, 178–179
  sample form, 181–182
  well-being promotion,
    177–178
Institutional Animal Care
    and Use Committee
    (IACUC), 244
intangible assets, 203
intellectual property,
    202–212
  data ownership, 202–203
  types of, 204
intellectual property law,
    204–207
  copyright, 204–206
  justification of, 207–212
  patents, 206
  trade secrets, 207
  trademarks, 206
  violations of, 207
interaction, 170
interests, 32–34
  categorical interests, 32–35
  diverse interests of students,
    21–22
  significant interests, 32
  trivial interests, 32

International Committee of
    Medical Journal Editors
    (ICMJE), 121
intervention, 170
Intuitive Level System (ILS)
    rules, 110–112
Isen, Alice, 70

Jefferson, Thomas, 209
Jobs, Steve, 206
Johal, G. S., 62
journal article refereeing,
    137–139
justice, 171
justification, 95–97
  codes of conduct, 108
  intellectual property law,
    207–212
  reason-giving contractualism,
    100–102

Kahneman, Daniel, 69
Kant, Immanuel, 160
Kentucky Fried Chicken, 207
Kington, Raynard, 199

land-grant universities,
    274–276
  funding issues, 275
  racial equality issues, 275
language, 98
LANGURE, 1
Lecky, William, 14
legal rights, 157–158, See also
    rights theories
Leopold, Aldo, 267
Levin, Paula, 70

MacLean, Douglas, 159
Macrina, F. L., 138
mammography effectiveness
    meta-analysis, 148
Martinson, Brian, 49
McCabe, Donald, 3, 23, 42, 55
McCutchen, C. W., 140
McDonalds, 206
McGinn, Robert, 2, 43
Mellon, Bill, 26
Mengele, Josef, 169
mentoring, 184
  benefits of, 193
  characteristics of good
    mentors, 184
  complexity of, 185–186
  dealing with problems in
    relationship, 193

ethics of, 188–189
importance of, 185
mentor interview, 194–196
mentor roles, 186–187
minority students and
    women, 189–190
on ethics and responsible
    research conduct,
    187–188
responsibilities of mentors,
    191–193
  allowing for personality
    differences, 192
  being available, 192
  learning about mentoring,
    193
  letting trainees make
    decisions, 192
  teaching by words and
    example, 192
responsibilities of trainees,
    190–191
  communicating needs and
    expectations, 191
  distinguishing between
    mentors and
    supervisors, 191
  identifying career plans, 190
  learning about mentoring,
    191
  locating prospective
    mentors, 190–191
rewards, 193–194
toxic mentoring, 188
MentorNet, 190
metaethics, 10
micrograph image
    manipulation, 84–86
Milgram, Stanley, 172
Mill, John Stuart, 76
minority students
  land-grant universities, 275
  mentoring and, 190
  racial disparity in grant
    awards, 199–201
misappropriation
  of ideas, 136
  of priority, 136
monists, 231
Monty Hall phenomenon,
    72–75
moral emotions, 97–98
moral judgments, 97–98
moral rights, 155–162,
    226–227, 234, See also
    rights theories

human pesticide toxicity testing case study, 163–167
negative rights, 161
of animals, 157, 249–250
case against, 247–249
positive rights, 161
respect for dignity, 162–163
Morrill, Justin, 274
Myers, Samuel, 200

Napster, 207
narrow contractualism (NC), 92
problems with, 94–95
National Cancer Institute (NCI) mammography effectiveness meta-analysis, 148
natural variability, 150–151
non-renewable goods, 268
Nordhaus, William, 270
normal, 150–151
normative ethics, 10–11
Nuremberg Code, 169

observation bias, 68–69
Office of Laboratory Animal Welfare (OLAW), 244
Open Source movement, 210
OpenSeminar in Research Ethics, 1, 8
ownership rights. See intellectual property, property rights

Padilla, Garett, 26, 41
patents, 206, See also intellectual property law
DNA patents, 212–216
commodification and, 214–215
human dignity and, 213–216
slavery and, 214
peer review, 133–140
carrots and sticks, 140
guidelines, 137–140
archival journal articles, 137–139
grant proposals, 139–140
problems with, 135–137
conflicts of interest, 136
innovation recognition and encouragement, 137

nonperformance of editors and reviewers, 135–136
publication bias, 137
reviewer variability, 137
role of, 134–135
pesticide toxicity testing case study, 163–167
Photoshop, 80, See also image manipulation
brightness/contrast adjustments, 81–83
cleaning up background, 83
enhancement, 84
linear vs. nonlinear adjustments, 84–85
splicing, 84
pixels, 85–86
plagiarism, 23
definition, 58–59
detection services, 61
getting away with, 61–62
identification of, 61–64
protection against charges of, 58–61
theft of ideas, 49–50, 66
theft of words, 64–65
plant patents, 206
pluralists, 231
Poehlman, Eric, 3
Pons, Stanley, 121, 135
Presidential Award for Excellence in Science, Mathematics, and Engineering Mentoring, 193
Price, M. V., 139
primary author, 123–124
prioritarianism, 271
probability ineptness, 72–75
professional codes of conduct, 105–106, 116
contents specification, 111–112
Ecological Society of America Code of Ethics, 108–115
justification, 108
types of rules, 106
common rules, 106–107
specific rules, 107–108
property rights, 203–204, See also intellectual property
publication, See also peer review
authorship issues, 118–124

case study, 124–129
coauthor acknowledgement, 121–124
guidelines, 130–131
primary author, 123–124
publication bias, 77, 137
Purcell, G., 139
pure discounting, 271
pushovers, 137

questions, 9

racial disparity in grant awards, 199–201
reason-giving contractualism, 100–102
Redelmeier, D. A., 124
Regan, Tom, 157, 160
Relman, A. S., 134–135
renewable goods, 268
Rennie, Drummond, 122, 124
research, 8–10
aims, 231
animal use in, 243, 264–265
case for, 247–253
critical thinking about, 246
difficulties in calculating benefits, 253
misleading results, 259
moral asymmetries, 255
reduction, 251–252
rules for humane treatment, 243–245
substitution, 251
as a vocation, 2–4
definition, 9
research misconduct, 22–30, See also cheating; departure from accepted practice
case study, 24–30
definition, 22–23, 39
prevalence, 23–24, 54
reporting. See whistle blowing
researchers, 1–2
Resnik, David, 6
resolution, 85–86
respect for persons, 171
Responsible Conduct of Research (RCR) training, 4–7
rhetoric, 69

Rhyne, Bill, 46
rights theories, 13, 155–157,
    226–227, 286, *See also*
    legal rights; moral
    rights; property rights
Riley, Wayne, 199
Ritchie, Bill, 120
Rosenberg, Alexander, 208
Rosenzweig, M. L., 139
Royal Society of London, 134
rule-breaking, 39–40
    See cheating; research
    misconduct
rules
    codes of conduct, 105–106
    Intuitive Level System (ILS)
        rules, 110–112
    types of, 106
        common rules, 106–107
        specific rules, 107–108

Sagoff, Mark, 2
salami publications, 61
Schatten, Gerald, 120
Schnieke, Angelika, 120
Schon, Jan, 10, 122
self-understanding, 71–72
Shamoo, Adil, 6
shared knowledge, 77
Sheridan, Alan, 59
significance, practical
    importance and, 147
Silen, William, 186, 188
Singer, Peter, 14, 249
slavery, DNA patents and, 214
social animals, 97
socialization, 186
Soulé, Michael, 113
speciesism, 249–251
Spier, R. E., 139
Spriggs, James, 42
statistics, 144, 146–152
    average versus normal,
        150–151
    biases in surveys, 148–149
    cause and effect, 147
    confusion of the inverse,
        149–150

data collection, 144–145
low power versus no effect,
    148
probable coincidences, 149
significance and practical
    importance, 147
Steneck, Nicholas, 6
Stern Review on the Economics
    of Climate Change, 270
Stern, Nicholas, 270, 272
Syphilis Study, Tuskegee,
    Alabama, 94–95

tangible assets, 203
Thacker, S. B., 123
toxic mentoring, 188
trade secrets, 207, *See also*
    intellectual property law
trademarks, 206, *See also*
    intellectual property law
Tuckson, Reed, 200
Tversky, Amos, 69
two-level utilitarianism, 235–238
    reservations, 283

United Nations Universal
    Declaration of Human
    Rights, 161
United States Patent and
    Trademark Office
    (USPTO), 206
Universal Copyright
    Convention, 205
university missions
    history, 276
    land-grant universities,
        274–276
    funding issues, 275
    racial equality issues, 275
    Wingspread Declaration, 281
    challenges, 279–281
    civic responsibilities,
        276–279
unwritten agreements, 93–95
US Public Health Service
    Syphilis Study,
    Tuskegee, Alabama,
    94–95

utilitarianism, 110–111,
    229–231, 286
    assigning equal weighting,
        232–234
    contractualism relationship,
        110–111
    maximization of good
        consequences,
        231–232
    problems with, 234–235
    sentient animal inclusion,
        238–240
    two-level utilitarianism,
        235–238
    reservations, 283
utility patents, 206
utility theory, 180

Valenti, Jack, 210
Varner, Gary, 236, 239

Waser, N. M., 139
Watson, James, 119
Watson, Peter, 47
Weber, Max, 2, 285
whistle blowing, 30–32, 41–43,
    54–55
    protection of whistle-
        blowers, 42, 54–55
Wilmut, Ian, 120
Wingspread Declaration,
    281
    challenges, 279–281
    civic responsibilities of
        research universities,
        276–279
women in science
    case study, 197–199
    mentoring and, 190
words, theft of, 64–65

Yalow, R. S., 135–136, 185
Yank, Veronica, 122, 124

Zacharias, Maria, 200
zealots, 137
Zimmer, Carl, 77
Zuckerman, Harriett, 186

Printed in the United States
By Bookmasters